AF686512

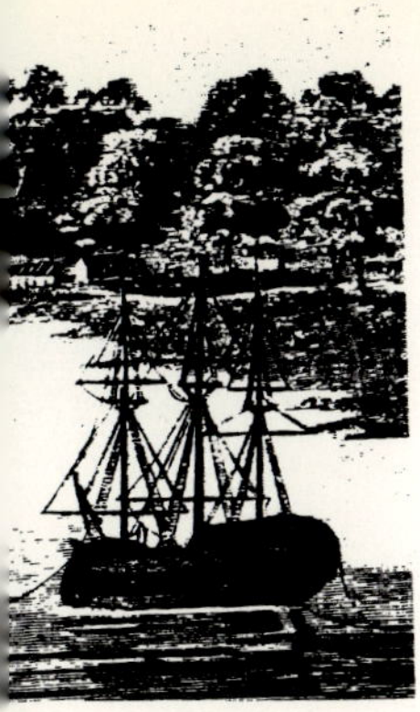

CONTENTS

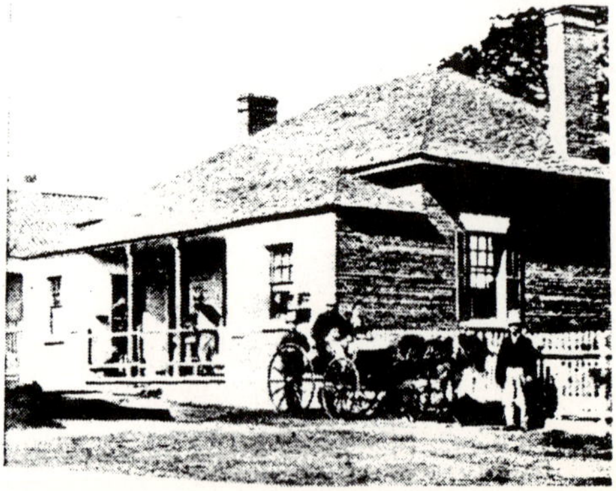

FEVERS AND FRONTIERS

Editors

John Pearn
Mervyn Cobcroft

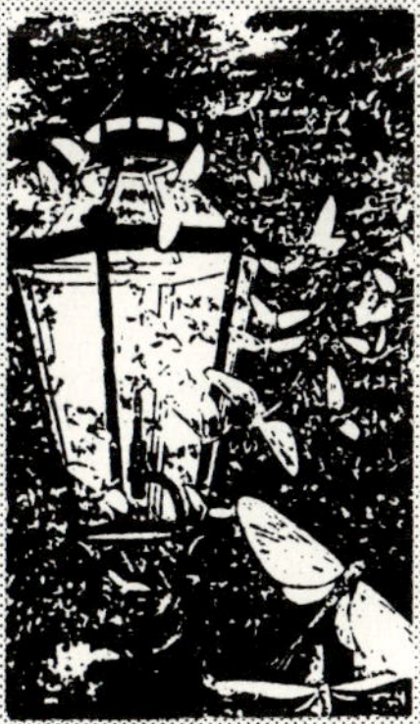

Amphion Press
Brisbane

FEVERS AND FRONTIERS

Bibliography
Illustrations
Notes and References
Tables
Includes Index

1st Edition (English)
First Published 1990

This book is copyright. Apart from any fair dealing for the purposes of private study, research, criticism or review, as permitted under the Copyright Act, no part may be reproduced by any process without written permission. Enquiries should be made to the publisher.

Editors: Professor John Pearn and Dr Mervyn Cobcroft

Typeset and Published by: Amphion Press, (Department of Child Health Publishing Unit), Department of Child Health, University of Queensland, Royal Children's Hospital, Brisbane, Q. 4029. Australia.

Printed by: Merino Lithographics, 18 Baldock Street, Moorooka, Brisbane, Queensland, 4105, Australia.

Cover by: Paul Ramsden and Bronwyn Searle

© The University of Queensland

CATALOGUING IN PUBLICATION DATA
National Library of Australia
Editors: Pearn, John Hemsley and Cobcroft Mervyn David

Fevers and Frontiers

1. Public health – Australia – History. 2. Medicine – Australia – History. I. Pearn, John. II. Cobcroft, M.D.

362 10994

NATIONAL LIBRARY OF AUSTRALIA CARD NUMBER AND ISBN
ISBN 0 86776 381 7

FOREWORD

There are frontiers on land and on sea, and in the minds of those who live and work at the edges of expanding worlds.

Aboriginal men and women had long conquered the frontiers of their home. When a new wave of usurpers displaced them, familiar territory became a new frontier. A friendly environment, itself unchanging, became hostile to the pioneers of a new frontier society. In turn, subject to new fevers and forces hostile to health, the new inhabitants reduced their rates of illness and trauma.

This evolution of better health in Australia can be traced on many fronts. Indeed, a true perspective of triumphs over disease can be obtained only by taking a multiportal approach to the evolution of health care. The contribution of health surveyors and inspectors, of nurses, of country general practitioners and of scientists has each been of the greatest importance. In many instances in the history of the European colonisation of Australia, it was the medical role taken by individual colonists themselves which contributed to survival itself.

Improved standards of health evolve because of the efforts of pioneers, of those who work at the frontiers of medicine and nursing. The frontiers are not only physical, but comprise also frontiers of society, of attitudes, and of the established ways of conducting our daily lives. Advances in community health do not always come from doctors. Rather, such steps into new territory often result from the work of social pioneers. In the colonial era, prior training in medicine and allied fields, however, so often produced an informed perspective of a novel yet hostile environment, and its threats. Prior training in nursing and in medicine, and experience in the basic sciences of botany and zoology afforded some protection against the climate and enzootic diseases of the new frontier.

These frontiers were in one sense a vanity of the European perspective. The land and its Aboriginal peoples were in symbiosis millennia before the latter day health frontiers of Western medicine were defined. Thus it is important, in any collection of essays on the history of health care, to include the perspectives of Aboriginal medicine. The lifestyles and medical practices of the Australian Aborigines had solved many of the problems which were to reappear, when new waves of emigrants (white skinned or yellow skinned) pushed into the unknown in the 19th century. Many of the lessons of preventive medicine, formally evolved over millennia, had to be relearned by the often paternalistic and patronising new chums who displaced the original inhabitants.

A feature of Australian medical history is its diversity of region and of diseases, and of the personalities and styles of those who worked at the medical frontier. It is this great variation in the personalities of Australia's medical and nursing pioneers which makes the nation's medical history so fascinating. Their characters, above all else, dominate the great centrifugal push which was the ethos of nineteenth century colonization. Nowhere has this been more dramatically shown than in the accounts of the exploration of Northern Australia.

This book includes some vignettes of several themes which have comprised the diverse frontiers of Australian medicine. A developed theme in this volume highlights the contributions of those who, from the perspective of many occupations and callings, have contributed to the high standard of health enjoyed by our contemporary population.

History exists so that we might see the perspective of the present, and that we might make better decisions for the future. History informs us and is written to entertain. There are few things more interesting and entertaining than the history of our own society.

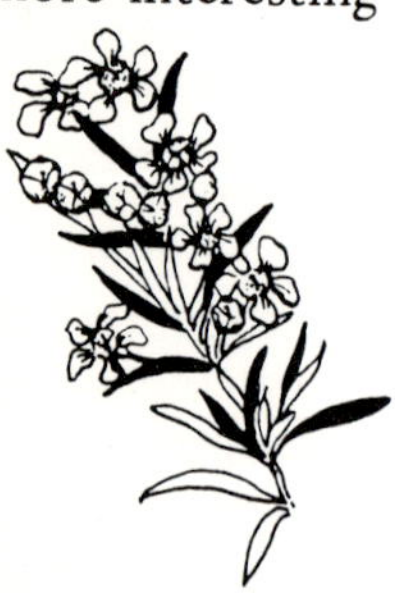

Professor John Pearn, AM, RFD
Vice President,
Royal Historical Society of Queensland

1990

CONTRIBUTORS

★

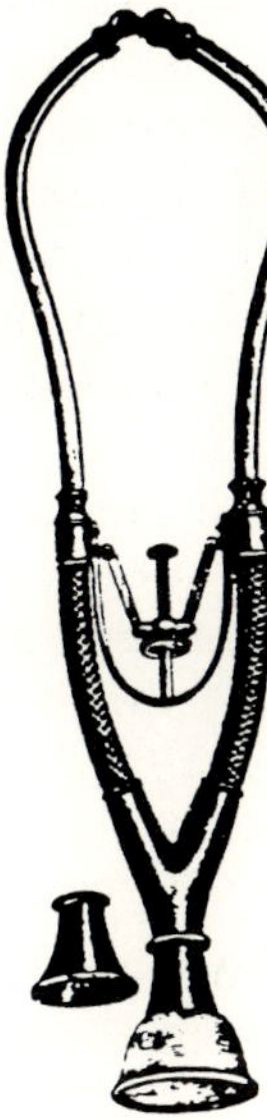

PAMELA CHICK, MB BS, has been the Medical Director of the Family Planning Association of Queensland since 1979. She is a member of the National Biological Sciences Committee of the Family Planning Federation of Australia, and sometime member of its Medical Task Force. She is a member of the Executive of the Australian Association for Adolescent Health (Queensland Branch) and has particular interests in adolescent and women's health.

★

MERVYN COBCROFT, MB BS, FFARACS, is a medical historian and specialist anaesthetist in private practice in Ipswich, Queensland. He is the Curator of the Marks-Hirschfeld Museum of Medical History at the University of Queensland. His historical interests lie with the maritime activities of colonial Australia, especially whaling, sealing, and pearling. His library of original published works relating to these times forms one of the largest private collections in Australia. He has published many articles and two books on these maritime themes of colonial Australian history.

★

JEANETTE COVACEVICH, BA, MSc, biologist and scholar, is the Senior Curator (Vertebrates) at The Queensland Museum, and the President of the Australian Society of Herpetologists. She has published extensively on the biogeography of rainforests. Other contributions have included interpretative studies of early navigators' maps, and the documentation and preservation of traditional rainforest Aboriginal lore. A noted conservationist, she is the author of books on some of Australia's unique coastal habitats, and its creatures. She was one of two scientists chosen by the British Broadcasting Commission to feature in the Australian component of *Great Walks of the World.*

★

RALPH DOHERTY, AO, MD, MPH, FRACP, FRCPA, FRACMA is the Pro-Vice Chancellor (Health Sciences) in the University of Queensland. He served as the Director of the Queensland Institute of Medical Research and Dean of the Faculty of Medicine (University of Queensland). He has a long-term interest in the infectious diseases of tropical Australia and in the people who contributed to their elucidation and control. He has published extensively, and in 1986 edited the book *A Medical School for Queensland*.

PETER FENNER, MRCS, LRCP, MB BS, D Obst, MRCGP is a medical practitioner in Mackay, Queensland. He is a member of the Medical Advisory Committee for the Surf Life Saving Association of Australia, Marine Stinger Officer for the Queensland Surf Life Saving Association, a member of the International Consortium of Jellyfish Stings, and member of the Queensland Government Task Force on 'Box Jellyfish'. He is the author of several articles and booklets on marine envenomation and its treatment and prevention.

★

LORI HARLOE, RN, BA (Hons) is an historian and nurse, formerly based at the James Cook University of North Queensland. Her research interests include the changing concepts of health, illness and lifestyle in tropical Australia. She is the Queensland convenor of the National Nursing Archives of the Royal College of Nursing, Australia. Her present clinical appointment is that of Registered Nurse in the Bone Marrow Transplantation Unit at the Royal Brisbane Hospital.

★

VINCENT LITTLE, SBStJ, is a medical representative for Roussel Pharmaceuticals (Australia). He is a former ambulance officer with the New South Wales Ambulance Service (from 1955) and a former Honorary and then full-time officer with the Queensland Ambulance Transport Brigade. He has served in the Royal Australian Army Medical Corps for 22 years. He was the founder and editor of *Emergency*,, and has been an editor for periodicals published by St John Ambulance Australia, in which body he is a Divisional Officer.

★

JOHN HEMSLEY PEARN, AM, RFD, OStJ, MD (Qld), BSc, PhD (Lond.), FRCP (UK), FRACP, DCH, Fell Amer Coll Trop Med, Fell Roy Hist Soc Qld, is Professor and Head of Department of Child Health, University of Queensland. Paediatrician and clinical geneticist, of Brisbane. His professional contributions include clinical research studies of neuromuscular diseases, toxicology and the prevention of child injuries; and works on the medical history of Australia, of which he is the author of several books. Formerly the Consultant Physician to the Australian Force in Vietnam (1970), he is Colonel Consultant (RAAMC), Army Office, Canberra; and National Director of Training for St John Ambulance Australia, and serves on a number of national medical bodies including the Australian Resuscitation Council and the Human Genetics Society of Australasia.

WENDY SELBY is an historian, formerly of Mackay, and Griffith University (Brisbane), and now resident in Port Moresby, Papua New Guinea. She has professional interests in the evolution of health care delivery systems in Australia, and has made special contributions to the history of obstetrics and paediatrics in this country.

★

M. JOHN THEARLE, MD, FRCP (Edin.), FRACP, DCH (Lond.) is a Senior Lecturer in Child Health, University of Queensland, and a medical historian. He is a co-author of two paediatric textbooks, editor of a medical history book, and has had many papers published on clinical paediatrics and medical history. As an active committee member of the Brisbane History Group, he pursues his interest in local history and the history of paediatrics in Queensland. He is an avid collector of infantilia, the archaeology of the nursery.

★

LESLEY WILLIAMS, BA, MSc, PhD is a Senior Lecturer in the Department of Anatomy, University of Queensland; and a member of the Marks-Hirschfeld Museum of Medical History within that University. She is an historian, writer and bibliophile, contirbuting to Australian colonial history. Her current interests include women's roles in the area of evolving health care in colonial and early post-Federation Australia.

★

BERENICE WRIGHT, BA, Dip Ed is a scholar, historian and librarian of Mackay, Queensland. She is currently Honorary Librarian, and Curator of the Historical Collection, Mackay City Library.

ACKNOWLEDGEMENTS

A book of this nature is possible only with the help and support of many colleagues who give their time and skills, and material support, unstintingly.

We thank particularly Dr Ian Chapple, Dr Duncan Robertson, Dr William Boyd and Dr Michael Williams (all of Mackay, Queensland) and the Executive of the North Queensland Medical Congress for their encouragement. Their advocacy, and the material contribution of the Congress Organizing Committee for 1990 have made this book possible.

We thank also Nestlé Australia Ltd, whose generous support for the concept of this book made its final publication a reality. We thank especially Ms Julie-Ann Okely and Ms Robyn Gosman for their special encouragement.

Special thanks are due to Mrs Peggy Carter, for her tireless and selfless efforts not only in the editing of this work, but also in its technical production. We thank also Mr Graham and Mrs Esther Jurott, and Joyce King, Maryanne Wade and Lisa Cooper, all of the University of Queensland, whose invaluable help contributed to the final work; and Mr Charles Scandrett and his staff at Merino Lithographics, Brisbane, for help with so many projects relating to the promotion of Australian history.

The cover of this book was the concept of Mr Paul Ramsden, and the graphics and artistry are the work of Ms Bronwyn Searle and Mr Paul Ramsden – we value so much their ongoing support and encouragement.

Mervyn Cobcroft
John Pearn

Editors:
Marks-Hirschfeld Museum of Medical History,
The Medical School, Brisbane, Australia.

PART I

FRONTIERS ON LAND AND SEA

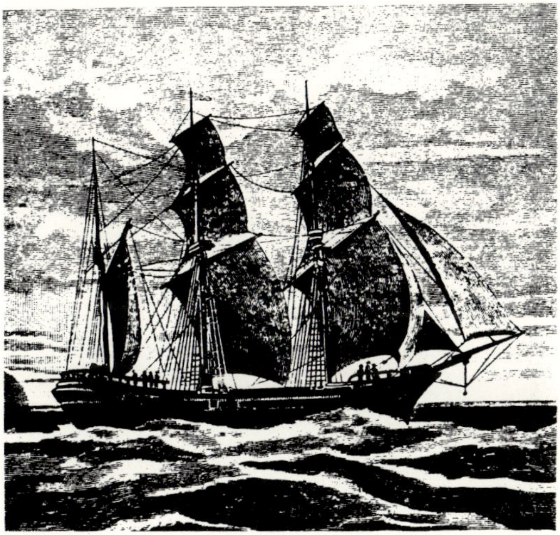

FEVERS AND FRONTIERS 1

EXPEDITIONS, SURGEONS AND FRONTIERS

John Pearn

Surgeons fulfilled a key role in the expeditions which pushed back the frontiers of colonial Australia. The doctor-explorer brought the promise of safety to the often tenuous existence of his colleagues who ventured into the unknown. He brought security to those who knew that fever, starvation and trauma were the legacy for many who ventured into the unmapped interior.

Many dozens of expeditions built up the map of Australia, prior to Federation in 1901. The first medical explorers were the English and French naval surgeons who accompanied such leaders as Cook (1770), Phillip (1788), D'Entrecasteaux (1791–93), Flinders (1798–99; 1801–03), Baudin (1801–03) and Owen Stanley (1846–50). They helped map the shores; and took part in the often hazardous foraging expeditions that ventured inland from the longboats left under guard on the beaches. After 1788, land parties pushed inland from Sydney, Hobart, the open air gaol which formed the first colony at the Moreton Bay Settlement, Port Phillip, Adelaide and from the settlement on the Swan River. Unlike the naval surgeons who had helped map the shore hinterlands, the doctors who volunteered as land explorers tended to be private citizens who sought adventure for the thrill and fame of discovery.

Doctors have always been a diverse lot, and the doctor-explorers of the colonial era were as different as the disparate terrains through which they rode and walked. Some were scholars, others not. Some were conservatives, others radical and at the forefront of constant change. Prior to their adventures in an unmapped Australia, some had lived their professional lives in their home cities, while others had already journeyed widely to the limits of the known world. These latter had already tasted that wonder which comes with the awareness that one was being a part of something that no forebear had experienced before.

The naval surgeon-explorers who had been so prominent in exploring Australian shores – Robert Brown, Deschamps, Peron, La Billardiere, the Forsters, Gaimard and Bynoe, for example – these men brought with them a background of system and of a disciplined experience of working in a team. They were, by the nature of their training and the disciplined naval service in which they lived and worked, trained at keeping records.

By contrast, a later wave of land-based doctor-explorers comprised those, almost always rugged individuals, who came to join both government-sponsored and private parties of exploration. They came not in a sense as passive members of naval crews, but rather themselves made the specific overture for exploration and adventure in the Australian outback. Some were recruited in England and Scotland, or came with single-minded purpose to explore the newly settled continent, from homes in Germany. This second wave of doctor-explorers usually took part in formal expeditions, and their writing and biographies are to be found in the official government records of the expeditions which they made possible by the medical security they brought to the team.

A third group of doctors comprised those who gave their medical skills to private enterprise exploration, often hastily conceived, and in which the preparation for and records of the journeys were often incomplete. This latter group of doctors were driven either by personal ambition, or by a personal daemon which craved adventure. Leichhardt's first journey from Moreton Bay to Port Essington is an example of this latter group, a journey which turned out to be one of the greatest epic adventures in the whole history of Australian exploration.

Popular history records the leaders of expeditions, and highlights the new knowledge that the team – as an entity or a whole – brought back to civilisation. The individual members of the team – the surveyors, horsemen or camel drivers, scientists and doctors – such tend to be forgotten in the greater perspective of the discoveries which they made. Most of the formally-established exploring parties had a surgeon in the team. Their legacies, often unsung, remain in the placenames of newly discovered rivers and mountains, and in the scientific names of animals, insects and plants which their journeys of discovery revealed to a wider world. This account records the biographic pre´ces of some twenty selected doctor-explorers – a group chosen to highlight a collectivity of courage and adventure which has so often been the handmaiden of scientific discovery.

Dr HERBERT BASEDOW (1881–1933)

Dr Herbert Basedow was a physician, conservationist and humanitarian before his time. One of the more significant Australian-born medical explorers, he was born in Adelaide and made his major life's contributions in South Australia and the Northern Territory. His early studies as a geologist brought to his later work as a doctor, a trained and enquiring mind – one which saw the relationship of men and women in the broader ecosystems and environments of which they are but one small part.

In 1907 Basedow went to Germany, and studied at the medical schools at Heidelberg (1909) and at Göttingen (1909-1910). Subsequently, he undertook research on the anatomical and pathological features of Australian Aboriginal skeletons which were held at that time in the Hunterian Museum, at the Royal College of Surgeons at Lincoln's Inn Fields, in London. Basedow had always evinced an enlightened attitude to the Aboriginal race in Australia, and in 1911 was appointed as Chief Protector and Chief Medical Officer for Aboriginals in the Northern Territory. Disenchanted with the paternalistic approach to Aborigines, he complained that the Aborigines Act of 1911 was unworkable, and resigned. He was one of the great medical linguists (another was Dr Joseph Lauterer, of Brisbane), who recorded details of Aboriginal tongues which even then (by the first decade of the twentieth century) had started to disappear. He compiled a detailed journal of some 1,500 words of the Aluridja and Aranda languages of central Australia.

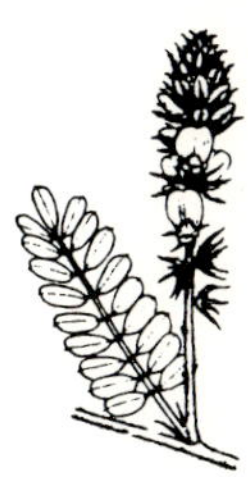

Indigofera basedowii

Basedow was an enthusiastic explorer. He had been a member of the 1903 South Australian Government's North-West Prospecting Expedition, during which he had compiled detailed geological, botanical and ethnological reports. In the period 1905 to 1907 he travelled to the north-west coastal regions of the Northern Territory. In 1916 he was the leader on an expedition to search for minerals which, it was hoped, would help the war effort, travelling in the northern Kimberleys in Western Australia. In August 1919 Basedow journeyed (with his wife, the nurse Olive Basedow) to the arid Queensland border region of South Australia; and in 1920, he undertook a medical relief operation funded by the South Australian and Commonwealth Governments –

> *... to tend, examine and report on the prevalence of disease amongst central Australian Aboriginals.*[1]

In 1926 Basedow led the First Mackay Exploration Expedition of geographical, geological, and biological investigations into the south-west desert region of the Northern Territory. The Expedition was a mixture of the old and the new, including for the first time a wireless-telegraphy apparatus and a phonograph recording system; but was camel-mounted. It was recorded that –

> *... to spell the camels, Basedow and Donald Mackay walked almost two fifths of the 2,092 kilometres which the expedition covered.*

His biographer, Ian Harmstorf, recorded that in 1928, when Basedow was forty-seven, he –

> *... made his most important piece of zoological-anthropological research when he led the Second Mackay Exploration Expedition towards the Gulf of Carpentaria into what is now the heart of Arnhem Land.*

Basedow was noted for his lean and powerful build, his 'great broad shoulders', and for 'the remoteness of his gaze' (*Figure 1.1*). He was one of the few Australian doctors to have been given an obituary in the scientific journal *Nature*. In 1934, the Australian Government bought Basedow's ethnological and anthropological collections, which today form an important part of the national heritage which is kept in the Australian Institute of Anatomy, in Canberra. Basedow was a very keen botanist, and was particularly

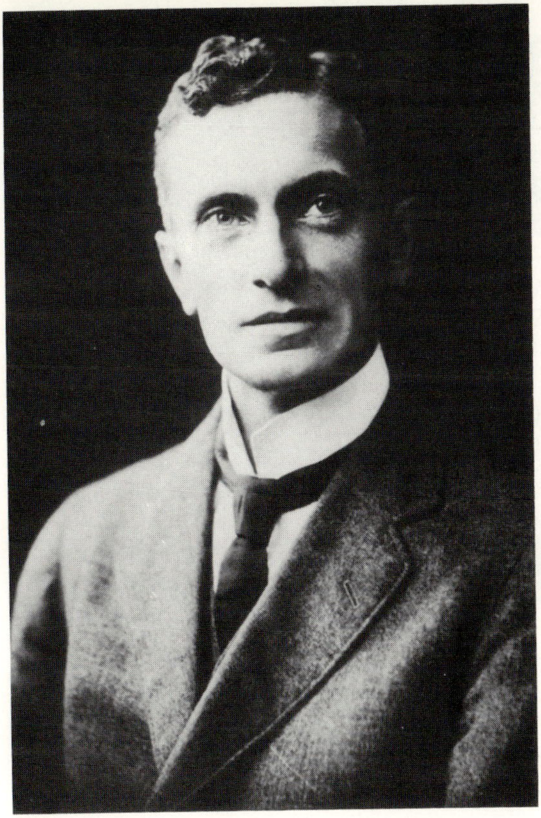

Figure 1.1:

Dr HERBERT BASEDOW (1881–1933).

Australian-born physician, anthropologist and explorer and Chief Protector of Aborigines in the Northern Territory.

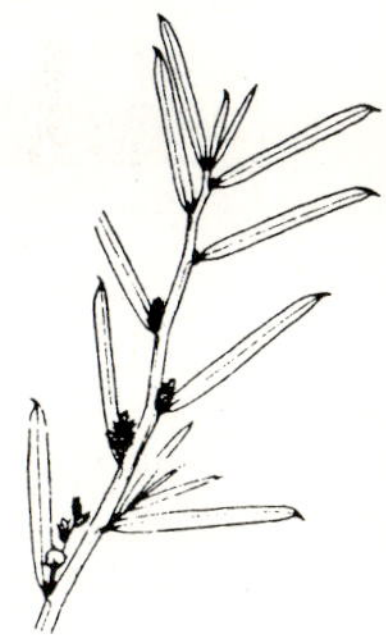

interested in plants of the dry central arid regions. The genus *Basedowia* records his life and works, as does the Australian spinifex *Triodia basedowii* which grows near the Olgas and Ayers Rock. The wattle *Acacia basedowii*, and the wild indigo of the Alice Springs region, *Indigofera basedowii*,[2] bear testimony to his journeys to the Red Centre.

Dr HERMANN BECKLER (1828–1914)

Dr Hermann Beckler (*Figure 1.2*) a native of Germany, spent but six years in Australia, but his exploration and discoveries advanced both biological and geographic knowledge of the unmapped continent. He was born in Germany, at Hochstadt near the Donau River, the elder son of Caspar and Franziska Beckler. As a schoolboy he attended the Gymnasium (High School) in Billingen; and commenced his medical studies in the Faculty of Medicine at the University of Munich in or

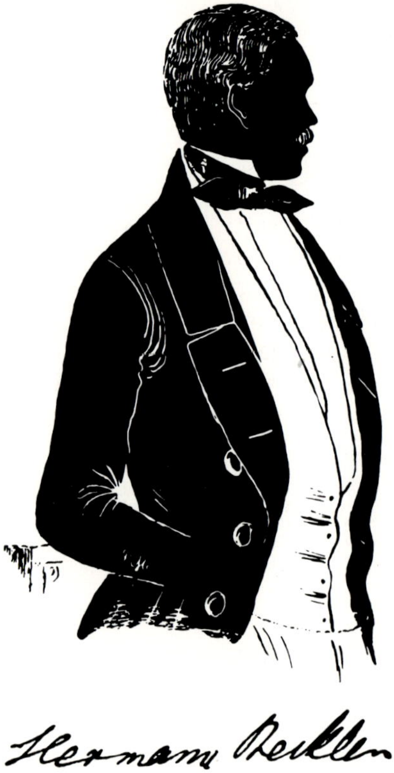

Figure 1.2:

Dr HERMANN BECKLER (1828–1914)

Physician, surgeon, botanist and explorer in Australia.

The Pencil Orchid Dendrobium beckleri, is one of eight plants whose scientific names commemorate him.

about 1850, graduating with his Doctorate of Medicine in 1855. There was little prospect of employment for young doctors in his home region of Bavaria. During his years of University study, there was revolution and political unrest in Europe. Perhaps because of this, Beckler became imbued with ideas of liberalism and freedom, and decided to emigrate to the free Moreton Bay Settlement, in Australia.

Hermann Beckler sailed from Hamburg on the 30th September 1855 on board the *Johan Cesar Godeffroy*, and arrived in Moreton Bay on the 2nd February 1856. He attempted to establish himself in medical practice, but had difficulty convincing the local colonists of his medical qualifications. It is known that he lamented the fact that he could not afford to go to Sydney to undertake the additional study which would have given him qualifications accepted more readily in the colonies.

Dr Beckler commenced medical practice first at Ipswich, and then (in the period 1857–1859) practised at Warwick. He took part in explorations in the Warwick region, particularly motivated by his love of botany. He brought a trained mind to this discipline and sent specimens to Ferdinand von Mueller, the Director of the Botanic Gardens in Melbourne. Unable to settle in medical practice at Warwick he tried again in Tenterfield, but finally in January 1859 went to Melbourne to work as a plant collector for von Mueller. He was a member of a number of expeditions in the Port Macquarie area (October 1859–February 1860); and took part in an overland collecting expedition from Sydney to Brisbane in the period March to May 1860.

Because of his medical and botanical skills and because of his experience as an explorer he was recommended by von Mueller to be the doctor and botanist on the Burke and Wills Expedition. There had been a huge rush of applicants to be considered for the ten places on the expedition (some 700 applications were received in Melbourne alone). It was a tribute to his character that he was

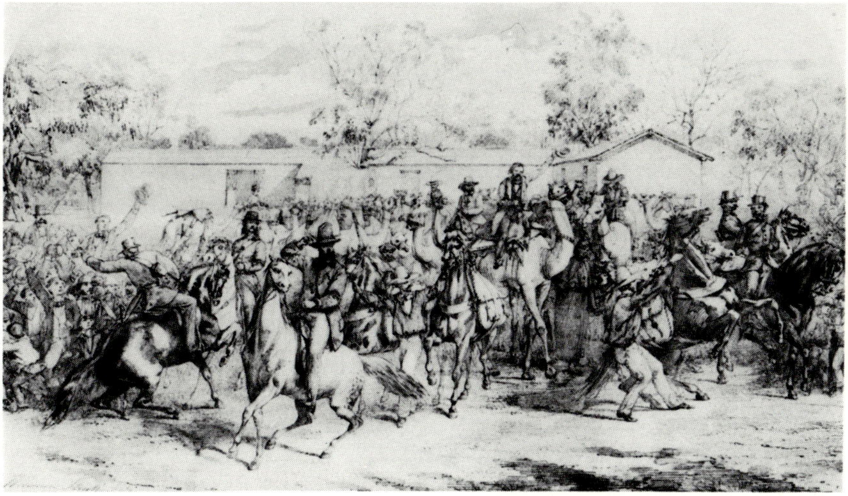

Figure 1.3: The departure of the Burke and Wills Expedition, from Royal Park, Melbourne on 10 August 1860. Dr Hermann Beckler (1828-1914) was the doctor-botanist in the party. From a tinted drawing (1861) by W. Strutt, in the Possession of the Public Library of New South Wales, with acknowledgements.

appointed as the third in charge when the expedition left Royal Park in Melbourne on August 10th, 1860.

In spite of the great promise of the expedition's success (*Figure 1.3*), Beckler became disillusioned and formally resigned when the team reached Menindie, on the Darling River in central west New South Wales. His decision proved to be a prudent one as subsequent events showed.

Beckler's last expedition in Australia was that undertaken at the instigation of the Director of the Observatory in Melbourne (Dr Georg Neumeyea) which in 1861 travelled from the junction of the Murray and Darling Rivers, to the estuary of the Murray where it enters the Southern Ocean in South Australia.

Dr Hermann Beckler left Melbourne for Germany in January 1862. After further medical studies in Berlin and Munich, he returned to medical practice as a general practitioner in Allgau, maintaining his interest in botany and other natural sciences to the end of his life. He died on the 10th December 1914, aged 86. Some eight Australian plants named after him[3] record his sojourn in the southern continent, including the wattle *Acacia beckleri*, and the delicate pencil orchid *Dendrobium beckleri*, of the rainforests of Queensland and New South Wales.

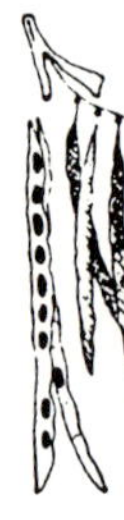

Dr HANS HERMAN BEHR (1818–1904)

Biographic entries of Professor Hans Herman Behr describe him as a physician, botanist, entomologist, lepidopterist, poet, writer, humorist and linguist. A native of Germany, he made two trips of exploration and discovery to South Australia, and the nation was enriched by his scientific contributions. Although many plants and insects have been named to honour his memory, his various biographies highlight above all else his humane and caring approach to sick and injured patients, by whom he was much loved.

Hans Herman Behr was born at Colthen in the Duchy of Anhalt, in Germany, on August 18th 1818. He was educated at the three Universities of Halle, Wurzburg, and Berlin, graduating with his Doctorate of Medicine on the 23rd March 1843. As a doctor in his later life in Australia and in the United States he was described –

> *... as a physician second to none in medical knowledge, and one who kept well posted on the progress of medical science. He did not understand the art, so highly developed among modern physicians,*

of making medicine pay. On receiving the Degree in Medicine, in accordance with the old medieval custom of his University (of Berlin), he had to take a Latin oath to help the needy sick without regard to remuneration. This oath he kept conscientiously.

He was friends, as a young man, with the great German naturalist and traveller, Alexander von Humbolt, who recommended to the young medical graduate in 1844 that he travel to Australia, and study the Aborigines; and to investigate the botany and insects of the newly founded colonies. He journeyed to Adelaide in 1844, and spent almost two years travelling and exploring in the Barossa Range region, at Gawler in the Mount Lofty Ranges and at the Light and Onkaparinga Rivers. He collected many new species of plants, corresponded with botanists in many countries, and in 1851 wrote a paper 'On the character of the South Australia flora in general'. He returned to his native town of Koethen in Germany in June 1846, and spent two years there classifying and writing about his botanical and entomological studies in Australia.

He was a courageous and humanitarian person, but his socialist sympathies (particularly towards the poor, and the poor sick) led him into trouble with the conservative local authorities. In 1848 his father had to arrange hastily for him to sail again for South Australia where he arrived in November. This visit was shorter than the first, but he visited the Murray River, and his old collecting sites in the Barossa and Mount Lofty Ranges. An explorer and adventurer, he left Australia in October 1849 and collected in the Philippines. His legacy and his works are best known now from the United States of America, for it was there, in 1850, that he decided to emigrate and to pass the remainder of his life. He lived in San Francisco, and was appointed Professor of Botany at the California College of Pharmacy.

Professor Behr became one of the leading authorities on insects and butterflies in the United States. He was appointed Curator of the Entomological Department of the California Academy of Sciences. He corresponded with and became close friends of the major biologists of his day, including the German pathologist Virchow, Louis Agassiz, Alexander von Humbolt, and Ferdinand von Mueller, the latter in Australia. Professor Behr was described as a true 'renaissance man'. He wrote German poems (of beauty and with a special sensitive feeling), a story of life in the Philippine islands which was published in *Atlantic Monthly*, and a novel of life in California. It was recorded that 'Greek

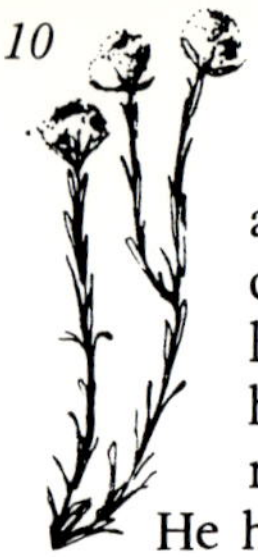

and Latin were about as familiar to him as English, he could quote from the classics indefinitely, and he understood every language in Europe'. He had been a student of Sanscrit, and he had learned Hebrew as a boy. He was one of the early members of the famous Bohemian Club of San Francisco.

He has many memorials in both the animal and plant world.[4] A beautiful gum, *Eucalyptus behriana,* and many wildflowers of the central deserts record his sojourn in Australia.

SURGEON GEORGE BENNETT (1804–1893)

One of Australia's most famous and influential naturalists and surgeons, George Bennett, was one of those who excelled at two simultaneous professions. It was said that —

> *... all Nature was his domain, and every moment he could spare from his medical practice in Sydney he gave to the study of the natural history and of the flora and fauna of Australia. He discovered many new species, many of which still bear his name.*

He was an insatiable voyager and explorer. Among the many illustrious Fellows of the Royal College of Surgeons of England, Surgeon George Bennett was described as the 'Nestor of the Australian Naturalists'.

George Bennett, originally a Devon man, was born in Plymouth on 31st January 1804. As a young teenager his personality was driven by wanderlust. Rather than embark on the apprenticeship which was then the mode of training for surgeons, he left home at the age of fifteen to seek his fortune across the world. He spent two years travelling, visiting and studying natural history in the islands of the Pacific Ocean, at Sri Lanka (then Ceylon) and at Mauritius. He returned home and commenced his studies in medicine at the relatively late age of twenty-one, studying both at Plymouth and in London, and was created a Member of the Royal College of Surgeons of England in 1828. The young George Bennett, already widely travelled, and already with a penchant for botany and zoology, was greatly influenced by Sir Richard Owen, the surgeon-naturalist and Conservator of the Hunterian Museum of the Royal College of Surgeons in London. In 1828, soon after his graduation as a surgeon, George Bennett left on another world tour on the sailing ship *Brothers* under Captain Towns, bound for New South Wales. The voyage lasted three years, and besides acting as its surgeon and physician, Bennett manifested an insatiable scientific curiosity. Following this voyage he published two volumes of his book

Wanderings in New South Wales, Batavia, Pedir Coast, Singapore and China; being the Journal of a Naturalist in those Countries during 1821–1833 and 1834. He described in detail his trip to Australia, and echoed the sentiments of many emigrants who even today sail across the world to make their new home in an antipodean wonderland of plants and animals.

He described his initial misgivings at the 'sombre appearance of the Australian coast' and his 'feelings of an immigrant in approaching it'. On arrival in Sydney, he stayed at Parramatta which he described as 'a pretty village situated in a vale'. He described midwifery practices amongst the Aborigines, much about the fish of Australia and wonderful descriptions of domestic life at the various colonial settlements which he visited. He made anthropological, botanical and medical observations. Everything interested him. He discussed the differences between the aboriginal physique and that of Europeans in a section entitled 'Impression of the Feet of Aboriginal Natives' and noted how these might be 'readily distinguished' from those of his native Devonians. He described plants which had been introduced into the Colony in its fifty years of existence, and recorded the vegetables that were being grown in the gardens of Sydney in the period 1832–1834. He captured a living animal of the pearly nautilius (1829) which excited the scientific world as none had been seen since the original description of the specimen in 1602.

After his return to London, with his world perspective, he decided to emigrate permanently to Australia and returned again to land at Sydney on August 25th, 1832. Springtime in Sydney is always a wonderful experience, and he recorded how –

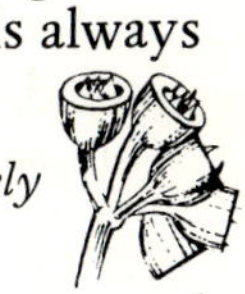

> *... the Beauties of the Kingdom of Flora are lavished so profusely in this Colony.*

He described the banksias, the boronias and the eucalypts and commenced a busy life of medical practice and of botany and zoology. He sent back numerous specimens of plants and animals and became interested in diseases of livestock (particularly sheep) and set about encouraging the introduction, cultivation and breeding of citrus trees. He wrote prodigiously on scientific and medical subjects, and undertook explorations to the Darling Downs in Queensland (in 1871), to Tasmania, to South Australia, to New Zealand, and Norfolk Island. He developed a large and lucrative medical practice, and his name appears extensively in *The New South Wales Medical Gazette*. He wrote about tetanus, and became a champion of the establishment of the Faculty of Medicine at the University of Sydney. He was appointed as one of the first members of the Faculty of Medicine at that University, and was a member of its first Board of Examiners. He lectured extensively on *materia medica* and on the science of the preparation of drugs with particular reference to their preparation from plants.

Dr Bennett was an ambassador between the world of clinical medicine and that of natural science. He wrote the *Snakes of New South Wales* which he published in the *Medico-Chirurgical Review* of London, in 1863. He was the first Secretary of the Australian Museum, and published *Gatherings of a Naturalist in Australasia* in 1860 (*Figure 1.4*).

GATHERINGS OF A NATURALIST

IN

AUSTRALASIA:

BEING

OBSERVATIONS PRINCIPALLY ON THE

ANIMAL AND VEGETABLE PRODUCTIONS

OF

NEW SOUTH WALES, NEW ZEALAND,

AND SOME OF THE

AUSTRAL ISLANDS.

BY

GEORGE BENNETT, M.D., F.L.S., F.Z.S.,

FELLOW OF THE ROYAL COLLEGE OF SURGEONS OF ENGLAND;
MEMBER OF THE MEDICAL FACULTY OF THE UNIVERSITY OF SYDNEY, NEW SOUTH WALES;
AND
AUTHOR OF "WANDERINGS IN NEW SOUTH WALES, SINGAPORE, AND CHINA."

LONDON:
JOHN VAN VOORST, PATERNOSTER ROW.
MDCCCLX.

Figure 1.4: Title page from a book (1860) by the surgeon and voyager, Dr George Bennett (1804-1893), of Sydney.

One of Bennett's greatest scientific contributions was his study of the platypus, and his unravelling of many of the mysteries surrounding the births of marsupials and of monotremes (the platypus and the echidna). He was the first of that great succession of scientists who tried to domesticate and breed the platypus, a feat only achieved in the 1940s by Mr David Fleay. Surgeon Bennett was the first to show that eggs could be found in the oviduct of the platypus, but nobody had ever found an egg in any of the platypus burrows. Bennett set out to establish the true details of platypus reproduction, but, 'in spite of years of endeavour

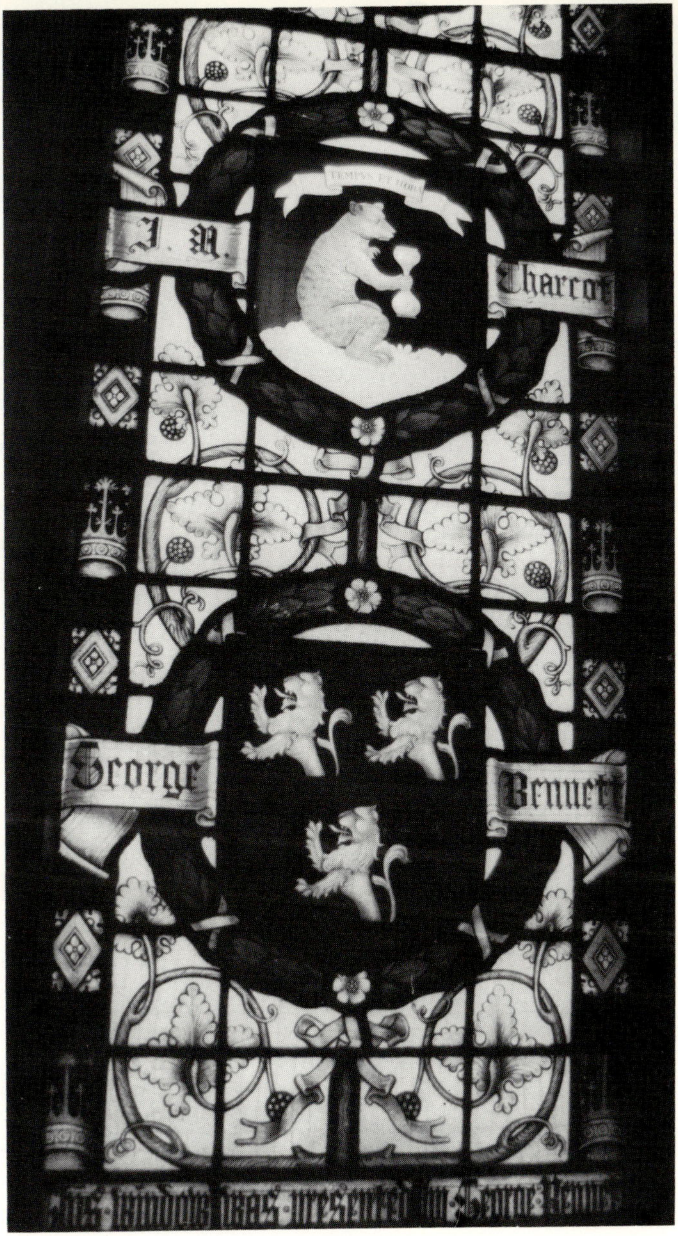

Figure 1.5 : The Memorial stained-glass window to Dr George Bennett (1804-1893) in The Anderson Stuart Building, Faculty of Medicine, University of Sydney. Bennett was a surgeon, explorer, anthropologist and biologist and a Founder of the Faculty of Medicine at the University of Sydney. Photo by the author, 1987.

Bennett was never able to bridge the gap between the eggs in the oviducts of living animals and the young he found in burrows'. The gossip remained, however, that the animal laid the eggs and many bushmen and aborigines supported it. No one however, had ever been able to produce a platypus egg and this problem obsessed him. It was not until 1884 that it was announced in the *Sydney Morning Herald* (September 6th) that the young English zoologist Caldwell had found the first egg outside the platypus body, thus closing one of the most interesting chapters in the scientific life of Australian natural history.

Many honours were bestowed upon Bennett. He was elected to an Honorary Doctorate of Medicine of the University of Glasgow in 1859, and was awarded the Fellowship of the Zoological Society of London, which also in 1862 awarded him its Silver Medal. He was elected President of the New South Wales Zoological Society in 1882, and in 1888 was elected President of the Natural History Association (later the Field Naturalists' Society of New South Wales). When he was eighty-six years of age, he was awarded the Clarke Memorial Medal of the Royal Society of New South Wales –

For meritorious contributions to ... natural history of Australia.

He died in Sydney on 29th September 1893, and he is commemorated in two quite distinct memorials. The memorial stained glass window of the old Medical School in Sydney portrays his coat-of-arms (*Figure 1.5*), but perhaps his greater memorials are *Eupomatia bennettii* and the beautiful Bennett's Ash of New South Wales and Queensland, *Flindersia bennettiana*.

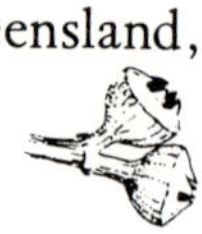

Dr DANIEL CURDIE (1810–1884)

Daniel Curdie was born on the 9th January 1810 at the village of Slidderie at Arran in Scotland. After secondary schooling, he studied at the University of Glasgow and graduated as a Master of Arts in 1832, thence commencing his medical studies at the University of Edinburgh from which he graduated in 1838. One of his classmates was David Livingstone, later to make his fame as an explorer in Africa. Daniel Curdie emigrated to Australia in the *Caledonia*, arriving in Sydney on the 29th September 1839. The rich grazing lands that Major Mitchell had recently discovered and called *Australia Felix* held the promise of fortune to those who were prepared to be pioneers. Curdie grasped this opportunity and the young doctor and his nephew over-landed to Port Phillip, acquiring stock *en route*. They camped in the spring of 1840 in what is now the site of the present Melbourne Botanic Gardens. Dr Curdie established a homestead at *Tandarook* twelve miles south of the present town of Camperdown, in Victoria, and it was from that base that he was to contribute much to the world of medicine, medical education, exploration and biology. It is recorded that he was distinguished for his uniform kindness to the Aborigines, many of whom he met on his various explorations. In 1845 he followed Curdie's River down to the sea – its estuary was named Curdie's Inlet after him. He was an enterprising pastoralist, and unselfishly devoted much of his time and means to the public good. A keen botanist, he was particularly interested in seaweeds, and the new genus *Curdiea* was named in his honour.

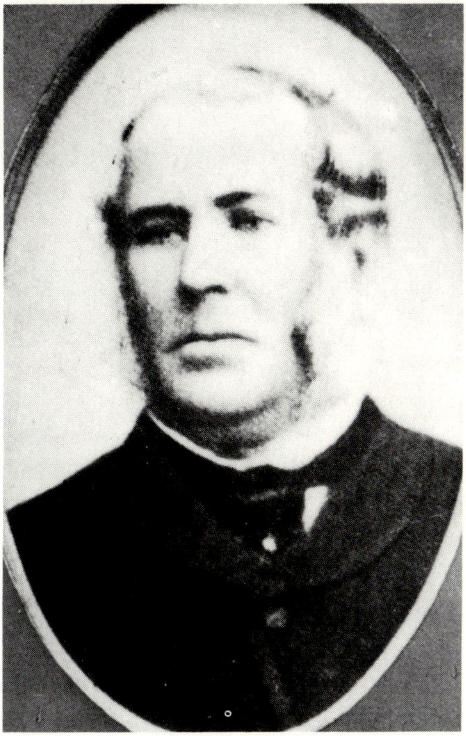

Figure 1.6: Dr Daniel Curdie (1810-1884), physician, explorer, botanist, pastoralist and Senator of Melbourne University. Curdie's River and Curdie's Inlet (which he explored) are named after him.

In 1857 he was elected as Chairman of the Hampden and Heytesbury District Roads Board, and in 1863 when the Shire of Hampden (in Victoria) was created, he was elected its first President, and remained a Councillor until 1877 (*Figure 1.6*).

Curdie corresponded with leading botanists of the day. He undertook excursions to the mouth of the Glenelg River in 1855 when another famous doctor–botanist, Professor William Henry Harvey visited Victoria.

Besides his explorations in Victoria, he was a member of the Government Expedition which was sent to observe the total eclipse of the sun at

Cape York in 1872, in the steamer *Governor Blackall*. He was a great promoter of tertiary education, and was influential in the establishment of many advances at Melbourne University, of which he was a member of the Senate for many years. He was admitted to the degree of Doctor of Medicine *ad eundem gradum* on the 23rd April 1870.

A memorial was erected to him in the town of Camperdown in Victoria, and his living memorials occur in the land plants and seaweeds[5] which bear his name.

Dr JOHN RAVENSCROFT ELSEY (1834–1857)

The sad death of the young surgeon, John Ravenscroft Elsey, at the age of 23 years brought to an end the eventful and meticulous life of one who, had he lived, would have been destined to contribute much to the benefit of mankind.

John Ravenscroft Elsey was born in London on 14th March 1834, and educated at Mill Hill School in north London. He trained in medicine at Guy's Hospital. A bright student, he obtained his Fellowship of the Royal College of Surgeons (of England) a few days after his twenty-first birthday, and was appointed as the naturalist and surgeon to the North Australian Exploring Expedition which was commissioned in London in 1855.

This expedition was planned by the British Government who proposed to establish a settlement in the north of Australia. The Colonial Secretary (The Duke of Newcastle) proposed to 'lay open' parts of the new land in the Australian tropics,* to explore in the coastal hinterland of what is now the Northern Territory, and to search for the hoped for inland sea. It was proposed that a base camp would be established at the mouth of the Victoria River in the north-west of the Northern Territory, and to explore this great river to its source. Two ships, the barque *Monarch* and the schooner *Tom Tough* were made available for it. The experienced surveyor and explorer A.C. Gregory was appointed as leader. Members of the expedition were the leader, A.C. Gregory, his brother H.C. Gregory (the second-in-charge), J.S. Wilson (as geologist), T. Baines (as artist and storekeeper), and (fifth-in-charge) John Ravenscroft Elsey as surgeon and naturalist. Sixth in rank was Ferdinand von Mueller, the botanist from Melbourne. Just before he left for Australia, Elsey learned that he was also to be the meteorologist for the expedition.

*From an Aboriginal perspective, the land was never closed! [Ed.]

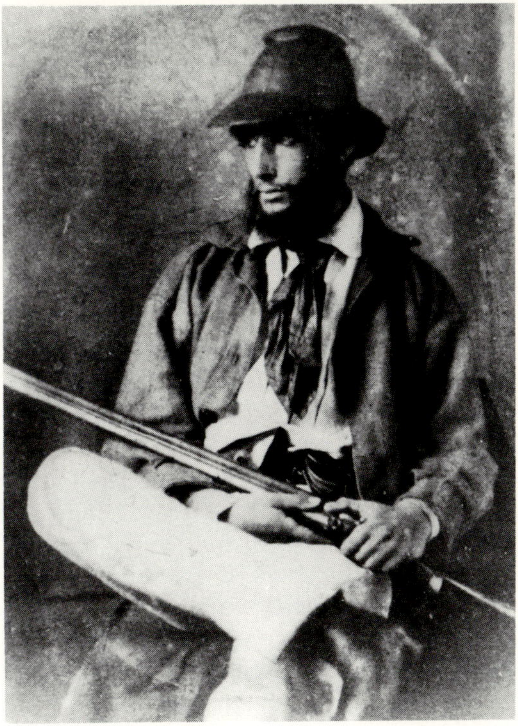

Figure 1.7.

Dr John Ravenscroft Elsey (1834–1857) surgeon, explorer and naturalist.

He spent nine months at the Victoria River in the Northern Territory in 1855-56, and trekked overland from there to Brisbane, a distance of 3,500 kms. in 1856 in one of the epic journeys of Australian exploration.

He died in the West Indies, of illness contracted in Australia, and at the age of 23 years.

Photo, courtesy of the National Library of Australia, with acknowledgements.

John Elsey travelled to Australia on the *Marco Polo,* and he reported to A.C. Gregory on the 30th June 1855, in Sydney. The exploring party travelled via Brisbane and Torres Strait to the mouth of the Victoria River, where they were to spend nine months. It was here that Elsey established his reputation not only as a doctor, but as an ornithologist, zoologist and botanist. He was aged 22 years at the time (*Figure 1.7*) and his research and contributions were indeed outstanding for one so young. One of his biographers, Mr A.H. Chisholm has written –

> *... what modern surgeon, young or less-young, would care to guard the health of a motley crew of humanity living under primitive conditions in a wild spot, and at the same time, collect, prepare, and classify from memory numerous types of fauna, carry out meteorological observations make dips into geology; take detailed measurements of crocodiles; breed out caterpillars in boxes, and on the domestic front, build 'gunyahs' [huts] and cultivate vegetables?*

He did all this and more. He discovered two new species of birds, recognised new plants, and collected animals and insects which were new to science. In June 1856, together with the two Gregory brothers, the botanist Ferdinand von Mueller, and three stockmen, he left on the great overland trek east and south that was to extend for 3,200 kilometres until Brisbane was reached. They took with them 34 horses (7 for riding and 27 pack carriers) and were to be out of contact with civilisation for six months. They accomplished in six months what it had taken Leichhardt 15 months to accomplish, in 1844–46. It was to be one of the great treks in Australian history.

Elsey's health was affected by the trip, and he left Sydney on the *Alnwick Castle* on the 15th March 1857 for England. He was created a Fellow of the Royal Geographical Society, but because of ill health he journeyed to St Kitts in the West Indies hoping to continue with his zoological and botanical studies there. He died within a few weeks of his arrival in the West Indies. It was tragic that whereas no lives had been lost during the 15 months that he had, as doctor, cared for the expeditioners in the most remote parts of Australia, he himself was to succumb within two years of his graduation as a doctor.

His name is immortalised for all Australians in the plants,[6] animals and birds which bear his name, and in the Elsey River (a tributary of the Roper River) on which stands Elsey Station, immortalised in Mrs Aeneas Gunn's *We of the Never Never*..

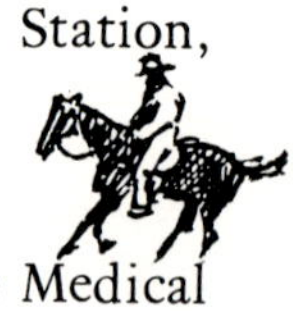

Dr WILLIAM HAIG (1823–1893)

William Haig, destined to become the President of the Medical Society of Victoria, was born at Regent's Park in London in 1823. After his early schooling in London, he accompanied his father and family to the United States where he studied medicine. He graduated as a Doctor of Medicine at the University of Maryland in 1848, and thereafter engaged in private practice in Baltimore. In 1850 he was appointed as the Assistant Resident Physician at the Penitentiary and Smallpox Hospitals, and at the Alms House on Blackwell's Island, New York. The year 1852 was the era of the great gold rushes in Australia, with men flocking from all over the world to the promise of new riches at Bendigo, at Eaglehawk and at Castlemaine. One such ship, the *Oreco*, brought 200 gold miners directly from New York. They had been attracted by reports of the recently discovered gold fields, with the stories as told in New York losing nothing in the accounts of untold riches which were picked up literally from the surface of the ground. The *Oreco* arrived in 1853 with Dr William Haig as the ship's surgeon and one of its potential gold miners.

William Haig established his practice at Emerald Hill, then a village of tents on the goldfield. His obituary noted that –

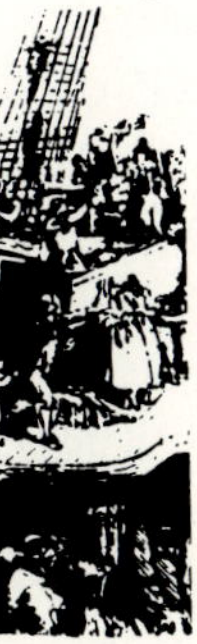

> *... like every other colonist in those days, he had, for some time, to battle with the difficulties and the roughness of that wild excited period, when ships crowded with enterprising emigrants, were every day discharging their living cargoes upon these shores. But he was then young, and had resolution, enterprise and patience and therefore he soon established himself in the position which he steadily held and continuously improved; so that at the time of his death he was not only the oldest medical man in that prosperous and popular suburb, but probably by a long way the oldest and most successful inhabitant ... he watched the steady growth of the locality from a collection of extemporised structures of canvas, weatherboard and corrugated iron, to a well planned city (now the city of Melbourne) whose present appearance makes it difficult for a newcomer to believe, that in two score years, it could have been so well appointed, so spacious and so substantial.*

Dr Haig was appointed as a magistrate and Medical Officer of Health for the town of Emerald Hill. He was commissioned to the rank of Surgeon-Major in the Victorian Artillery and in 1871 was appointed as Outpatient Physician at the Alfred Hospital in Melbourne. He served the Alfred Hospital as a Consultant Physician for fourteen years (1871–1884). He was initially auditor of the Medical Society of Victoria, and in 1884 was elected as its President.

Dr Haig was a pleasant, good natured man, one who enjoyed very much the company of fellow doctors and scientists, and one who –

> *... was always ready to take part in any movement having the common good of the profession in view.*

He was a friend of Ferdinand von Mueller, and was imbued by him with a love of botany. He collected on the Warrego River in Queensland and New South Wales, and sent specimens of new plants to von Mueller for classification and naming.

It is fitting that one of these, the beautiful sunray, Haig's Everlasting (*Helipterum haigii*) commemorates his pioneering life in Australia.

Dr WILLIAM EDWARD HEARN (Flourished 1866, Died 1893)

One of the cucumber-like vines of the north Queensland rainforest commemorates a father and son bearing the same name, William Edward Hearn. They were pioneers in Melbourne.

William Edward Hearn (1826–1888) was a political economist, jurist, politician and university teacher, from County Cavan in Ireland. He was one of the four original professors at the University of Melbourne –

> *... probably having been attracted to Melbourne by the high salary of £1,000 with accommodation in the University building.*

He emigrated to Melbourne in 1855, and in 1873 was appointed Dean of the newly established Faculty of Law. When he died in Melbourne on the 23rd April 1888, it was recorded that –

> *... Victoria had lost a scholar who attended the rawness of colonial life with learning and intellectual distinction and brought lustre to the name of its young university – one who was black bearded and bespectacled, he was witty and courteous, although ambitious and sometimes devious in controversy.*

His son, Dr William Edward LeFanu Hearn, became a traveller and pioneer. One of the earliest graduates from the University of Melbourne, he gained his Bachelor of Medicine degree in June 1876, and established a practice in the goldmining town of Inglewood, some 170 kilometres from Melbourne. He practised as 'Resident Surgeon' in the goldmining areas of Inglewood and Hamilton, and was the doctor at the Pleasant Creek Hospital –

> *... almost certainly another goldmining institution but one too small to appear in the Medical Gazetteer even of the 1880s.*

He was appointed as one of the Public Vaccinators and Health Officers for the region. He travelled widely, and for a time established a practice in Robe in South Australia. He was active in local affairs and was made a Justice of the Peace.

Many young doctors of Irish ancestry returned to Dublin for further training, and William Hearn made this pilgrimage in 1885, sitting for and receiving his Licentiate of the King's and Queen's College of Physicians and of Midwifery in Ireland. In 1891 he transferred his practice to Bellair Street in Kensington, in Melbourne. In the year before his death he shifted to Carnarvon in Western Australia, and was registered as a doctor there before he died.

His colleague, Ferdinand von Mueller, mindful of his work and the signal contributions to colonial Melbourne life made by his father, named a rediscovered rainforest plant after the family. *Trichosanthes hearnii* is a cucumber-like climbing plant, found in the hot tropical regions of far north Australia. The specimens which came to von Mueller's notice had been collected both in the region of the Endeavour River, and from Rockingham Bay. The plant grows to several metres, and is a vine of the rainforest.

Dr FREDERICK MAURICE HOUSE (1865–1936)

Frederick Maurice House was born at *Privett* in Alverstoke, England on July 16th 1865. This home had a particular sentimentality for him, and at the end of a fulfilled life of medicine, exploration and natural history, he called his Australian property at Gnowangerup (in Western Australia) *Privett* to establish a life's continuity.

As a teenager, he studied medicine at St Thomas' Hospital in London, graduating in 1890. He emigrated to Western Australia in 1891, and was appointed District Medical Officer in the township of Beverley on January 1st 1892. His life was to be spent in the western outback of the Australian continent.

He was a keen naturalist, and collected plant, bird and insect specimens in Western Australia. He was appointed as District Medical Officer at Katanning on March 1st 1893, and District Medical Officer at Derby in November 1895. He was held in high regard, and in 1899, Frank Hann, the explorer, named Mount House in his honour. He was appointed as the naturalist and surgeon to the West Australian Government Expedition of April 1901 (under the leadership of F.S. Brockman) to –

> *... explore the extreme north end of the State, lying between the 17th and 14th parallels of latitude, and west from the 128th meridian.*

The exploring party traced the course of the Sale River and its tributaries, correctly surveyed the Glenelg River, discovered and traced the source of the Calder River and identified the headquarters of the Prince Regent River; located the positions of tidal waters extending inland from Collier and Doubtful Bays, and discovered the Moran River. The Durack River was traced to its entrance into the tidal waters of the Cambridge Gulf. It was recorded that –

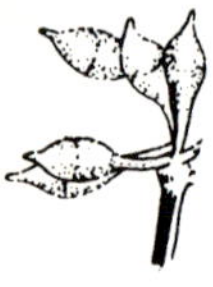

> *... the practical results of this expedition consisted of the discovery of a large area (six million acres) of basaltic pastoral country, covered with blue grass, Mitchell and Kangaroo grasses, and many varieties of top feed ... many objects of scientific interest among the flora and fauna of the district were discovered and brought back by the party.*

Dr Frederick House was a keen ornithologist and discovered the Black Grass Wren, (*Amytornis housei*) subsequently named in his honour.

Dr House was appointed Resident Magistrate at Katanning on September 24th 1902. He enlisted with the Australian Imperial Force in 1915, and served on active duty as a military surgeon in Egypt. After peace was declared, he retired to Gnowangerup and devoted himself to his stud sheep farm which was to become notable throughout Western Australia for its genetic contributions to the national merino flock.

Of the many records which note his contributions to Australian society, perhaps none is more fitting than the beautiful gum, *Eucalyptus houseana*, which commemorates his life and explorations.

Dr GODFREY HOWITT (1800–1873)

The beautiful Australian wildflower, the Blue Howittia, *Howittia trilocularis*, is the enduring memorial of one of the great Australian doctor-naturalists and collectors of the 19th century.

Godfrey Howitt was born into a Quaker family on the 8th October 1800, at Heanor Wood, in Derbyshire. He was tutored by his elder brother, William Howitt, who went on to achieve fame as an explorer-naturalist in Australia. It was William Howitt who was to find King, the survivor of the Burke and Wills Expedition, in the centre of Australia, fifty years later. Godfrey enrolled as a medical student at the University of Edinburgh, and graduated with a Doctorate of Medicine in 1830. He practised thereafter in Leicester and in Nottingham, and was appointed as Honorary Physician to the Nottingham General Hospital and to the Nottingham City Infirmary.

He married in a Quaker ceremony in 1831, and in 1839 left to start a new life in the infant colony at Port Phillip Bay. The family arrived on the *Lord Goderich* in April 1840. He established a busy medical practice in Spring Street, at a site very near what is now the imposing building of the Royal Australasian College of Surgeons. Dr Howitt joined the staff of the Melbourne Hospital, and in 1847 was appointed as President and Honorary Physician of the Melbourne

Benevolent Asylum. He was a great scholar and for almost two decades served on the Council of the University of Melbourne, and on its Faculty of Medicine, originally formed in 1861. The Medical School Committee consisted of six people (under the Chairmanship of Dr Brownless) including Dr Howitt. He was the first Vice-President of the Philosophical Society of Victoria, and a noted member of the Royal Society of Victoria which succeeded it.

Howitt had a particularly high professional reputation amongst physicians and surgeons of the day, but it was as a collector and a patron in the area of botany and entomology that he achieved his international fame. He was regarded as the foremost entomologist in Victoria for many years and made many collecting trips and expeditions to document the arthropod fauna and the natural flora of his adopted country. Dr Howitt's private surgery garden, at the corner of Spring and Collins Street in Melbourne, was a feature of that colonial town. In 1852, his explorer brother, William Howitt, described the features of the garden as –

> *... a beautiful garden scene – our European trees are in full blossom; the plums, cherries and hawthorn are in full flower. The balance of flowering shrubs, large masses of arums, beds of mesembryanthemum and borders of thyme were all brilliant with florescence. The cacti and cereuses were in full blow in the conservatories ... tall clusters of bamboos, the tobacco tree, the native indigo, the date palm, and various types of primulas, flourish side by side. The arrowroot plant, African and French olives, the prickly pear, the fig and guava, the New Zealand flax, the pomegranate, the oleander and the English hawthorn grew in other parts of the garden, while multitudes of beautiful Cape heath roses, geraniums and strange shrubs and plants from the Murray and Plenty Rivers flourished luxuriantly. The honey bird came to the honey plant in numbers, and swallows with cinnamon coloured breasts built under the eaves.*

Dr Godfrey Howitt was a founder of the Entomological Society of London. Prior to his emigration to Australia he had already published two works on botany – *Exsiccatae–muscologia Nottinghamiensis* ('A collection of Nottingham mosses'), and his *The Nottinghamshire Flora*, the latter published in 1839. He was a good friend of Ferdinand von Mueller, and when a new beautiful native blue-flowered mallow was discovered, von Mueller raised the new genus *Howittia* 'in acknowledgement of his devotion to botany', to commemorate his life and works.

Dr JOSEPH LAUTERER (1848–1911)

The contributions of Dr Joseph Lauterer to Australian medical botany have remained unsung. Such is time, that great obliterator of good and bad alike, that although his obituary recorded that 'he was well known in scientific circles some years ago', Lauterer's name is virtually unknown today. How fitting that his monument should be the Corduroy Tamarind, *Arytera lautereriana,* of the Queensland rainforests.

Joseph Lauterer was born on the 18th November, 1848, at Freiburg in Baden, in what is now West Germany. He studied medicine at the University of Freiburg and whilst still a student was a keen botanist and amateur geologist, travelling and recording field observations near his home. He graduated as a doctor in 1872 at the age of 24 years, and passed his registration examinations to practise clinically as a doctor at Carlsruhe nearby. Two years later (in 1874) he was to publish his major work on botany *Excursions flora von Freiburg und seine Umgebung*, a book of some 224 pages with 24 text figures.

The region of south-west Germany where he lived had been for centuries the uncomfortable border region between Germany and France. Indeed, after Lauterer's death the battles of two World Wars were to continue this tragic theme of international conflict. Lauterer lived at the time of the events which led to the Franco-Prussian War of 1870. He was a senior medical student at the time, and enlisted and served as a Surgeon, or Surgeon's Mate, one in a succession of later Australian doctor-botanists who have rendered altruistic service to the wounded in war. The Franco-Prussian war (1870-71) was the end result of mutual jealousy which had existed between France and Prussia for at least a decade. It was recorded that 'the war was welcomed by both sides with equal enthusiasm'. Whatever were his experiences in that war, he left the region soon afterwards, never to return.

Lauterer had wide interests in medicine and natural history and travelled widely. It is known from his later writings that he made a pilgrimage to the grave of Linnaeus, the Swedish doctor-botanist who lived and worked in Uppsala. Lauterer visited his garden and his grave in 1879. Lauterer was interested in wine-making, and also recorded that he travelled extensively to all the major wine-making centres of Europe. Subsequently he was to make detailed suggestions about a proposed viticulture and distilling industry in Brisbane. He finally left Germany in 1882, and emigrated to Australia. The reasons for this emigration, to the very outpost of civilisation across the world, will forever remain unknown. He settled for some six months in the Blue Mountains, in New South Wales, but then moved to Brisbane in Queensland in November 1885 to start a new life.

Lauterer brought a truly scientific and enquiring mind to the botany and zoology of pre-Federation Queensland. At his home and surgery in Woolloongabba (South Brisbane) he established a laboratory to identify the chemical constituents of local plants and trees, and investigated their chemical and medicinal properties. He practised as a general practitioner and surgeon for twenty-five years in the South Brisbane region. Besides his medical practice, Lauterer contributed to knowledge in four particular areas – botany, phytochemistry, entomology, and the study of Aboriginal languages. In the history of early scientific medicine in Queensland, his importance ranks second only to that of Dr Joseph Bancroft, another doctor-botanist who had preceded him in Brisbane by some two decades.

Lauterer studied and wrote about Sassafras Trees, about *Macrozamia* poisoning in stock, and about the Bunya Pine, *Araucaria bidwillii*, of south-east Queensland. One of his major scientific contributions was a doublet of two papers entitled 'Native Medicinal Plants of Queensland', read before The Royal Society of Queensland in 1894. He wrote about the astringent effects of juice from some of the local wattles (especially from *Acacia cunninghamii*), and believed that this burning juice was one cause of 'Sandy Blight', the blinding eye disease now known to be the viral condition of trachoma.

He was acutely aware of the untouched and uninvestigated wonderland of potential drugs and medicaments from Queensland plants. He ventured two reasons why the medicinal properties of Australian plants should be studied with vigour –

(a) *the commercial value must for the first reason be utilised for a country where money is scarce, and*

(b) *a second reason for investigating our native remedies is given by the fact that we can always obtain them at a lower price and in a fresh state, and besides we might have the good luck to find something which might prove more helpful than the drugs of the old country.*

His detailed and careful experiments with plant properties were partly driven by the lure of finding a new treatment, in an era where antibiotics had not been dreamed of, when there was still no effective chemotherapeutic agents other than arsenic and topical zinc preparations; and where the distinction between viral illness and other causes of infection were undreamed of. He quoted his long-renowned countryman, Paracelsus, who wrote –

> *Every country has its diseases and every disease has its best remedy growing near the place, where it occurs.*

His contributions in the area of phytochemistry were great. In his laboratory he experimented with extracts of local eucalyptus and angophoras, and local wattles. He discovered the chemical properties of their gums and extracts, measured their components of tannin and organic acids (such as ellagic acid and arabic acid and gallic acid), and described in detail the differences between the components in these Australian species and other plant extracts which had been used extensively throughout Europe. He used solutions of copper acetate, ferric chloride and calcium hydroxide to develop tests which would identify the components of these Australian species. One of his major papers 'Queensland Native Astringent Medicines, Illustrated by the Chemistry of the Gums of Eucalyptus and Angophoras' was published following his major presentation to the newly formed Australian Association for the Advancement of Science in 1895. This was the forerunner of some six major papers in the area of phytochemistry.

This expatriate German doctor brought a trained scientific and disciplined mind to bear on many of the undescribed natural wonders of the Queensland region. He was interested in all living things, and described a new species of Scorpion which he named *Charon annulipes*. He had found it under the deciduous bark of one of the local gum trees. He noted this new creature was distinctive in that its first pair of walking legs had evolved into 'a physiological pair of feelers', and that 'this highly interesting animal possessed legs which are quite without a parallel in the whole class of *Arachnidae*'.

Besides his interests and contributions in phytochemistry, medicine and natural history, Lauterer was one of the significant pioneer linguists of Aboriginal languages in this country. He appreciated the need to record the details of a dying dialect of the local Aboriginal tribe in the Brisbane region. He published one excellent paper 'Outlines of a grammar of the Yaggara, the Language of Yerongpan Tribe on the Sandy Country between Brisbane and Ipswich'. He recorded a small lexicon for this tribe, and gave lists of Aboriginal words which he had analysed and found had been descended from those used by the local English and German settlers. He discovered the form of syntax used by the local tribe, noting that 'the adjective is, as in the English language, unchangeable. it has no gender, no number, no case'. He listed the different tenses of common verbs, and wrote about interrogatives and negatives. His research on this Aboriginal language of the Brisbane region had an urgent frenetic quality to it, and he recorded formally that the tribe and its languages were quickly dying out. He travelled and explored widely. Lauterer was a public spirited man and took an active part in the Royal Society of Queensland, serving as a councillor in the period 1893-95 and was elected to the Presidency of that body in 1896.

He worked closely with the Queensland Government Botanist, Dr F.M. Bailey, and it was Bailey who named a newly discovered rainforest tree after Dr Lauterer in 1891. In that year, in the rainforest at Eudlo (north of Brisbane), a magnificent new rainforest tree was identified, called in local vernacular the 'Corduroy Tamarind'. Its scientific name *Arytera lautereriana* records the medical life and scientific contributions of this fine doctor. It was described as growing

> *... sometimes to 30 metres in height with a 50 centimetre girth, it is sometimes buttressed ... with leaves glossy green, and the flowers ... white and perfumed ... .*

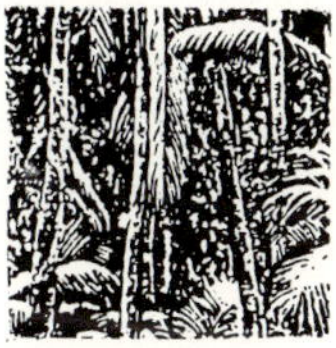

It grows in the rainforests of Northern Australia from Mt Glorious in the south to Cape York, and each year spreads its perfume and influence to remind the passerby of Dr Lauterer's life and works.

Dr FRIEDRICH WILHELM LUDWIG LEICHHARDT (1813–1848)

Leichhardt's name symbolises so much that is paradoxical. His memory recalls both courage and folly, adventure and tragedy, and the hardship yet success that is the history of Australian exploration. Driven by an internal fire for discovery, Leichhardt's contributions to science were enormous. Following in the mould of some other great doctor-explorers of Australia – Solander, Anderson, Bass, Peron, Leschenault, Gaudichaud and Wilson – Leichhardt mapped vast tracks of the new Continent. and contributed significantly to the delineation of the living world which inhabited this most ancient land.

Dozens of Australian plants and trees have been named after Leichhardt,[7] and for one whose official biographies record his passing in the poignant phrase, 'lost in Australia, 1848', there are perhaps no more fitting memorials.

Ludwig Leichhardt was born on the 23rd October 1813 in the village of Trebatsch, near Beeskow in what is now the centre of East Germany. Then a part of Prussia, his village was near the Schwielochsee, a beautiful inland lake. He was the son of Christian Leichhardt, farmer and Royal Inspector of Peat. The young boy was educated at his village school in Trebatsch and then at boarding school at Zaue and at the Gymnasium School at Cottbus. As a university student he studied philosophy and languages at the University of Berlin, enrolling in 1831. In 1833, he transferred for a time to Göttingen University, where he met with an English medical student, John Nicholson, whose family friendship and support of Leichhardt was to alter the course of Australian history. At Göttingen, Leichhardt became passionately interested in natural history – botany, zoology and geology – and after returning to the University of Berlin (1834-1836) he became the closest friend of William Nicholson, the younger brother of John whom he had met at Göttingen. At the end of 1836 he decided to abandon his university studies in Germany, and he accompanied William Nicholson to England.

Leichhardt spent an incredible five years in zealous personal study. Between 1837 and 1842 Leichhardt and his friend William Nicholson 'lived frugally on William's small income whilst they studied medical and natural sciences at the Royal College of Surgeons in London, and at the British Museum'. From the base of the Nicholson home at Clifton (then a village on the outskirts of Bristol in Gloucestershire), the two scholars travelled to Paris to study at the Jardin des Plantes, and to travel to France, Italy and Switzerland. It was William Nicholson who 'finally paid Leichhardt's fare to Australia, provided clothes and necessities for the journey, and gave him £200'.

Leichhardt's fame was achieved in the six years of life, in Australia, that remained to him. He emigrated to Sydney, arriving on the 14th February 1842 in the *Sir Edward Paget* with an expressed personal intention of exploring inland Australia. Governor Gipps, however, was unimpressed and Leichhardt was not given any official appointment or commission. Alone, and at the age of 29 years he made personal collecting trips northwards in the Hunter River hinterland (1842), and explorations northwards from between Sydney to what had until recently been the convict colony at Moreton Bay in the years 1843 and 1844. Leichhardt's great inland journey, on which his fame rests, was made from Brisbane to Port Essington, the inlet at the northern-most part of Arnhem Land, in what was to become the Northern Territory.

Leichhardt made that epic expedition as a privately-sponsored enterprise, unauthorised by the government of the day. When the party – long given up as lost – reached Sydney in the *Heroine* on the 25th March 1846, there was public rejoicing and Leichhardt was hailed as the 'Prince of Explorers'. This feat – 5,000 kilometres across unmapped and unknown territory on foot and horseback across some of the most difficult terrain, earned him instant recognition. In 1847 he was awarded the annual prize of the *Société Géographique de Paris*, and the Patron's Medal of the Royal Geographic Society of London, the latter citation reading –

As recognition of the increased knowledge of the great Continent of Australia.

His official Australian biographer, Dr Renee Erdos, also recorded that –

> *Prussia recognised this achievement also by the King's Pardon for having failed to return to Prussia when due to serve a period of compulsory military training.*

In 1848, he staged through Brisbane to begin what was to be his last great journey from east to west, across the Australian Continent. The party left the Condamine River in March 1848, staged through McPherson's Station (called *Cogoon*) on the Darling Downs, and moving west or north-west was never seen or heard of again. No trace has ever been found of Leichhardt's end.

In spite of his university studies in Göttingen and in Berlin, and his medical studies in London, no formal degree in medicine was ever conferred upon him. He was universally titled 'Doctor' in Australia, and it is believed that this arose from his scholarly demeanour, from the knowledge that he had been a medical student, and the fact that he encouraged the use of this appellation. Leichhardt's field journals and diaries, and his published work reflect his personal integrity and honesty, and are a legacy of his scientific training in medicine and in natural history. In the *Australian Dictionary of Biography* it is recorded that –

> *Botanists and geologists have valued Leichhardt's collections of specimens and the records of his observations which, in an age accustomed to extravagant travellers' tales, were remarkable for their restraint and accuracy. He believed that as long as the traveller*

> *was truthful the scientists at home would be thankful to him. Leichhardt was a most dedicated servant of science and from this very dedication sprang a singleness of purpose which shaped his life, and made him somewhat ruthlessly regardless of all but his research. With perseverance, energy, courage and complete disregard of discomfort, and of the physical handicap of poor eyesight, he pursued his goals as an 'Explorer of Nature'.*

Leichhardt's fame as an explorer has tended to overshadow, at least in the public mind, his great significance as a botanist. He collected thousands of plant specimens and forwarded these to Sydney and Melbourne, to Kew and to the British Museum. He gave botanical lectures in Sydney. On his epic trip from Brisbane to Port Essington (on the northern tip of the Northern Territory) it was said that –

> *After the lapse of two years and two months, when everyone had given up all hope of seeing the Doctor again, he and his party managed to reach Port Essington in an almost starving condition, after their terrible journey of 3,000 miles. Having a considerable knowledge of botany, Leichhardt's narrative is by far the fullest public detailed account of the tropical vegetation of the interior of Australia.*

It is a nice turn of history that it should have been Surgeon Robert Brown who raised the new genus *Leichhardtia*, to be the memorial for the explorer whose remains were never found. When the news of Leichhardt's apparent disappearance reached London, Brown (who as a doctor-botanist also had first circumnavigated Australia with Matthew Flinders half a century before) was working in London on the new plant species which were constantly arriving from Australia. In the year following Leichhardt's disappearance in 1848, Brown named the new genus to commemorate him, the two men being some of the very few Western explorers who had ever set foot in the Northern Territory.

The *Leichhardtias* are slender climbers, found throughout the drier and subtropical parts of Australia. *Leichhardtia australis*, the native 'Doubah', and known to the early settlers as the 'Native Pear' is often found near watercourses. It is prized as an edible fruit. Of the many species commemorating Leichhardt, the beautiful Wattle *Acacia leichhardtii* gives to his memory an annual golden glow. Several trees are called 'Leichhardts' in laymen's vernacular – the Soft Leichhardt (*Nauclea orientalis*), and the Hard Leichhardt (*Neonauclea gordiniana*) also commemorate his achievements. Perhaps there is no more poignant memory to Leichhardt's days as a medical student, than the naming of *Duboisia leichhardtii*, one of the Australian native corkwoods, which as 'Pituri' has been used as a mood altering drug by Aborigines for millennia. Hybrids from this tree are now the source of much of the world's scopolamine, which is used as a pre-medication for everyone who has an anaesthetic, and is a major ingredient in travel sickness tablets for those who suffer from the miseries of seasickness.

Dr JOHANN LHOTSKY (1800–*c.*1861)

The beautiful Australian Snow Myrtle and several species of Fringe Myrtle commemorate the turbulent colonial life of Dr Johann Lhotsky – physician, explorer and naturalist in the Australian Alps and in Tasmania. His restless and unfulfilled life in Australia typified that of a group of troubled scientists who came to the early colonies, who were not encouraged by any official support, yet who achieved scientific advances because of their internal fortitude and determination. Johann Lhotsky was one such – a man who was eccentric and disorganised, combative and persecuted, yet one whose inner driving force made him one of the colonial personalities. He died unknown and impoverished, in London, and no known gravestone marks his passing. Rather, each year the beautiful Snow Myrtle blooms in alpine New South Wales and Victoria to record his life.

Johann (christened Jan) Lhotsky was born on the 27th June 1800, in the village of Lemberg (modern day L'Vov) in Eastern Poland, in what is now Western Russia. His parents were Czech, but his former ancestors almost certainly came from the Baltic region. The details of his early life are unknown, but the evidence of his later life in colonial Australia and in London lead one to believe that his early life was also full of want and discontent. It is known that he moved to a number of places for his education, and his university studies were completed in Prague, Berlin, Vienna and at Paris. He studied medicine, and graduated with his Doctorate in Medicine from the University of Vienna in 1830. Initially a surgeon, his restlessness led him to a life of exploration and travel, and natural history in all its forms became his great passion. He had an insatiable hunger for knowledge about animals and plants, minerals and geology, and the customs and ways of the indigenous populations of countries in which he travelled. In 1830 he persuaded the King of Bavaria to fund a collecting trip to Brazil, and he spent 18 months based at Bahia and at Rio de Janeiro, collecting natural history specimens in that country. He collected extensively in the Province of Matto Grosso and it is probable that he funded at least part of his travels by selling mineral specimens and natural history specimens to the great museums of Europe. Johann Lhotsky 'turned up' in Sydney in 1832, in what was to be the start of six turbulent years both for him, and the community in which he resided.

Lhotsky spent only six years in Australia. He established a private 'museum' at his home in Elizabeth Street, Sydney. He sold specimens of minerals, curiosities of natural history, bones, stuffed birds and shells. It appeared that he maintained himself from the sale of these for several years. Within a few months of arriving, he conducted in February 1833 –

> *... an interesting sale of a collection of 8,000 specimens of plants, insects, zoophytes, minerals, tympanum, bones of a whale, Brazil snakes, mosses, the various woods of the Colony, lizards, fishes and other curiosities ... Captains of ships and persons proceeding to Europe were specially notified.*

He gave public lectures on geology, botany and zoology, charging a fee for these to provide him with some income, as his medical practice in Sydney was very small. His lectures however 'were not a success even when illustrated by specimens'. His personality and style antagonised people. He was far ahead of his time in that he gave his lectures informally, and did not read them from a prepared text, as audiences of the day expected. The *Sydney Gazette* reported that 'unlike most other lecturers, Dr Lhotsky addresses his audience almost wholly *viva voce* – merely referring occasionally to notes ... the auditory [audience] was not so numerous as we hoped it would be'.

Lhotsky is best known for a three month expedition that he made (January – March) in 1834, to the Australian Alps. Like so many of his other endeavours, he was unable to persuade any of the official authorities to support him, and the expedition was conducted at his 'own private and very circumscribed means'. The expedition however yielded a priceless collection of zoological and other scientific information, but his notes and the formal narrative of the trip 'was plentifully interspersed with pungent diatribes against the authorities, as was his wont'. He published an account of his expedition under the title –

A Journey from Sydney to the Australian Alps, undertaken in the months of January, February and March 1834. Being an account of the geographical and natural relation of the country traversed, its Aborigines, etc., together with some general information respecting the Colony of New South Wales.

Again, an unsympathetic Colony was unimpressed by his credentials, his presentations, his collections or his enthusiasm, and he became more and more paranoid. He wrote that –

> *I was marked with the guilt of two capital offences which very few in the Colony (spoiled as it is by two bad and corrupted administrations) will ever forgive. I was a man without fortune and unconnected with Government.*

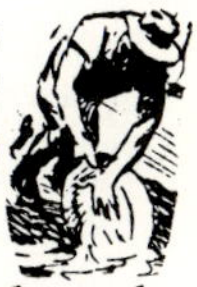

It was on this trip that Lhotsky found some gold-bearing sand, and history is the judge that he was one of the first discoverers of gold in Australia. On the great journey during which he explored Mount Kosciusko and Mount William, he collected some 3,000 specimens of insects and over 100 birds and mammals. He collected rocks and minerals and fresh water shells, and made ethnological observations on the lifestyles of the Aboriginals whom he encountered on the trip. He journeyed to Limestone Plains which is now the federal capital, Canberra. With an uncanny prophesy, he said that at Limestone 'at no distant period a fine town will exist ...' . In the Monaro district he took a particular interest in the residual 60 or 70 Aboriginals who comprised, as he recorded it, the 'Menero Tribe'. From them he obtained a vocabulary of some 160 words, and five years later (when he was impoverished and unknown in London), he published in the Journal of the Royal Geographical Society of London a paper entitled 'Remarks on a Short Vocabulary of the Natives of Van Diemen's Land and Menero Downs'. He was also one of the first musicologists in Australia, and published the *Song of the Women of the Menero Tribe*. He published this using formal musical notation and it forms an extremely valuable early record of music that had probably existed for many thousands of years.

Lhotsky remained a well known figure in Sydney for another two years (until 1836), undertaking several further explorations, and becoming more involved in personal political activities. He published pamphlets and tracts, one particularly intemperate one in 1836 being entitled 'Another Dose for the Reverend Doctor L...g [Lang] of

Slanderous Colonist Notoriety Applied by an Invalid Botany Bay flagellator'. Another account, published in the *New South Wales Literary Political and Commercial Advertiser* (in 1835), was entitled 'Illustrations of the present state and future prospects of the Colony of New South Wales by an Impartial Observer'. Above all else, Dr Johann Lhotsky yearned for the post of Keeper of the Colonial Museum in Sydney. The post had remained vacant since the death of its previous incumbent in 1831, and although provision for the salary of a new Director (£150 per annum) had been made ever since the death of the previous Keeper, the authorities were totally unwilling to appoint the intemperate and turbulent Dr Lhotsky. In the end, in 1836 he went to Tasmania, followed by the scorn and vituperation of the Sydney establishment and press. It appears that Lhotsky also left with some unpaid bills, because on November 1st, 1836 the *Sydney Gazette* having previously denounced him as the 'Prince of Humbugs' announced that Dr Johann Lhotsky –

> *... this celebrated literary character, has we are happy to announce to our readers, arrived at Hobart Town. As the enquiries after the Australian traveller have been numerous, we are glad to appease the excited feeling, which his premature and unexplained absence* [from Sydney] *has given rise to.*

In January 1837, such is the power of the press, that Lhotsky still felt the venom of the journalist's hand –

> *We don't like the man's principles. He left our office without paying us a farewell visit, much to our annoyance, for his name, unfortunately for the proprietress, stands conspicuously upon our ledgers. We also hear of the very disinterested way in which he bestowed his patronage and distinction, by borrowing from his friends a trifle of 30 shillings or so, which we suppose slipped his memory before he left for Hobart Town ...* .

Dr Lhotsky's turbulent and abrasive life continued in Hobart. He was recommended by the Surveyor General to be appointed Colonial Naturalist. The Acting Lieutenant Governor refused, but allowed him rations and three assigned servants to collect specimens. A particularly ugly episode centred around a belief, probably true, that he had misappropriated a manuscript relating to New Zealand (Maori) grammar. When Lhotsky then returned to London (in 1839), it was written that his behaviour in Hobart was such that –

> *Lhotsky narrowly escaped the justly merited fate of obtaining from Her Majesty's Judges, letters of denization to render him fully entitled to all the privileges of those for whose accommodation Her Majesty's Penal Settlement at Port Arthur was established!*

No-one doubted his enthusiasm, and whilst he was in Tasmania the doctor made a complete geological map of the Tasman Peninsula, and collected specimens indefatigably. Much to the relief of the Tasmanians, Lhotsky left Hobart in 1838, and sailed for London in the *Emu.* He became destitute and his health deteriorated, and he was last heard of, still pitifully applying for recognition and material support, in 1861.

The memory of this tragic doctor is perpetuated in the beautiful genus of plants, *Lhotskya*, many growing in the Australian Alps, which was the scene of one of his genuine exploring and collecting triumphs.[8]

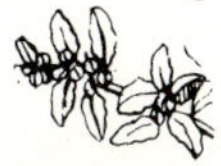

JOHN MacGILLIVRAY (1822–1867)

So often does the irresistible seduction of adventure come to students before they have completed their medical course at university. Some break away from their studies but fate smiles softly on them; for some life's circumstances allow them at some later date to take up again the threads of their medical course. Others break away, thankful to start a new life remote from the demands of hard work and the enormous self discipline that a medical course requires. Others interrupt their medical studies to grasp some never-to-be-repeated opportunity, and then fall prey to life's circumstances which forever deny them the joys of doctoring. In this latter group falls John MacGillivray – sometime senior medical student, then world explorer and adventurer, and later an esteemed natural historian.

John MacGillivray was born on the 18th December 1821, the firstborn of twelve children of Professor William MacGillivray, Regius Professor of Natural History at Marischal College, at the University of Aberdeen. He grew up in a family in which the living wonders of nature were given great respect. His father was a famous ornithologist, and his brother Dr Paul Howard MacGillivray went on to become a famous surgeon and naturalist in Bendigo, Victoria.

John MacGillivray studied medicine at Edinburgh University, but shortly before he was to graduate, one of those 'irresistible seductions of adventure' came his way. The British Government was sending out a major history expedition to the South Seas, in H.M.S. *Fly*, and

MacGillivray was offered the position as a naturalist on the scientific team. His mentor was the Thirteenth Earl of Derby, a powerful patron of zoology of that time. Thus it was that MacGillivray left England in H.M.S. *Fly* in April 1842. Apart from further periods in England, he was to spend the remainder of his adventurous life in Australia and the South Seas.

The *Fly* expedition spent three years in the waters of Australia and New Guinea. It engaged in a major survey of the Great Barrier Reef and Torres Strait, and the northern shores of the Northern Territory. MacGillivray collected extensively on this trip, and many of his specimens now reside at The British Museum and at Kew Gardens in London. MacGillivray spent ten months in England, but when the next great scientific expedition to Australian waters was being planned later that year – the H.M.S. *Rattlesnake* expedition commanded by Captain Owen Stanley – he was again appointed as one of the three naturalists on the staff. One of these was Dr T.H. Huxley, a surgeon and naturalist,

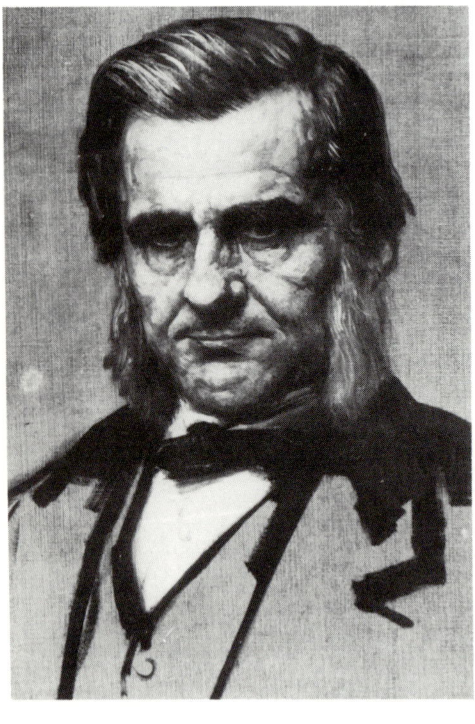

Figure 1.8.

Dr Thomas Henry Huxley (1825–1895), the surgeon, explorer, biologist and scholar who became President of the Royal Society.

One of the great doctor-biologists, he explored and collected at Lord Howe Island, on the Darling Downs of Queensland and in Papua New Guinea.

Portrait by Alphonse Legros in the possession of The Royal Society, London, with acknowledgements.

who was to become one of the most famous biologists the world has known. The *Rattlesnake* expedition lasted almost four years, and it was during this time, when the ship was in Sydney, that John MacGillivray married Williamina Gray, a Scot whom he met in the young Colony. The *Rattlesnake* survey was one of the great hydrographic surveys in the history of the Pacific, and much of our detailed knowledge of the Great Barrier Reef and southern coasts of New Guinea dates from those endeavours. MacGillivray was with H.M.S. *Rattlesnake* when it visited Port Curtis, Rockingham Bay, Port Molle, Cape York, Lizard Island and Moreton Islands. He was part of the team which examined Hervey Bay as the site for a new settlement. The ship returned to Sydney between its surveying and collecting cruises, and we know much of the detail of his voyage from MacGillivray's own work, *Narrative of the Voyage of H.M.S. Rattlesnake* which was published in 1852. One of his biographers, Dr J.H. Calaby, has recorded that –

> *John MacGillivray's zeal and energy as a field worker were unsurpassed, and it is obvious that he enjoyed collecting and observing in the field above all else. He had a remarkable facility for gaining the confidence of native people and took a great interest in them and collected vocabularies. His published work, notebooks, and effusive writings, show him as a critical and intelligent observer and demonstrate an excellent knowledge of systematic zoology and animal distribution. He made large collections of specimens of all kinds of animals, especially birds and mollusc shells, and plants ... among his collections were the typed specimens of many new species described by John Gould, George Bentham and others.*

After the *Rattlesnake* voyage, he stayed in England, writing his *Narrative* for some two years.

A third voyage of exploration and scientific discovery left England in 1852, in H.M.S. *Herald* under Captain H.M. Denham, but MacGillivray was dismissed from service, because of his 'intemperate habits'. Little is known about the next five years of his life, but it is recorded that during this time (1853–1860) –

> *... he spent ... years among the savage inhabitants of the South Sea Islands, where he had many strange adventures, and hairbreadth escapes. He had a wonderful power of gaining the confidence and adapting himself to the manners of the cannibal tribes among whom he lived.*

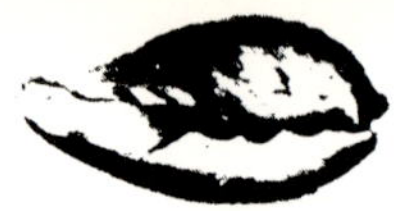

In 1861 he reappeared in Sydney, and worked arranging the shell collection of Dr James Cox, a doctor and well known shell collector in Sydney at that time. In 1864 he settled for two years at Grafton in what was then northern New South Wales where he spent his time collecting and selling natural history specimens. He returned to Sydney and died unexpectedly on the 6th June 1867. John MacGillivray was a very human person, and his memory evokes mixed responses from those who have studied his life and his works. Some, like his publishers, despaired that he did not have the self discipline to annotate and write up his collections. His companion on the *Rattlesnake* voyage, Dr T.H. Huxley 'found him an amiable companion, but later developed almost a contempt for him'. On the other hand, there are those that identify perhaps with his less-than-perfect rigid self control. One of his biographers has recorded that –

> *... his lapses have largely been forgotten ... because of his great contributions to Australian natural history.*

It is fitting that MacGillivray's memorials are found in the forests and shores of northern Australia, particularly in tropical north Queensland where he collected and explored. The Native Kapok, *Cochlospermum gillivraei*, records his passing, as does the native MacGillivray's Gardenia (*Gardenia macgillivraei*).

SURGEON JOSEPH MILLIGAN (1807–1884)

Scottish surgeons developed a strong tradition not only for medicine in the new Australian Colonies, but also for exploration and discovery, and botanical collecting. Surgeons Robert Brown, Archibald Menzies, Thomas Braidwood Wilson and Sir William MacGregor were but several of that Scottish band whose names are recorded in Australian plants. To this group one must add Dr Joseph Milligan, Surgeon to the Van Diemen's Land Company, and one of the founders of the Royal Society of Tasmania. He spent thirty years in Tasmania, and as a doctor and voyager, superintendent of Aborigines, scientist, geologist and botanist, his three decades in the new Colony were marked by intense scholarship and industry. Sir John Dalton Hooker referred to him as 'one of the most indefatigable and able of Tasmanian botanists'. He contributed very significantly to discoveries in botany, zoology and geology in the new continent, and his period as a doctor to the Tasmanian Aboriginals at that time of great shame in Australia's history, was accompanied by great concern for their welfare.

Joseph Milligan was born at Dumfriesshire in Scotland, and was apprenticed as a surgeon. He studied surgery at a time when university qualifications were not only not required, but were not normally undertaken by those aspiring to a career in surgery, as opposed to that of medicine. He obtained his Membership of the Royal College of Surgeons of Edinburgh in January 1829, and in the following year made the decision to leave Scotland forever and travel to what was then the farthest limit of the known world.

In June 1830 he was appointed as Surgeon Superintendent to the Van Diemen's Land Company, and in February 1831 arrived at Surrey Hills in Tasmania to take up his appointment. He remained in that position for eleven years and during that time explored widely, pursuing his passionate interests in botany and geology. He sent many specimens to Sir William Hooker (another surgeon-botanist) in London and it is there that many of the new species which he collected repose today. He took part in a major overland expedition to Macquarie Harbour (March–May 1842) as the surgeon and naturalist. In September 1842 he was appointed Inspector of Convict Discipline and a member of the Board for Distributing Convicts.

The 1830s and 1840s were a turbulent time in Tasmanian and Australian history. It was the time of caring for great numbers of convicts at Port Arthur and at the penal settlement at Macquarie Harbour, well remembered by all who have read *For the Term of His Natural Life.* It was also a time when relations between the indigenous Aboriginals and the Colonists deteriorated horrendously. Atrocities were committed on both sides, and it is indeed a point of shame in Australia's colonial history that the decision was made to 'collect the Aboriginal peoples and remove them from their homelands'.

In December 1843 Joseph Milligan was appointed by the Lieutenant-Governor, Sir John Franklin, as Superintendent of the Aborigines Establishment at Flinders Island. He was stationed there as their doctor for twelve years between 1843 and 1855. This was a time of personal tragedy for him also as his bride of one year died in childbirth on the 31st July 1844, at Flinders Island. There were five European males and their wives on the Island, one hospital nurse, and by 1843, only 54 Aborigines remained. In 1855, only 44 Aboriginals were left at Flinders Island – twelve men, twenty-two women, and ten 'young people'. The little colony, under Dr Joseph Milligan was ordered to move again to Oyster Cove in D'Entrecasteaux Channel.

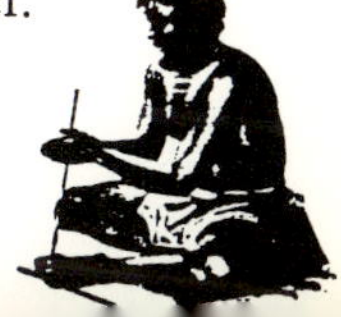

The Hobart *Town Courier* of October 20th 1855 reported –

> *Arrived in the schooner Sisters Gill, from Flinders Island with Dr Milligan and lady, 22 female, 15 Aborigines and 10 children which he landed at Oyster Cove in D'Entrecasteaux Channel.*

The settlement soon decayed, but besides being their doctor, Milligan compiled a dictionary of the Aboriginal language entitled 'Vocabulary of dialects of the Aboriginal tribes of Tasmania'. This is the largest and most complete vocabulary of that now extinct language.

Milligan was one of the founders of the Royal Society of Van Diemen's Land, and was its secretary in the period 1848–1860. He bequeathed land at Georgetown and Bicheno to the Royal Society of Tasmania after his death. His extensive explorations and his detailed knowledge of geology facilitated discoveries of coal, copper and gold in various parts of the Island. He collected numerous fossils and shells, and was particularly interested in chitons. The chiton *Ischnochiton milligani* records his interests in marine zoology. He had the respect of the two Governors whom he served, and was commissioned by Lieutenant-Governor Denison to survey the entire coal resources of the Island. He saw the great opportunities for business expansion in Tasmania, and in April 1855 he became Chairman of the Douglas River Coal Mining Company, and undertook explorations for the Fingal Gold Exploration Company.

After his retirement in April 1860, Milligan returned to England and died in 1884. His achievements brought wide recognition. He was elected to the Fellowship of the Linnean Society in 1850. His correspondent and botanist-surgeon friend in London, Sir William Hooker, raised the new genus *Milligania* in 1853 to honour his contributions. This genus is comprised of four species of fine plants, all appropriately found only in Tasmania. Besides these, many species of plants were named after him, including one of the beautiful Snow Everlastings *Helichrysum milliganii*, one of the most beautiful wildflowers of alpine Tasmania. Of the many other species that record his work, *Pimelea milligania*, Milligan's Rice-flower, exquisitely recalls his life of adventure and scholarship in the Tasmanian bush.

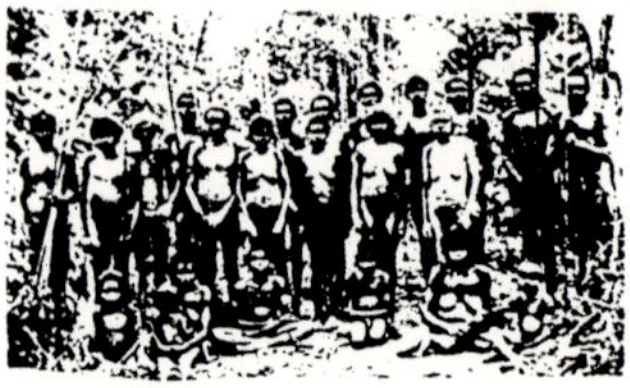

SURGEON JAMES PATRICK MURRAY (1839–*c.*1885)

Not all fine plants record the lives of fine people. The beautiful wattle, *Acacia murrayana*, is named after one of Australia's most infamous doctors, the psychopath and murderer James Patrick Murray. Surgeon Murray was an Irish doctor who spent 13 years in Australia and New Zealand. Like most psychopaths he had an appealing personality. The record of his life is one of adventure, poor impulse control, infamy, and final condemnation by a society which initially accepted him as a worthy member of the medical profession.

James Patrick Murray was born to a family of merchants in Roscommon in the County of Connaught in Ireland. He commenced his studies as a medical student, at the age of 17 years, on the 25th September 1856 when he entered Trinity College in Dublin. The circumstances of his life as a medical student are unknown, but he was admitted as a Licentiate of the Royal College of Surgeons of Ireland and immediately emigrated to Melbourne, arriving in November 1860. He was also elected to Membership of the King and Queen's College of Physicians of Ireland.

Like all scoundrels, Surgeon Murray was totally lacking in humility, and from the first week of his arrival in Australia, established a pattern of self-promotion. He stayed at Prince Georges Hotel in Swanson Street and offered his services as a surgeon with Howitt's Expedition, then being planned to rescue Burke and Wills who were overdue from their journey from Melbourne to the Gulf of Carpentaria. Dr Murray wrote in his letter –

> *... that the enterprise is one involving the greatest personal sufferings and dangers, these however I accept, being animated by an honourable desire for fame – and an ardent love of science.*

Whilst awaiting this venture, Murray was appointed as a Staff Surgeon to the Melbourne Hospital in 1861, but he served in that position for barely 12 months before he was given 'six months leave' to take part in the Burke and Wills Search Expedition. It is noted that 'he did not return from his six months leave for over a year' and was formally removed from the staff list of the Melbourne Hospital in March 1863.

Murray was only 23 years of age when he went as 'Surgeon and Collector' on Howitt's Expedition in search of the remains of Burke and Wills. There is no record of Murray's behaviour being a problem on that journey. The party rode north to Cooper's Creek where vegetables were grown which prevented scurvy – a scourge to previous Australian exploring parties. He was stationed in the base camp at Cooper's Creek but travelled in some of the surveying and exploring parties which radiated from it. Howitt gave the name Mount Murray on the edge of Sturt's Stoney Desert to a ridge discovered on one of these side-exploring journeys, and Murray's Creek (since renamed Candradecka Creek) to a local watercourse in the area. The party brought back the bodies of the dead explorers (Burke and Wills) to Adelaide. The return of the Expedition to Adelaide (on December 11th 1862) was a poignant and moving moment. It is recorded that –

> *A large ... course of the citizens of Adelaide assembled near the Newmarket Inn, to show their respects to the remains of the dead Victorians, being conveyed in ... a best hearse, drawn by four black horses ... the hearse preceded by the Mayor and the city officials and followed immediately by Mr Howitt, Dr Murray and South Australia's own Dr John McKinley.*

Murray returned with the Expedition on the *Haviah* to Melbourne.

Unsettled, Murray emigrated to Invercargill in New Zealand, where he spent two years in medical practice in which the basic unethical overtones of his personality again became apparent. He was appointed as Resident Surgeon to the Southland Provincial Hospital. However, there was soon increasing discontent about his practice and letters of disapproval were published in the local newspapers. He was described as –

> *... a young man of neat, rather dandified appearance, good looking with any amount of assurance and self-confidence, suave and ingratiating manner which 'went down' particularly well with the ladies ... .*

In 1864 and 1865, the Melbourne botanist, Dr Ferdinand von Mueller had kept the public conscience alive concerning the unresolved question of Leichhardt's disappearance (in 1848). After an impassioned public meeting, a Ladies' Committee raised funds for a further search exploration, and when the question of the surgeon for the party was raised, Murray's name was considered. Dr Ferdinand von Mueller appointed him second in command of the party, and the surgeon.

The Ladies' Leichhardt Search Expedition, for which £4,000 had been raised, was a tragic failure. The party reached Cooper's Creek on November 26th, 1865. Surgeon Murray, second in charge, was left in camp while Duncan MacIntyre (the leader) went ahead to look for water. Subsequent accounts and correspondence reveal that Murray's conduct at the time was scandalous. He showed gross cowardice and poor judgement, and on one occasion opened out the brandy and he and the party became drunk. The stock roamed free. The *Daily Telegraph* of Adelaide (3rd August 1866) noted his behaviour as '... debased, cruel and cowardly desertion of one in whom the leader of the party had first reposed implicit confidence'.

Murray returned immediately to Melbourne, undaunted by any factors of conscience. He received appointments as Resident Surgeon to the Benevolent Asylum, to the Immigration Hospital and to the Western Jail. Murray fancied himself as a clinician also, and in the July 1868 issue of the *Australian Medical Journal* he wrote an article suggesting that scarlet fever and diphtheria were the same disease. Like all convincing confidence tricksters, he was well received by his peers. In January 1869 he was elected to the Committee of the Victorian Medical Association. In November 1869, to the eternal shame of the traditions of artillery, he was gazetted as Assistant Surgeon to the Brighton Royal Victorian Volunteer Artillery Corps. To the chagrin of his professional colleagues, he advertised in the local newspapers, using such language as —

> *Clearly understand I do not wish to urge any member of the public to have me as his surgeon, unless he is perfectly satisfied that my qualifications are superior to any other surgeon about here, being a physician as well as a surgeon ... .*

In 1870, Murray saw the opportunity for making a quick fortune. It was the height of the Fijian cotton boom, and the new cotton establishments in Queensland desperately needed labour. 'Black-birding' became a disgusting but lucrative practice, and in early 1870 Murray sold his medical practice at Brighton in Melbourne, and on the 25th April 1871, purchased the Brig *Carl* of 280 tonnes. Murray undertook two voyages in Fijian waters, as part of his new enterprise. On the first voyage, he quarrelled with two of the planters and forcibly put them and their party ashore where they were eaten. On the second voyage he went to the New Hebrides where in September 1871, he seduced 160 indigenous men aboard. It was recorded that —

> *... this kidnapping cruise was unique even amongst the annals of blackbirding, in many ways. There was an exceptionally large number of prisoners ... they posed as missionaries to entice the*

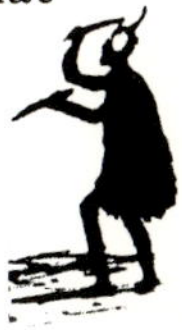

> *natives aboard ... and the crew took the boats on a wide excursion ... to round up natives at gunpoint. ... their final haul, extending over three days, took place in the Buka Strait between the islands of Buka and Bougainville, and more than 60 natives were captured. On the night of September 14th, in one of the most tragic sagas of an already tragic story, Surgeon Murray led his crew in a bloody massacre of some 70 of the prisoners who were held below decks.*

Surgeon Archibald Watson was also on the voyage, and it was Watson's evidence which subsequently led to Murray's downfall. Like the scoundrel he was, Murray turned Queen's evidence and escaped the gallows.

In spite of odium cast upon him by all society in Melbourne, Surgeon Murray returned there and obtained a local government appointment and was involved with a vaccination campaign following a Smallpox outbreak in 1872. His hypocrisy was unbounded, and on the 18th November 1872, he wrote to the Melbourne *Argus* that –

> *... it is true I was one of the humble instruments employed by God in stamping out the Smallpox in your city ... my object from the date of my conversion has been the suppression of South-Sea slavery.*

An editorial in the same newspaper did not encourage Surgeon Murray to submit any more letters to the Editor, in the following terms –

> *... at all events we hope we shall not be nauseated by any more communication from this murdering mawworm.*

Attempts were made to prevent him from practising medicine but he continued until he was last seen in Australia, in Sydney, on January 20th 1873. Little of his further life is known. He returned to England and practised at least for a period in Manchester, from which address he wrote (on December 28, 1878) to *The Lancet*, about his experience with Pituri, the extract from one of the Australian cork-woods, which contains atropine. Murray impressed Dr Ferdinand von Mueller, in the former's early days in the Colony. Von Mueller named three beautiful Australian plants after him – *Acacia murrayana, Ptilotus murrayi* and *Polyscias murrayi*. Thus are the sins of the wicked sometimes perpetuated.

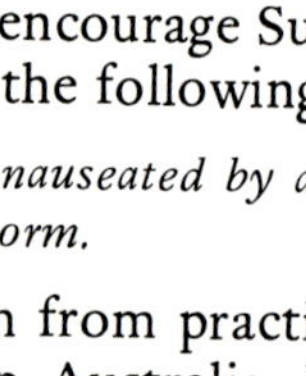

Acacia murrayana

Dr CHARLES BRIGHTLY PRENTICE (1820–1894)

Medicine, botany, entomology and public service – a full life, and one commemorated in the names of two beautiful Queensland ferns, and an Australian grass. These permanent memorials record the life of Charles Brightly Prentice, a surgeon and natural historian of Woolloongabba in Brisbane.

Charles Brightly was born the son of Charles Prentice, in Southwold, Suffolk in England in 1820. After apprenticeship as a surgeon, he was admitted as a Licentiate of the Society of Apothecaries of London at the age of 25 years. It is probable that he practised in Exeter, in Devon, where his first wife died. In 1857 he was admitted to Membership of the Royal College of Surgeons of England, and soon after (1859) remarried Eliza Dunn, also of Exeter. The reasons for his emigration to Australia are unknown, but *circa* 1865 he settled at Woolloongabba on the south bank of the Brisbane River and practised there as a physician and surgeon for some 30 years until his death.

Charles Prentice was well respected by his medical peers, and was chosen as a member of the Queensland Medical Board, a body established to supervise the registration, ethics and behavioural practices of Queensland doctors. He was also a member of the Board of Emigration, and the Central Board of Health.

Prentice is best remembered for his contributions to natural history. A keen botanist and zoologist, he was an avid explorer and collected throughout Queensland. He became a regular contributor (particularly in the years 1892 to 1894) to the meetings and publications of the Royal Society of Queensland. During his 30 years as a doctor in Brisbane, it was said that –

> *... during the whole of that time he was always a ready helper to those working in the branches of scientific research of which he was a master.*

His special areas of interests, and where he made his most significant scientific contributions, were in the study of ferns and grasses. His beetle collection (in the field of entomology) was also well known. To commemorate his work and contributions to the study of grasses, the new species *Panicum prenticeanum* was named in his honour. He had a particular love of ferns, of which the Queensland tropical and sub-tropical flora is so rich. A newly discovered species on Thursday Island, *Cheilanthes prenticei* was named in his honour. He

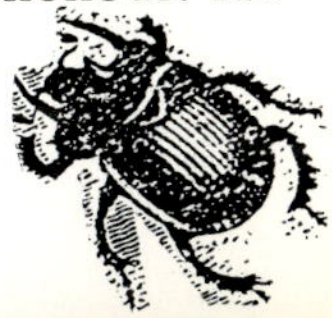

was a particular friend and colleague to the Queensland Government Botanist, Dr F.M. Bailey, and as an acknowledgement of Prentice's contributions to botany, Bailey named another particularly beautiful new fern, discovered at Trinity Bay in North Queensland, *Asplenium prenticei*, in his honour.

Dr WALTER EDMUND ROTH (1861–1933)

Walter Edmund Roth was a doctor, pioneer of public health, ethnographer and anthropologist, described in a contemporary newspaper of his day as –

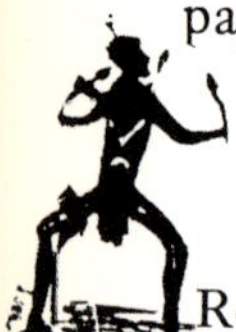

> *A big genial fellow in the very mid-summer of his manhood, earnest above all things in the work with Aboriginals that he has undertaken, but with the modesty and frankness of a schoolboy.*

Roth's particular talent consisted in the meticulous collection and recording of anthropological data. His wide interest and hobbies enabled him to bring a particularly broad perspective to all that he did. He explored widely both in Australia and in South America (he was the leader of three scientific expeditions in British Guyana), and his great accuracy for recording detail gave him a worldwide place among the ranks of famous anthropologists.

Walter Edmund Roth was born the son of Dr Mathias Roth, a surgeon, in London on the 2nd April 1861. He was educated in France (at Boulogne and Paris), in Germany, and in London. He was a resident at Magdalen College (Oxford) from which he graduated with his Bachelor of Arts with honours in biology in 1884. He studied medicine at St Thomas' Hospital in London, and by the time he was 27 years he had published two works relating to preventive medicine and public health. The first of these was a pioneering work – *The elements of school hygiene: for the use of teachers in schools*. He was interested in the transmission of disease in densely packed spaces in the context of Pasteur's discoveries of the germ transmission of disease. He published in London, in 1888, his book entitled *Theatre hygiene: a scheme for the study of a somewhat neglected department of the public health.* This latter work contained details for the safety, sanitation, ventilation, lighting and fire protection, and safe construction of public theatres. In 1888 he emigrated to Australia, and was appointed as the Director of the Government School of Mines and Industries, in Adelaide, an apparently strange appointment for someone whose background was in arts and medicine. However, his already manifested interest in safety and ventilation gave him particular credentials in this discipline.

In 1891 Dr Roth was appointed as a schoolmaster at the Brisbane Grammar School and he developed a special *camaraderie* with his pupils, now well accepted but a style less common in those former conservative Victorian times. In a newspaper interview in 1901, he recalled –

> *... it is a point of pride that some of my best friends of today have come from the ranks of my old Grammar School pupils, all of whom have gone well in life.*

Dr Roth explored and travelled extensively. He wrote meticulously and many of his records form the only formal direct observations of many ethnological practices that are now forever lost. A major publication (in 1901) entitled *Food: its search, capture and preparation*, gave detailed reports of Aboriginal life in northern Australia. He described in detail the preparation of many Aboriginal foods, the use of clay and minerals by Aborigines, details of ritual surgery, and detailed observations on sickness and disease amongst the Aboriginal population. He travelled widely to Normanton, to Cooktown, to the Northern Territory and to Western Australia. In 1894, he was appointed as the surgeon at the Cloncurry, Boulia and Normanton Hospitals in Queensland, and it was there that he first manifested his special interest in the local Aboriginal languages of the Mitakoodi and Kalkadoon tribes. His *Ethnological studies among the north-west-central Queensland Aborigines* was published in 1897. In that year he was appointed as Chief Protector of Aborigines in Queensland. He worked well with his contemporaries, and was a particular collaborator with Mr Parry-Okeden, the Queensland Commissioner of Police, who also had extensive experience of work with the Aboriginal population. In 1905 Dr Roth was appointed as a Royal Commissioner to enquire into the conditions of Aboriginals in Western Australia.

Roth's life was one of constantly seeking new interests and diversions. He was a passionate collector, not only of plant's and animals and shells, but of coins and medals as well. He wrote a series of articles on numismatics for the Queensland Press.

In 1906, Roth left Australia and went to South America, being appointed as Government Medical Officer, Magistrate and Protector of Indians in the Pomeroon District. Three major works on the *Arts, Crafts, Customs of the Guinee Indians* were published in the period

1924–1929, He died on the 5th April 1933, widely recognised and admired internationally as an anthropologist. Honours have been showered upon him, including (in 1902) the Clarke Medal of the Royal Society of New South Wales. His memorials are in his published work, and in three plants of the northern Queensland rainforest which bear his name. One of these is the native pepper, *Piper rothianum*, and another is the fungus *Anthurus rothae*. The Australian wattle, *Acacia rothii*, is perhaps his most appropriate living memorial, its yellow blooms in the arid regions of Australia symbolising his sunny disposition, and the many explorations to the outback which he successfully completed.

SURGEON WILLIAM STEPHENSON (*circa* 1790–1863)

Mr William Stephenson, A Medical Gentleman who will also act as Naturalist to the Expedition.

Thus was described the surgeon and botanist who accompanied Sir Thomas Mitchell on his 1845 Expedition from Sydney to Bourke (then Fort Bourke). Governor Gipps, in commissioning the expedition, held that its main aim was the discovery of the supposed great inland river or rivers which flowed northwards to the Gulf of Carpentaria. Stephenson's legacy, besides his place in the annals of Australian Exploration, and his clinical service to his patients in northern New South Wales, resides also in the plant *Platysace stephensonii* which bears his name.

The early details of Surgeon Stephenson's life are shrouded in mystery. He was born *circa* 1790, possibly in Ireland, and was early apprenticed as a surgeon. He joined the Army, and saw service as a military surgeon in both India and China. In one of those Campaigns, he sustained a leg wound, which forced him to ride side-saddle thereafter, a not inconsiderable feat when one considers the thousands of kilometres he traversed through unmapped and unknown country on his subsequent explorations in Australia. He arrived in Sydney at an unknown date prior to 1845, at a time when there was a great hunger to explore the great unknown interior of Australia. Governors Darling, Burke and Gipps were commissioning exploring parties to map the continent. Leichhardt's private expedition was overdue (long overdue) at Port Essington at the northern tip of Arnhem Land, and Charles Sturt was exploring in central Australia. Sir Thomas Mitchell, at 53 years of age was in Sydney 'growling in frustration' at not being commissioned to explore further. Finally, in late 1845 Governor Gipps allocated £2,000 for an expedition to proceed from Sydney, through north-western New South Wales to the Gulf of Carpentaria, and appointed Mitchell as leader. In December 1845 the party assembled at Boree, with instructions to proceed overland by way of Bathurst to Fort Bourke and thence to the Gulf.

Gipps instructed the party particularly to respect the Australian Aboriginals whom they would surely meet, and (as his specific instructions stated) —

> *... to endeavour by every possible means to conciliate their goodwill from which the most important assistance may be derived, and in the event of any hostile demonstration on their part, the utmost forbearance is to be shown by all persons composing the Expedition nor is the use of firearms or force of any kind to be resorted to unless the safety of the party should absolutely require it.*

Surgeon William Stephenson, obviously with a life already full with the adventures of military medicine and surgery, assembled at Boree with the rest of the party. His remuneration was to be 7 shillings and 6 pence per day. There were 30 men comprising the party, of whom 23 were convicts. Edmund Kennedy, the Assistant Surveyor, was second in command.

Governor Gipps specific instructions noted to Sir Thomas Mitchell, the Expedition leader were that —

> *... you will of course afford every facility to Mr Stephenson in the prosecution of his researches and for the preserving and conveying the collections he may be enabled to make of Animals, Plants, Roots, and Seeds. Specimens of every kind obtained during the Expedition are to be considered the property of the Public and lists to be made of them from time to time as they are collected setting forth the places where they have been found and any facts that may tend to elucidate their natural history and character.*

Stephenson discharged this duty well and plants from his collection made during that Expedition, reside in a number of major herbaria. He exhibited some of his collections in the New South Wales Exhibit at the Paris Exhibition of 1855. After the Mitchell Expedition (which discovered the Maranoa River and some of its tributaries) he took up property at Cundle near the Richmond River, and thereafter moved to the Manning River at Taree, where he established medical practice. He was universally liked by his colleagues on the Mitchell Expedition of 1845 – he rode a black pony which took him through all the Expedition, and it was known that he had a peculiar habit of whistling 'in season and out of season'. His death in 1863 robbed the district of a practical experienced surgeon and a keen naturalist, but the plant which bears his name, Stephenson's Platysace, blooms in New South Wales to perpetuate his memory.

Dr THOMAS TATE (1842–1934)

A number of doctors there are who left the ranks of clinical medicine to seek adventure, and whose exploits in other fields form their epitaphs. Most doctors lead conservative lives and the adrenalin of high adventure is not their lot. One exception was Dr Thomas Tate,

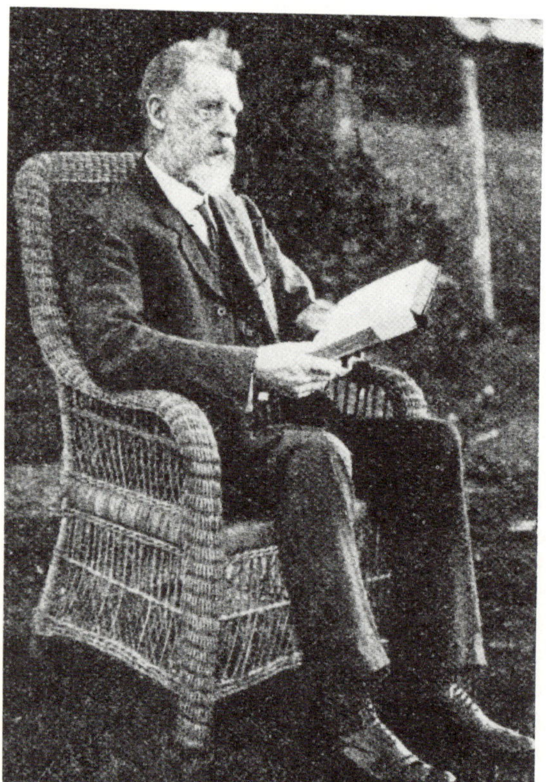

Figure 1.9

Dr Thomas Tate (1842–1934).

'Surgeon' to the ill-fated 'New Guinea Prospecting Association' of 1871, he survived sharks and Aboriginal attacks following the shipwreck of the 'Maria' near Cardwell, in north Queensland.

He was subsequently appointed as surgeon to the Hahn Expedition (1872) which discovered the Tate, Daintree, Walsh and Palmer Rivers on Cape York.

Photo by courtesy of Cummins and Campbell's Monthly Magazine (Townsville) of March 1934.

Queensland explorer and adventurer, whose life was a quest for travel and learning, far from the beaten track. A survivor of one of Queensland's most tragic shipwrecks, his spirit of exploration was undaunted. Mount Tate in North Queensland records his role as the surgeon on Hahn's Northern Expedition, and his contributions to botany are acknowledged in the small rainforest shrub, *Premna tateana*, which grows near the Walsh River of which he was a co-discoverer.

Thomas Tate was born on 25th June 1842 at Alnwick, north of Newcastle-Upon-Tyne in Northumberland in England. The children in his family received a good education, and no-one growing up in that beautiful part of England can escape the wonders of natural history that are to be found on the Northumberland Moors. The family milieu in which he developed was one in which studies of botany and zoology were encouraged. His elder brother, Ralph, also became an eminent botanist in Australia. Thomas was apprenticed as a surgeon, but the details of his training are unknown. In the middle 19th century, many English and Scottish doctors did not take formal degrees, nor were they required to do so until the passing of the *Medical Act of 1858*, when formal university based training was required. Tate's apprenticeship was such that he was caught up in the year of that changeover. Until that time –

> *... a large number of students were content to learn their profession as apprentices to some practitioner, and to take a few classes at some medical school such as Edinburgh, without proceeding to graduation.*

Many who completed their articles of apprenticeship went to medical school for several years, to 'top up' their medical training – Dr William Redfern, Australia's first medical graduate, and Dr Walter Scott, Queensland's first doctor, went to Edinburgh University as mature age medical students after completing their apprenticeship as surgeons. Thus also did Thomas Tate who, like so many Northumbrian lads aspiring to medicine, went to Edinburgh University. Like so many of his medical contemporaries of that era, he was not awarded any formal degree in medicine. There was some speculation after his death, whether in fact his medical training was ever more than that of a medical student. He was, however, universally known as 'Doctor Thomas Tate', and his initial appearance in Australia was as Surgeon to the ill-fated 'New Guinea Prospecting Association', formed impulsively as a wild scheme in Sydney in November 1871.

The events leading to Dr Tate's emigration to Australia are shrouded in mystery. After his medical studies at Edinburgh he joined the crew of a whaling ship; and thereafter was appointed as Ship's Surgeon on a ship bound for New Zealand. He arrived in Sydney from New Zealand at some period before 1871, and became caught up in the promise of gold in what was then the shadowy island of New Guinea, then a land unknown except for its coastline, and two of its major rivers, to the western world. At that time –

> *New Guinea with its reputed material wealth in gold, copper and other materials, in ebony ... and other valuable timbers, in tortoise shell ... and pearls ... spices and medicinal barks ...*

was almost wholly unexplored.

Gold was the talk of Sydney Town in the early 1870s. Tate attended several public lectures held in the Temperance Hall in Pitt Street, Sydney in late 1871. One was given by the Reverend John Dunmore Lang 'who pointed out the wonderful resources of New Guinea and stated there was an abundance of ebony, of sandalwood and other timbers which would be extremely valuable if placed on the market'. The Reverend William Clarke (1798–1878) the renowned geologist, spoke at these lectures of the probability of New Guinea being rich in gold. He said, 'that the four great gold-bearing lodes of Australia undoubtedly dipped at Torres Strait, and in all probability would be found to reappear in New Guinea'. [Neither gentleman had actually been to New Guinea!] A missionary from the Fly River stated that 'the cooking pots used by the Papuans showed traces of gold'. That was enough for the young men of Sydney.

> *These lectures naturally inflamed the young and adventurous* [Dr Thomas Tate, and Lawrence Hargreaves, later the renowned aviation pioneer, among them] *with a desire to visit this wonderful new country and a meeting was called at Princes Hotel. The result was the New Guinea Prospecting Association with a membership of 70. Everything was hurried for the members of the Association were not wealthy, and most of them put everything they had into the Association and could not afford to wait idly in Sydney.*

The New South Wales Government was distrustful of this so-called expeditionary Association. One member (Mr Thomas Ingham) later recounted 'We were all armed and had plenty of ammunition. It afterwards came out we were regarded as a filibustering expedition and Captain Moresby [in *H.M.S. Basilisk*] was instructed to keep a sharp watch upon us'.

The 70 young men commissioned the rotting brig, the *Maria,* ('a crazy old brig of 167 tonnes') in Sydney Harbour, to take them to New Guinea. Captain Moresby, who later rescued the survivors under amazing circumstances, later summed up the group as '75 hare-brained young men from Sydney who attempted a prospecting expedition to New Guinea ... they were wrecked on the *Maria* on Bramble Reef, about 30 miles from Cardwell, in North Queensland'.

The ship was overloaded, and a number of crew places were taken by the men of the exploration party, so that all 70 could go. In all, there were 75 on board with only the Captain and four other crewmen who were experienced sailors. When the *Maria* struck a coral reef in far North Queensland at 3.15 a.m. on 26th February, 1872, it was realised that there were not enough lifeboats. Confusion reigned. To his disgrace, the Captain 'made off in the whaleboat with 5 or 6 men' and was shot at by those left deserted on the wreck. Only two whaleboats remained, and two rafts were hastily fashioned. Dr Thomas Tate took command of one of the two boats, and with some 5 or 6 men reached Hinchinbrook Island. The survivors lived on 'shellfish and pulp biscuit' for five days, and then made for Cardwell (then the most northern port on mainland Australia) which they reached three days later, with the news of the disaster. The majority of the initial expedition perished in the wreck itself, others were taken by sharks, and some on the rafts which reached land were murdered by the Aborigines. In all 34 of the original 75 survived, Tate among them. The rescue was effected by Captain Moresby, in *H.M.S. Basilisk*. All the survivors, except Tate, returned to Sydney.

At that time (1872) a Government Expedition to Cape York was being planned, and no surgeon was available. Undaunted by his brush with death, and perhaps stimulated by it, Tate enlisted to explore the unmapped territory of the interior of the Cape York Peninsula. The Expedition, 'a well organised official party' was given in charge of William Hahn (1837–1889) 'a daring horseman and whip, and a first-class bushman' with Tate commissioned as the surgeon and botanist.

The party assembled at Fossilbrook, and proceeded northwards. They discovered the Tate River (named after Tate as the surgeon to the Party), the Daintree and the Walsh Rivers and the Palmer River where traces of gold were found. Although Tate was not to benefit, it was poignant that the great Palmer River Gold Rush was the scene of dramatic wealth for so many.

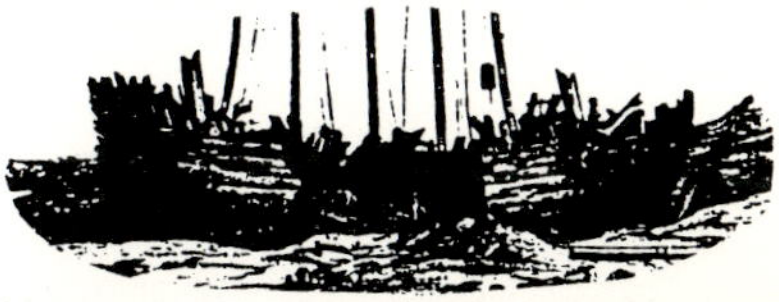

Tate sent specimens of plants from the Expedition to Kew Gardens in London, and some of the specimens were subsequently returned to Dr Maiden, the Colonial Botanist in Brisbane twenty years later. At Kew, Tate's specimens were examined and classified by Dr George Bentham, and were included in his great work *Flora Australiensis* which was then in preparation. Dr Tate's interest in natural history was not limited to botany. It was on that trip that Tate discovered the bones of the Tree Kangaroo. It was not formally described until 1884, in the *Proceedings of the Zoological Society*. The Expedition followed a grand circle, and 'was back at its starting point on the 10th November 1872'.

Tate then left the practice of medicine. There is some evidence to indicate that he was concerned that he did not have a formal degree in medicine, and at the age of 30 years (having already lived life to the fullest!) he probably felt he had time to use his formal training in biology in other pursuits. He became a school teacher, joining the Department of Public Instruction in Queensland. By 1903, he was teaching at Georgetown (at the Gulf of Carpentaria) and at Normanton. Subsequently, he taught at Pialba, Thursday Island, Cardwell, and finally at the State School at St Lawrence in 1913. He retired to Peak Vale at Clermont near Rockhampton in 1914, and died aged 91 years on January 27th 1934, at Rockhampton. Tate's legacy is an inspiration to those who make decisions, traumatic at the time, to change course in their professional lives and start a new career. Tate's memorials exist not only in his discoveries, and in the Tate River named after him, but also in one of the North Queensland rainforest plants which bears his name. Dr Bailey, the Colonial Botanist in Brisbane, wrote in 1890 that 'finding no plant named after this collector, I have given a lately received plant from that district his name, *Premna tateana*.'

PROFESSOR ARCHIBALD WATSON (1849–1940)

Archibald Watson, a legendary Professor of Anatomy at the University of Adelaide, was one of Australia's great medical teachers and adventurers. He published little, but kept a wealth of recorded observations as a diarist. His charismatic personality was such that many of his pupils (who went on to become eminent international medical figures themselves) remember the special significance of his influence and teaching upon them.

Archibald Watson studied surgery in Scotland, working under Dr Jonathan Hutchinson Snr., the famous Quaker Surgeon of widespread interests. Whilst still a young man of 23 years, Watson suffered the traumatic experience of sailing in the South Seas with the infamous Dr James Patrick Murray, in the blackbirding voyage of the Brig *Carl*.

Universally known as 'Watty' by the medical students whom he taught, Archibald Watson's special interest was surgical anatomy, and the way in which new interpretations and discoveries of human anatomy could help the practising surgeon. He was particularly interested in gynaecological anatomy, and his students recall his many dissertations on hysterectomy for various benign tumours of the human uterus.

In the Second Archibald Watson Memorial Lecture (delivered before The Royal Australasian College of Physicians on the 11th November, 1949, in Melbourne), Sir John Burton Cleland (himself an eminent doctor-botanist) noted that –

> *He gave no set lectures in anatomy, but his demonstrations and talks, illustrated by sketches, on points of anatomical and particularly surgical importance impressed us more lastingly than could any lecture or textbook. He would approach his subject of instruction with some anecdote or experience having often, as far as one could see, no possible connection with anatomy. He would seemingly ramble on discursively and we would wonder what his talk was leading up to, and finally would come to its application to an anatomical fact or surgical procedure.*

He enjoyed adventure and travel in many parts of Australia, including the Queensland outback. He was an organiser of the Elder Exploring Expedition (of 1891) from northern South Australia to Wiluna in Western Australia. His care and enthusiasm in this venture was such that the leader of the Expedition, (David Lindsay), named a 750 metre mountain, Mt Watson, in his honour.

It is fitting that a beautiful fringe-myrtle *Calytrix watsonii* (Watson's Fringe-myrtle) should bear his name.

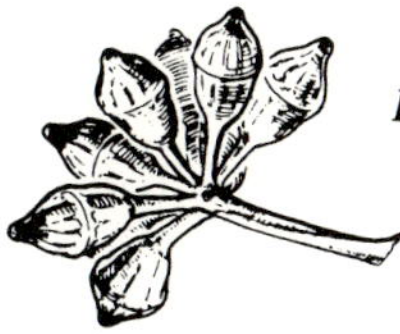

Eucalyptus clelandii

SURGEON WILLIAM F. WHEELER (Flourished 1861)

Surgeon Wheeler remains a doctor about whom little is known. He was appointed as the surgeon and botanical collector of the Victorian Relief Expedition, sent by the Royal Society of Victoria's Exploration Committee to search for the lost Burke and Wills, in 1861 and 1862. This expedition under the command of a William Howitt left Melbourne in 1861, and followed the known course of the lost explorers through Swan Hill, Pamamaro Creek, to Menindie, and thence to Jacob's Station at Parallana. This latter point was reached on 4th June 1862.

Surgeon Wheeler collected botanical specimens in the interior of Australia, and two of the hardy plants of that dry area forever record his passing. *Euphorbia wheeleri* is one of those uncommon plants which honours two medical practitioners – in this case two doctors who were literally poles apart not only in place, but in time. Euphorbus was the physician to King Juba II of Mauritania (in north Africa, *c.* 48 B.C.–23 A.D.). Euphorbus wrote about the treatment of plant poisonings, and was an advocate of the use of cold baths to treat mania. The genus *Euphorbia* bears his name. Both Euphorbus and Wheeler practised as doctors and botanists in desert regions. Their names, linked across two millennia, portray the continuity and universality of medicine.

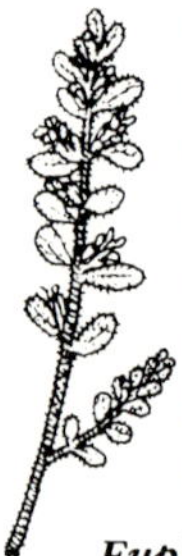

Euphorbia australis

SURGEON THOMAS BRAIDWOOD WILSON (1792–1843)

A 'thoughtful, upright and energetic man credited with the introduction to Australia of the honey bee, lilac and many other plants, being also a surgeon in the Royal Navy, from 1821 Surgeon Superintendent of some nine convict ships, and a vigorous explorer of Western Australia'– thus was Thomas Braidwood Wilson, an esteemed pioneer and colonist of Australia. These events occurred almost two centuries ago, recalled in tangible form whenever one sees the beautiful *Grevillea wilsonii*, which perpetuates his name.

Thomas Wilson was born in Braidwood, Lanarkshire, in Scotland, on April 30th 1792, and given the nameplace of his birth. In turn, he was to give his name to the town of Braidwood in New South Wales where he settled and died as a much loved colonist at the age of 51 years, in 1843.

Thomas Wilson was also named after Dr Thomas Braidwood of Edinburgh, who had achieved much fame as the first to teach the deaf to speak, and had had founded one of the first hospitals for abandoned children in the Western World. Thomas Braidwood Wilson studied as a medical student at Edinburgh University (1810–1813), but abandoned his studies there because of the national fervour to fight the French in the Napoleonic Wars. He joined the Navy, and was apprenticed as a Hospital Mate in 1813, at the Royal Naval Hospital at Haslar, in Gosport in Hampshire. On August 17th 1815, at the age of 23 years, he was promoted to the rank of Surgeon on H.M.S. *Trident,* and served in the Mediterranean. He subsequently accompanied King George IV on a trip to Ireland and to Germany.

Navy and Military Surgeons feared peace in those times, and the end of the Napoleonic Wars that would force retirement on many. Those who were fortunate enough to remain on active service had little hope of promotion. At the time the toast of the officers ward room at naval hospitals was 'a bloody war or a sickly season'. One avenue open for employment to naval surgeons was to become Surgeon Superintendent on the convict transports plying between Port Arthur (in Van Diemen's Land) and Sydney Cove. Among the tragic stories of convict transportation to Australia, the establishment of the office of Surgeon Superintendent of Convicts stands out as a wise and humanitarian decision. Those fine doctors did much to protect convicts from much of the helplessness and brutality potentially inherent in that system. Surgeon Thomas Braidwood Wilson made nine voyages in this role, between 1821 and 1840. After the disasters of the Second Fleet (when almost one half of the convicts who left England did not survive the voyage or the first weeks after arrival in Sydney Cove, so extreme were their privations), the Surgeon Superintendents were given the absolute authority and responsibility for convicts' welfare on those voyages. Surgeon Wilson himself wrote that he was required —

> *... not only to officiate as physician, surgeon, and apothecary, but also as clergyman, schoolmaster, justice of the peace and inspector of provisions.*

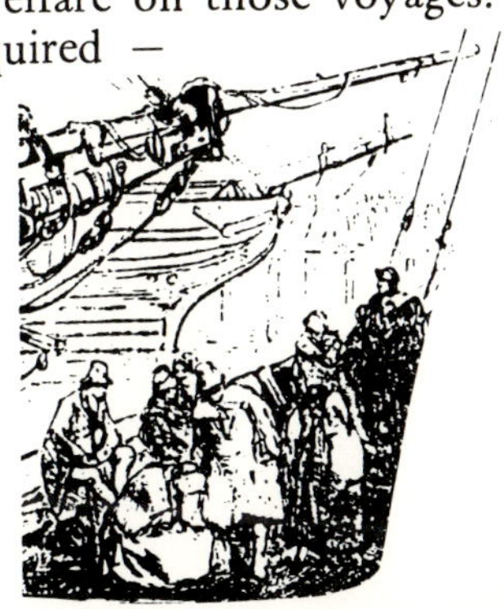

Some 2,000 convicts were protected, by his care, from the potential harassment and abuses of a system in which harassment and abuse was, if not below the surface, always potentially below decks.

The *Sydney Gazette* of July 22nd 1824, noted that Dr Wilson –

> *... has not only anxiously attended to the bodies of the unfortunate exiles committed to his care, but also studied by every possible means to enlighten and improve the nobler part – the mind. To the lasting fame of Dr Wilson, be it recorded, that several men not only now can read, but actually write – all owing to the establishment of schools on board at the insistence of the doctor.*

He suffered privations on these voyages, and was twice shipwrecked. On one occasion he was cast away in Torres Strait and eventually visited the northern settlement of Melville Island (off what is now the Northern Territory, and reached Java in the ship's boats). In 1829, Wilson commenced some of his most significant exploration work, exploring in the south-west of Western Australia, particularly in the region of King George Sound. He discovered the Denmark River and named this after one of his many naval surgical colleagues, Surgeon Alexander Denmark. It is appropriate that both Denmark and Wilson now have their names commemorated in fine West Australian plants. Wilson wrote about the land and its people, and in his book published in London in 1835 *Narrative of a Voyage Around the World*, he described much valuable anthropological information about the Aborigines whom he encountered on his explorations.

Wilson was a keen botanist, and brought seeds and plants to Allan Cunningham, King's Botanist and later Curator at the Sydney Botanic Gardens.

In 1826 Wilson was given some 5,000 acres of land in New South Wales, which is now the site of the town of Braidwood.

The life of a naval surgeon albeit one of travel and adventure, is one of separation from one's family. Finally, in 1836 he brought his wife and two children to New South Wales where the family settled on his property at Braidwood. Tragically, his wife died two years later, his business affairs declined in his depressive state which followed, and he became bankrupt. Rich however his memory is, in the beautiful red *Grevillea* which bears his name.

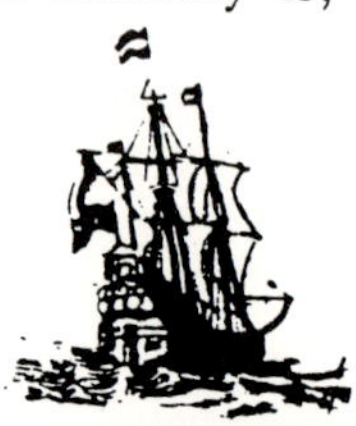

REPRISE

What profiles can one draw from these lives of adventure, medicine and service? What common themes enmeshed them in a window of history – a century the opportunities of which can never return?

These doctor-explorers had three special themes in common. Perhaps the most striking and consistent was a love of natural history, of plants and animals and birds and minerals. They saw the living world as an entity, and in many cases the fact that they studied medicine as their first discipline was a manifestation of their interest in the living world. Almost without exception they were passionate collectors, interested in the discovery, classification and naming of new plants and animals, and the development of a better perspective of the world of living things of which human kind is but one part.

A second theme which identified them as a group is their special interest in and interaction with people. Almost without exception their explorations brought them into very close contact with the special personalities of those who comprise exploring parties. Their relationships were those intense ones of individuals who are interdependent one upon the other for their safety and sometimes survival. They sought out small groups and spent months (and in several cases years) in their close company, isolated from the world of civilisation by great distances of unmapped space. They were interested in the Aboriginal peoples whom they encountered, and at least five of them recorded the languages of the Aboriginal people whom they met. These linguistic activities have formed, in several instances, the only record of the vocabulary and syntax of languages now forever lost.

The final theme which distinguished this group of doctor-explorers is their manifest love for adventure. From their homes in England, Germany, Scotland, and from Ireland and Poland, they came across the world to stand in places where Western man had never stood before. Their apprenticeships as surgeons, and their studies as medical students had given them a *carte de visite* to new colonial societies in an ancient land. Thus has medicine always been a passport to adventure and to a wider world.

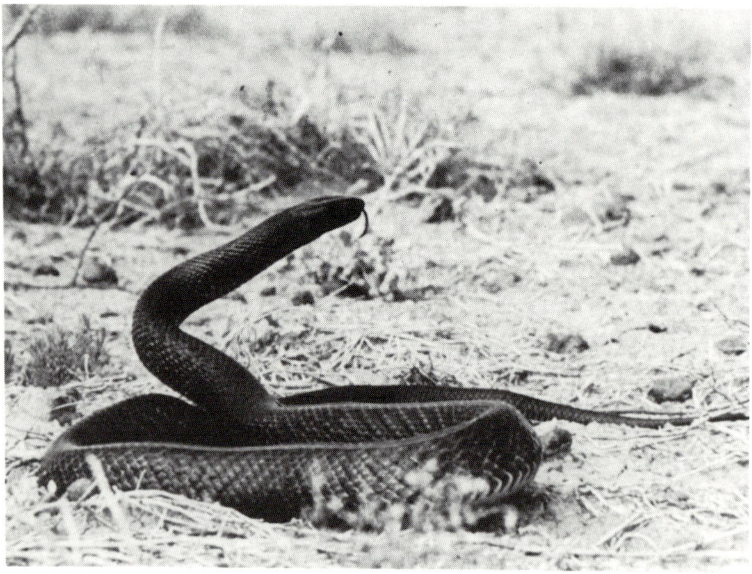

Figure. 2.1. 'Dandarabilla' to traditional owners of the country between Coopers Creek and the Diamantina River.

'Oxyuranus microlepidotus' (the Western Taipan) to European scientists.

Potentially very dangerous because of its highly toxic venom. Survival of a full bite by a large specimen of this species without the modern European approach would have been impossible.

FEVERS AND FRONTIERS 2

PHANGS AND PHYSIC
40,000 years of Risky Business

Jeanette Covacevich

Australia has a rich Aboriginal history of at least 40,000 years. Contemporary oral history of surviving Aboriginal lore provides a glimpse of the world's longest surviving medical practices. All evidence suggests these medical procedures predate the teachings of Hippocrates and Galen, not by centuries, but by millenia. Ancestors of today's traditional owners of this country entered 'Australia'* from Southeast Asia, via the Indonesian Archipelago. They quickly adapted to colonise the whole country.

Two hundred years ago Europeans came to Australia. At that time, there were some 600 Aboriginal language groups on this continent, not newly found (because they had not been lost), but first brought to European awareness. Populations were concentrated in coastal areas, where the combination of ocean foreshores and diverse, well-watered forests provided seemingly inexhaustible resources of food, water and shelter in generally benign climates. The Aboriginal people adapted also to the apparently waterless deserts of the centre and to all the habitats between those arid regions and the coast.

*The coastline of this continent has changed many times as sea levels have alternatively risen and fallen in response to climatic changes. During the Pleistocene, when Aboriginal people first set foot on what is presently Australia, sea levels were low. 'Australia' was much larger than it is now and there were extensive land connections between the southeast Asian mainland and 'Australia'.

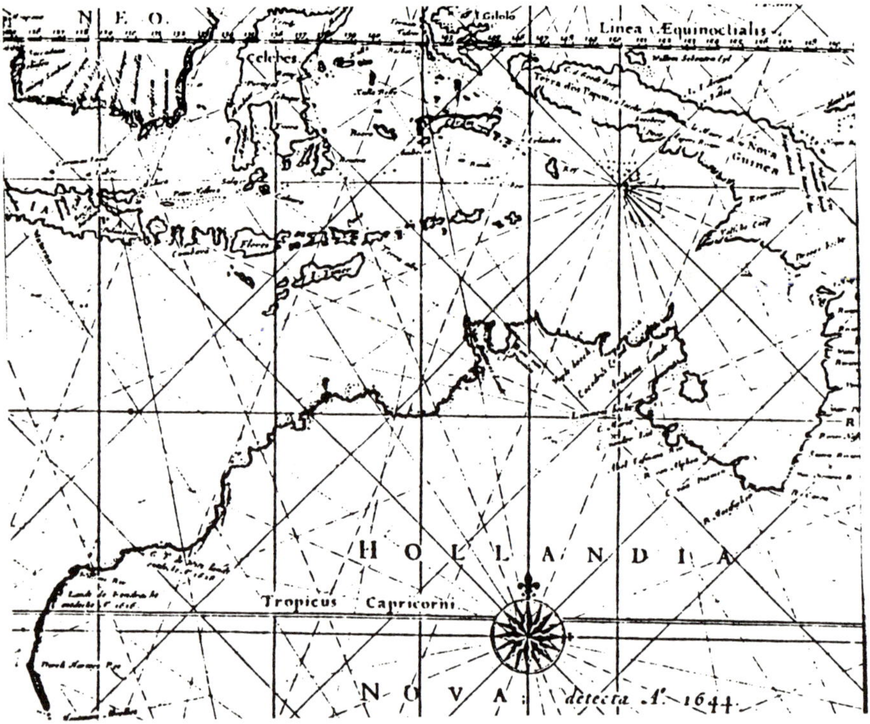

In any setting (steamy rainforests, cold alpine meadows, and arid niches) – Aboriginal people developed unique strategies for a superbly successful nomadic life.

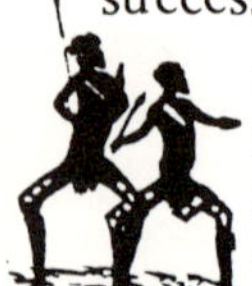

> *The Aborigines ... seemed primitive to the settlers, but it is now known that their life-style in relation to their environment was of high order, and their treatment of the sick more advanced in some ways than eighteenth century* [European] *practice.*[1]

In each language (?=tribal) group, a *materia medica* – diverse, extensive and apparently successful – evolved. Myth, magic and sorcery played important roles in sickness and recovery from it. There was heavy reliance on medicines derived from plants. Both the Aborigines and Europeans had contact with snakes in their daily lives and, in both societies, a plethora of procedures, preparations and potions were used to deal with the problem of snakebite, always something of a medical *cause célèbre.* This short account summarises Aboriginal approaches to the first aid and medical treatment of snakebite.

Australia's snake species command special attention. Amongst the elapids (i.e. the front-fanged species) are the world's most venomous and dangerous land-dwelling species, the Western Taipan (*Oxyuranus microlepidotus*) and the Coastal Taipan (*O. scutellatus*). There are 136 land dwelling snake species in Australia. Of these, seven species (Common Brown, *Pseudonaja textilis*; Tiger, *Notechis scutatus*; Death Adder, *Acanthophis antarcticus*; Rough-scaled Snake, *Tropidechis carinatus*; Mulga Snake, *Pseudechis australis*; Small-eyed Snake, *Cryptophis nigrescens*; Taipan, *Oxyuranus scutellatus*) are known to have inflicted fatalities since European records began.[2] A further nine species are capable of doing so by virtue of their relationship to those known to have been responsible for at least one fatality (Western Taipan, *Oxyuranus microlepidotus*; Collett's Black Snake, *Pseudechis colletti*; Black Tiger Snake, *Notechis ater*; Western Brown Snake, *Pseudonaja 'nuchalis'*, Copperhead, *Austrelaps superbus*, Spotted Black, *Pseudechis guttatus*; Butler's Black Snake, *Pseudechis butleri*; Red-bellied Black Snake, *Pseudechis porphyriacus*; Dugite, *Pseudonaja affinis*). The remaining species include those snakes whose bite may cause local (but sometimes very severe) effects, as well as many whose bites are of no consequence medically.

Snakebite has apparently been a not inconsequential cause of death and concern in Australia. There are no reliable records, of course, of the incidence of snakebite here before European settlement. Several authors refer to it as a rare event in traditional Aboriginal society, yet the treatment of snakebite figures prominently in much of the early literature on Aboriginal societies. It also figures prominently in European medical records and literature. This may reflect the often spectacular nature of snakebites and the fear they engender in the victim, those treating him/her, and everyone else involved either as a spectator, or as a supporter or relative of the victim. On the other hand, such prominence may reflect a truly frequent incidence. The latest figures on the incidence of snakebite in Australia show that there are approximately 3,000 cases of snakebite each year.[3] Somewhere between 200 and 500 of these bites are treated with antivenom, although no data are available on exactly how many bites really require treatment in this way. Figures on fatalities reflect recent improvements in both first aid and medical treatment of the problem, and there has been a steady decline in the number of deaths since the development of antivenom.

Between 1910 and 1926, 198 fatalities were recorded, while for roughly the same period between 1968 and 1982 there were 56 fatalities.[3]

Methods of treatment for snakebite in 18th, 19th and even mid 20th century medical-scientific circles were no less bizarre or useless than those that had evolved and were in use in Aboriginal societies where spirits controlled states of well-being and disease, and where sorcery played a major role in cure. Bearing in mind the extremely high toxicity of the venoms of the dangerous snakes which occur here, and the utterly devastating effects they can wreak on a victim (e.g. coagulopathy, cerebral haemorrhage, renal failture, paralysis, muscle destruction, anaphylaxis and cardiac problems), it is clear from a review of all treatments in use in this country through 40,000 years until the last decade, that survival of a serious case of envenomation must have been an extremely rare event. The *vis medicatrix naturae* has obviously been important, central in fact, to survival of both envenomation and the treatments promoted and practised vigorously to counter or cure its effects.

Different cultures are framed by different perceptions, classifications and concepts. There are no detailed early analyses of environmental concepts in pre-European tribal groups, but recently-gathered data highlight Aboriginal concepts of dangerous snakes which differ markedly from those of European science/natural history. On Mornington Island several species of snakes 'dangerous' to European eyes occur, along with a host of other harmless or nearly harmless species. Also on the island are many species of lizards, all of which are non-venomous and quite harmless. The King Brown, *Pseudechis australis;* the Common Brown, *Pseudonaja textilis*, have inflicted fatal bites elsewhere, and are on Mornington. The highly dangerous Taipan, *Oxyuranus scutellatus* may also be there, although there are no specimen records from the island. Also on the island is the Black Whip Snake, *Demansia* (?) *atra*, a species whose venom is poorly known, but considered a potential problem where large specimens are concerned. None of these species, even today in the face of heavy European influence on the cultures of the Mornington Islanders, is of more than passing concern to the people whose beliefs are strongly rooted in tradition. Of major concern, greatly feared, is a species whose language name translates loosely as 'Flying Snake'. This 'snake' can, it is believed, inflict a bite that is both certainly and rapidly fatal. The Flying Snake of Mornington Island is a Burton's Legless Lizard, *Lialis burtonis*, to European scientists. This is one of the pygopodid lizards and, like all Australian lizards, quite harmless, being adapted to feed on small skinks. These it captures and holds in a series of needle-like teeth, rather than by immobilisation with venom.

The Western Taipan, *Oxyuranus microlepidotus* was first described scientifically in 1879, but remained virtually unknown to science until the 1970s when work began on its taxonomic affiliations, venom and medical significance.[4] This is the species acknowledged by European science to have the highest known lethality index (= a ratio between venom yield and venom toxicity) and one measure of potential danger.[5] Of course, *dandarabilla,* as this snake was known to the traditional owners of the vast open ashy downs country of Goyder's Lagoon, South Australia and beyond, was well known to be capable of inflicting a fatal bite. Whether it was known by the people that the means of inflicting harm was by venom or not, is unknown. Mrs Linda Crombie, who now resides in Birdsville and who is one of the traditional owners of the country of *danarabilla* provides the following legend about this snake ...

> *An old lady was coming up Goyder's Lagoon way. She met an old man who had with him some snakes in a bag. He gave her the bag in exchange for some strings made of hair. The bag was not tied up properly and her little boy, who was being carried in a hair shoulder bag, was bitten by a snake. The old lady knew that little boy should have cried to be fed because he would be hungry for the breast around lunch-time, but he didn't. The old lady looked in the bag and found he was dead, poor little fella.*

> *She came from Mount Gayson. She came past Toowell, past Putabutna. Went straight pass Kulpitathoolta, got to Yapawarrilina, and that's where she buried her little boy, then she came down to lagoon waterhole. She started to collect wood and cry at the same time, when a needle from a needle bush poked in the eye. She was blind for awhile. She then went home to Duck Egg Sandhill where she left some duck eggs. She flew back to lagoon waterhole where she tipped all the snakes out on the ground. She went back to Coongie and stayed there until her death.*

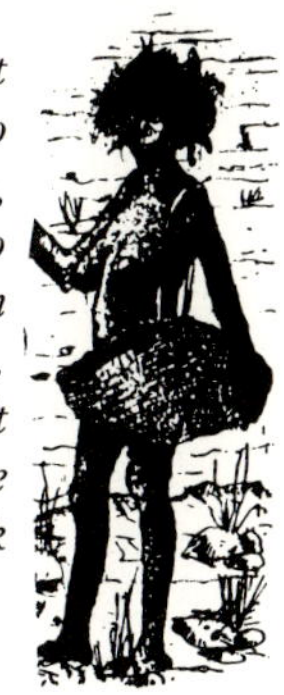

TABLE 1. TREATMENT OF SNAKE BITE IN TRADITIONAL ABORIGINAL SOCIETY

1. *... tying a tight ligature above the part and scarifying and sucking the wound ...* (? Sydney area)[6]
2. Bark of *Eucalyptus microtheca* is beaten up and heated and used as a poultice. (Queensland)[6]
3. 'Drill' into the wound with sharp pieces of bark. In the cavity soft wool from a possum is placed. Then fur is singed smooth with the skin. (Sydney area)[7]
4. Scarification, suction and forced exercise, until the effect of the poison had passed away. (Clarence River, NE N.S.W.)[8]
5. ... *continuously beating the bitten part by a small rod, or rods, till the vitality of the tissues was entirely destroyed ...* . (Tasmania)[9]
6. Rub the wound with emu fat. 2 adult deaths only. No deaths in children noted. (Western district of Victoria)[10]
7. No knowledge of snake bite deaths. Snake bite is treated by putting ligatures some distance above and below the wound, and then opening the largest artery in the vicinity of the bite with a stone, shell, or other sharp instrument; several incisions are made until copious bleeding is the result. The ligatures are not removed for two or three days, when the patient is all right. (Port Darwin district)[11]
8. Snake bite most common cause of death (with sunstroke). (Cloncurry River, NW.Q.)[12]
9. No remedy. (Herbert River, NE.Q.)[13]
10. *Lobelia purpurascens* deconcoction reported as an antidote. Maiden appears sceptical. (Macleay River District, NE. N.S.W.)[14]
11. Apply ligature above puncture, then suck the wound. (Central Australia)[15]
12. Two treatments, one for fatal, the other for non fatal snake bite.

(i) Death from snakebite 'only rarely happens ... the purely natural cause and fatal effect are are not reconciled ... a variation of the superstition of the death-bone is brought into requisition ... no effort, in fact to apply a remedy, loses heart, gives way and dies ...'

(ii) *... the sufferer would see the creature gliding away after it had bitten him, and would carefully watch the hole into which it hides: This he immediately blocks up, and makes a careful note of the exact spot. With his hair belt, or any other convenient twine, he next ties two ligatures around the limb bitten, above and below the knee if on the leg, or above and below the elbow if on the hand, 'to stop the blood come up': if possible, he applies suction to the wound. His gin, or any other mate who may be present, would rush back to consult the nearest doctor, and returning, dig a largish hole in close proximity to where the accident took place, kindle a fire in it and heat some big stones and lumps of rock: when these have become sufficiently hot and the flames somewhat subsident, a lot of fresh leafy boughs and branches and leaves, sprinkled with water to prevent ignition, are placed on top. Upon this smoking mass of foliage the bitten individual now lies, and what with the smouldering embers and hot steam arising from the leaves he soon becomes enveloped in perspiration, falls asleep for two or three hours, wakes up refreshed, has a 'spit', and is quite recovered. In the meantime, however, the medicine-man has not been idle, for he of course has had a share in the cure. when the messenger first came to report the accident, he would, after cross-examination, look up at the sky and declare that he could see 'Mulkari' spitting, and that therefore the patient would be all right if he went under the prescribed treatment. Furthermore, the doctor himself comes to the place where the accident happened, is shown the identical spot where the snake lies imprisoned, digs it out and lets it travel away a few feet before commencing to pelt at it with stones. During this process the snake gradually becomes smaller and smaller until, from an original length of 3 or 4 feet, it may dwindle down to 12 or 10 inches: the creature, thus rendered harmless, is carrid back to camp, where the medicine man, turning its skin half-way inside out while still alive, throws it into the water, and so makes an end of it. It is needless to say that no lay-man is allowed to witness the process of causing the ophidian to diminish in size ...*
(Boulia District, NW.Q.)[16]

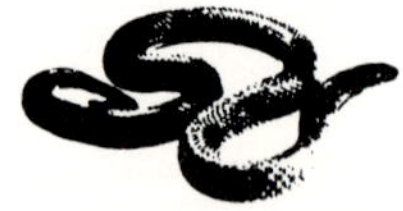

TABLE 1 (contd)

13. No 'tricks' were used by the doctor ... 'suction, with or without scarifying by knife or stone, and ligature, followed by sweating over heated leaves, especially if the particular species is believed to be a dangerous one ... ' (Mitakoodi, ? Boulia District)[16]

14. Seldom bitten/one informant had never heard of a fatality from snake bite '... cut the skin at the site of the wound until it bled freely. Then all the doctors sucked it. No ligature was applied ...' . In addition, above the wound a ligature of the skin of a possum was applied. (Yukumbul, New England area, NE. N.S.W.)[17]

15. 'Recourse to running water of a stream ... ' even stagnant water poured on wounds for an hour or more.[18]

16. No cure, fatalistically yielded and died. (? northern tribes)[18]

17. Ligature, incision, bleeding, mud plaster. 1 death recorded. (Daleburra, northern Qld)[19]

18. A man who has been bitten is made to sit down beside a fire while another man blows smoke through a hollow branch or dry pandanus stem on to him. As the smoke emerges at the other end of the tube another man carefully watches, and if in the smoke he sees the *mali* (non-material form) of a snake, it is known that a *ragalk* (sorcerer) has brought about the misfortune and the man will die. If no such form is observed the man will recover. Frequently this ceremony is performed after the man has died, and so merely serves to corroborate a conviction which has already been definitely reached. In such a case imagination never fails to create the *mali* of the snake.
Another very curious procedure is as follows – If a person has been bitten and he is able to capture the snake he does so by pressing a stick upon it just behind the head and then binding the snake to the stick at that point. With the snake thus held he returns to camp. There the snake is left until it is seen to pass all the blood it has extracted from the person bitten. When this occurs the person begins to recover, and soon all ill effects have passed away. The snake is now released not killed. If it were killed the person would undoubtedly die also. (Eastern Arnhem Land)[20]

19. Know nothing of ligature, but cut the area to make the blood flow and then make the person sit in water. (Cape York, NE.Q.)[21]

20. Treated by immediately pinching the part between finger and thumb to squeeze out the blood. As soon as the blood ceased to flow, a possum skin which had been heated as hot as possible without being spoiled was applied. As soon as it was cool it was removed and the puncture was sucked while the skin was being reheated. This procedure was repeated for three-quarters of an hour. A death-adder bite was considered hopelessly fatal and no treatment was undertaken.[21]

21. Singeing by the medicine-man is the method chiefly relied upon, but ligatures are also tied above the bite.[21]

22. Sucking the wound to draw out the young snakes which had been injected and cauterizing with a fire stick. (Euahlayi, NE. N.S.W.)[22]

23. *Capparis lasiantha*/plant and roots is macerated and soaked in water. Liquid applied to snake bites ... (Broome area, NW. W.A.)[23]

24. *Dodonaea lanceolata* (Carnarvon, Onslow and Roebourne area)[23]

25. *Haemodorum corymbosum* (Charters Towers, NE.Q.)[23]

26. A cut was made across the bite in the form of a cross – the sharp head of a spear was often used to make the cut. A nest of the Green Tree Ant was picked from a tree and twisted to kill the ants, and the liquid dripping from the nest was allowed to run into the wound until the liquid stopped running. Meanwhile, a *Yuwara* vine was cut, hammered between two stones to soften it, and wound firmly around the limb above the bite to stop the pain going up the limb. The treatment was repeated until it was felt that all the poison was out.
Another method was to cut open the bite, as described above, and apply hot leaves or a hot stick to the wound. Leaves of Purple Beach *Convolvulus* were used if the patient was at the beach. Most bites were on the leg as Aborigines have very good eyesight and are unlikely to pick up a snake in mistake for a stick. (Eastern Arnhem Land)[24]

27. Assiduously avoided. If bitten, no cure. (Yidinyji, NE.Q. rainforest)[25]

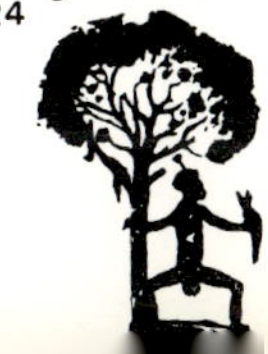

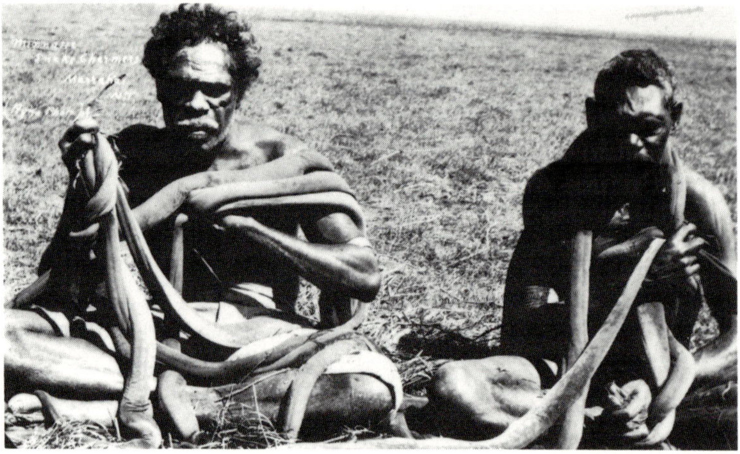

Figure 2.2. 'Aboriginal snake charmers, N.T.' says the old caption. More appropriately, it would read ...'Aboriginal men posing with harmless File Snakes (Acrochordus arafurae), a favourite food item for some of the people of the Northern Territory. (Photo, Ryko Collection, Queensland Museum.)

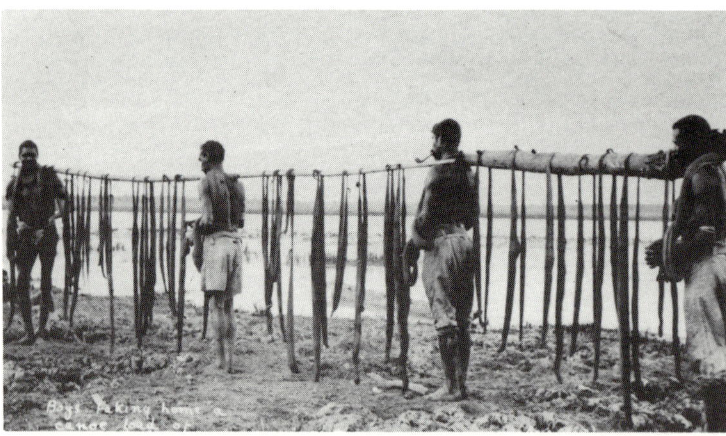

Figure 2.3. A successful hunt. File Snakes (Acrochordus arafurae) are harmless, aquatic snakes which are extremely common in many northern freshwaters. Both traditional Aboriginal and early European methods would have 'treated' bites by A. arafurae specimens very successfully.
(Photo, *Ryko Collection, Queensland Museum.)*

Knowledge of traditional Aboriginal perceptions of snakes, snakebite, and its treatment is poor, and accurate information of the incidence of snakebite in traditional Aboriginal societies is non-existent. Table 1 is a summary of a range of treatments, cures, and practices reportedly used by a wide range of Aboriginal people in the early days of European contact, and in more recent times. Some of the practices listed seem very unusual by today's standards but are not so unusual when matched with early European medical approaches here. Some methods, cutting the wound or applying a tourniquet, were in use in both Aboriginal and European societies. Whether they evolved independently or were exchanged between the cultures is not known.

European knowledge of the elapid snakes of Australia has accumulated slowly. Prior to 1800, only one species of elapid had been described (the Red-bellied Black Snake, *Pseudechis porphyriacus* White 1790). The nineteenth century saw a further 55 species described, with description of the majority of these coinciding with the era of great exploration and settlement of the latter part of the century. The remaining 24 species were described this century, mostly before 1950. Only 3 species have been described since 1980. Included in these is *Pseudechis butleri* Smith 1982, a close relative of the Mulga Snake, *Pseudechis australis*, a well-known dangerous snake responsible for many fatalities.

The first major review on Australia's snakes was published in 1869.[26] At that time 35 species of elapids were recognised. At present 80 species of elapids are known and it seems unlikely that many species remain undescribed. Detailed knowledge of their life histories and habitats is emerging largely through recent work on specimens held in museum reference collections. It was not until early this century that the mechanism by which some snakes could kill their prey – immobilising them by powerful neurotoxins and other toxins – was known certainly, although it was the dominant theory. A virus transmitted by the snake, fear following a bite, alcohol drunk before or after a bite were also blamed for fatal snakebites.[27]

The early methods of treatment of snakebite in Australia by European medical practitioners and others are almost as diverse and certainly as ineffective in the face of serious envenomation as any of those used by Aboriginal doctors. They have been a subject of curiosity and amazement and have been written about quite extensively.[7,27,28]

In regard to treating snakebites Agnew[29] gave his colleagues in the medical establishment some sound advice –

> *In calculating the value of a remedy, it is to be borne in mind, that a bite of a snake is by no means invariably fatal to man even when no treatment is adopted ... .*

With the retrospectoscope it is easy to see how victims survived *some* bites by snakes and how 'cures' now known to be absolutely useless could be seen as effective remedies. There are many more harmless snakes in this country than dangerous ones, and most bites are inflicted by harmless Tree Snakes, Pythons and other near harmless species. A victim of a bite by a harmless or near harmless snake would, of course, 'recover' following Aboriginal treatments like the application of body fluids of Green Tree Ants (which was also used as a tonic and to 'cure' constipation by some of northern Queensland rainforest people), or possum skin, or a concoction from *Capparis lasiantha, Dodonaea* spp., or *Haemodum corymbosum*, or squeezing or sucking the wound. About equally 'effective' against harmless snakebite would have been the European methods of cautery, suction, excision, or injection of potassium permanganate, strychnine, ether or ammonia; or consumption of ether or copious quantities of alcohol; or the application of arterial tourniquets, a practice strongly endorsed by the medical profession until the 1970s. At the time that Agnew[29] could write so patronisingly of Aboriginal approaches to snakebite –

> *... the treatment ... had no effect ... I do not deny that in some cases it may have been beneficial in an indirect manner. The confidence of recovery it may have inspired in the case of a man man being bitten* [by a snake], *would, by removing the depressing effects of terror, be a very likely means of bringing about a result, in which the curative qualities of the application itself had no part whatever ... .*

he (and his colleagues) were treating snakebite in this country by forcing alcohol (brandy and whiskey 'a wine-glass full every half hour to an adult', were recommended) or ammonia on the hapless victims. He conceded that neither agent could be looked on strictly speaking as an antidote, but that they were effective because –

> *... they acted ... not by rendering inert or destroying the poison itself, but by rousing and exalting the nervous system, and so by*

> *itself, but by rousing and exalting the nervous system, and so by keeping the vital forces active, prevent*[ing] *the occurrence of that fatal coma, which so depresses all physiological action as to render impossible the elimination of poison from the system.*

Respect for the healing profession and the confidence with which medical advice was dispensed seem to have been important, too, in cures –

> *... I think the recovery in all cases was mainly due to my telling them at once that there was not the slightest danger or cause for alarm....*[30]

The first objective experimental work on the venoms of Australian elapids was not undertaken until late in the 19th century when it was shown[31, 32] that the venom of *Pseudechis porphyriacus* (the Black Snake) contained several components which affected not only the blood (causing intravascular clotting), but also the heart, and the medullary respiratory centre. At roughly the same time, it was reported for the first time that a snake could withhold venom in a 'dry' bite (based on work with *Acanthophis antarcticus*, the Death Adder).[33] Early this century it was demonstrated that 'anti-venin' was effective against snakebite,[34] but it was not until 1930 that the 'modern era of snakebite management' began.[3] The Commonwealth Serum Laboratories produced the first antivenom – for *Notechis scutatus* (the Tiger Snake) – in 1930, following experiments by Fairley.[35] That work demonstrated that attempts to remove venom from the bite site (by cautery, suction, excision or chemical denaturation) were ineffective.

Arterial tourniquets had been *de rigueur* in the procedure for treating snakebite for many years and continued as standard at the first aid level until just over a decade ago. (Such practice was based, it seems, on 17th century work in Europe, which suggested some protection against the effects of snakebite).[27]

The work of Sutherland[36, 37, 38] and his colleagues at the Commonwealth Serum Laboratories, Parkville, Victoria saw the development of the present, very effective management of snakebite. Building on previous studies, Sutherland developed his hypothesis. He then tested it on experimental animals, and trialled it clinically. Primarily as a result of this research, snakebite need no longer be a major cause for alarm. Management is now so efficient and effective that the death rate averages only 4 per annum,[39] notwithstanding a population of 16 million largely concentrated on the eastern seaboard where many of the most venomous land snakes known are found.

Anthropologists have observed[40] that in all societies methods of restoring good health fall into one (or more) of three classes –

> ... *faith healing, where an attempt to remove the morbid state is made by means of influences exerted on the mind; secondly, by hygienic therapy, founded on recognition of the fact that the body tends to cure itself and this should be aided as far as possible; and thirdly, by the use of drugs, a relic of poison lore ...* .

For 40,000 years of Aboriginal history and for most of the 200 years of European history in this country the treatment of snakebite has been based largely on faith and the body's ability to recover. Full bites by large specimens of any one of a dozen species of the dangerous snakes must invariably have been fatal in both Aboriginal and European societies for most of their history in Australia. This situation changed only when research began to establish how venom affected a victim and how antibodies could be transferred passively by the use of antivenom.

Acknowledgements

Dr John Thearle generously provided me with many references useful in preparing this paper, and Professor John Pearn and Mr Richard Robins constructively criticised the manuscript.

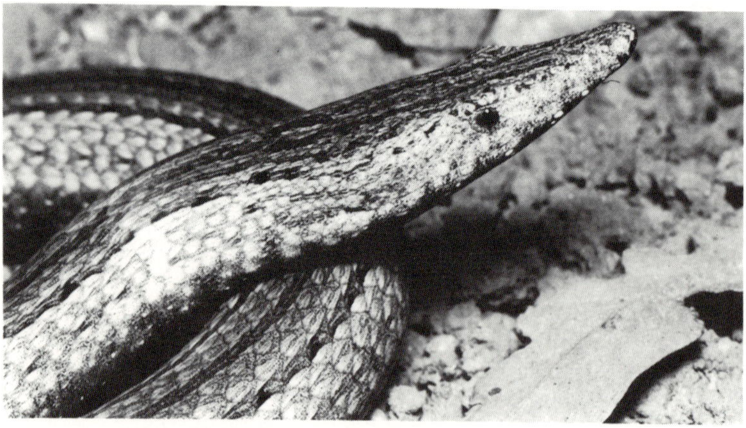

Figure 2.4. For Aboriginal people on Mornington Island a bite by the Flying Snake is rapidly and certainly fatal. To European scientists the Flying Snake is the harmless Burton's Legless Lizard, Lialis burtonis.

FEVERS AND FRONTIERS 3

MEDICAL FRONTIERS IN AUSTRALIAN SEAS

Peter Fenner

One of the last frontiers to be explored in Australia has been its extensive tropical coastline, extending from Broome in Western Australia, along the North Western Coastline (only now being opened up by oil and gas companies), over the sparsely populated northern coastline of the Northern Territory and round to Cape York. Here, on the eastern coast of Queensland, the Great Barrier Reef extends southward for some two thousand kilometres.

These areas are rapidly becoming 'discovered' by tourists, particularly those with such an idyllic setting as the Great Barrier Reef with its clear tropical waters, coral cays and Island resorts. In such areas, particularly when the weather is hot and humid in the summer, people love to go swimming. Unfortunately, at this very time during the summer months, and in the same surrounding waters of Tropical Australia, is *Chironex fleckeri,* the most deadly jellyfish in the world. *Chironex* has now been responsible for almost 80 recorded deaths in Tropical Australia[1, 2] – more than the total Australia-wide numbers having died after a shark attack.[2]

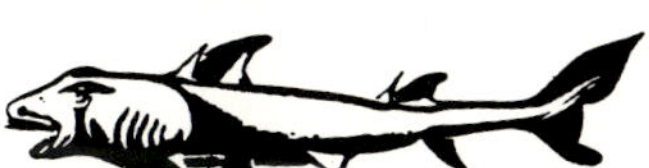

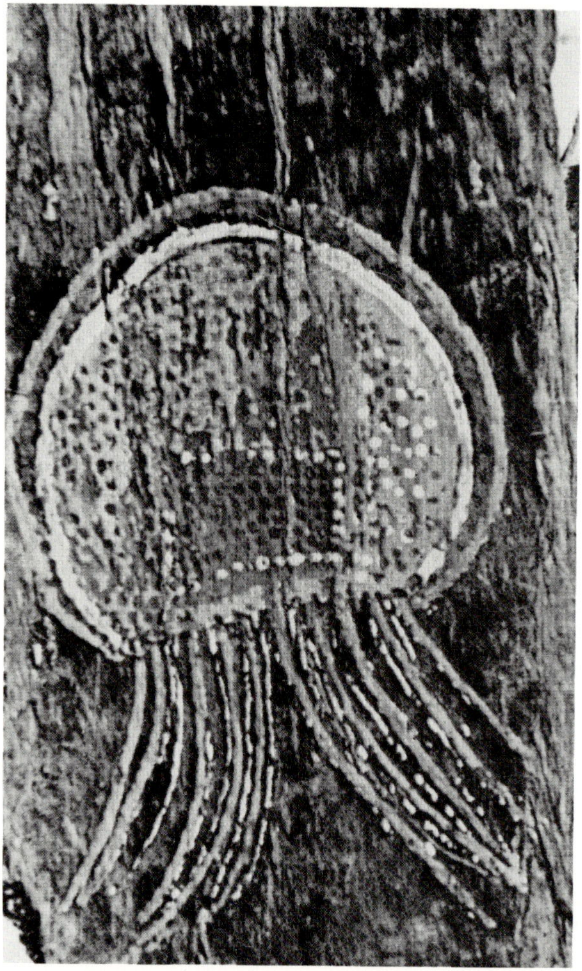

Figure 3.1. Aboriginal bark painting at Liverpool River, Arnhem Land. Believed to represent the lethal north Australian Box-Jellyfish.

Photo courtesy of Dr Ronald Southcott (From – Injuries to man from marine invertebrates. Cleland and Southcott, with acknowledgements)

Also found in these same tropical waters during the summer season are at least two other dangerous jellyfish, *Carukia barnesi* which produces a classical syndrome with severe systemic, and potentially lethal, effects[3,4,5,6] and *Chiropsalmus quadrigatus* (Australia) which is very similar in appearance to *Chironex* and produces a severe skin reaction, but which has not yet proved fatal.[7]

Despite the fact that the first death actually recorded as being due to a jellyfish sting was only in 1884 in Townsville,[1] Aboriginals in north Australia knew of this problem possibly hundreds of years beforehand. There is an aboriginal painting (*Figure 3.1*) which, although not an exact illustration of *Chironex fleckeri*, shows a jellyfish with groups of tentacles arising from separate areas (corners?).[1] As accurate records of deaths from marine stings have only been kept in the last century, and then mainly for the European settlers, it is probable there have been well in excess of the 80 odd people whose deaths have been documented to date. These would be amongst the Aboriginal population in whom deaths have probably occurred for many hundreds of years. Even today there are on average two deaths per year, usually in aboriginal children in remote areas.[2]

Since 1884 there have been regularly documented deaths in north Queensland from jellyfish stings. However, originally the cause of death was often given as 'drowning', or 'allergic reaction to a jellyfish sting'. It was often believed that an allergy to the sting of *Physalia* was the cause of death, or death was due to a heart attack after a *Physalia* sting, as this jellyfish was readily seen at all times of the year.[1] No explanation was given to the fact that deaths occurred only in the summer months, despite *Physalia* often being seen in most months of the year.

Australia has been fortunate to have medical men of great tenacity. Despite the fact that they were far from major cities with medical research facilities, in true pioneering spirit, through meticulous thinking, great practical skills and an indomitable will, they first described many serious marine envenomations syndromes. Further to this they caught and identified the animals responsible for this mortality and morbidity, then suggested treatment principles and methods of preventing, reducing or treating the effects of these serious stings.

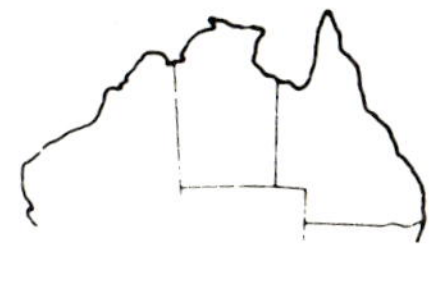

THE DOCTORS

Dr Ronald Southcott

Dr Ronald Southcott (*Figure 3.2*) was a doctor in the Australian Army stationed in the Cairns area in 1944. During this time he had to treat many stings on soldiers stationed in the area and he recognised that there were two distinct types of marine sting, even though at that time nobody was aware of the cause of the problem. He divided the stings into two categories, naming them Type 'A' stings and Type 'B' stings.[8]

The Type 'A' stings usually presented with a very small and insignificant skin mark which was followed a short time later (usually between 20 to 30 minutes) by a number of severe systemic symptoms which often caused prostration, even in the fittest of troops.

Type 'B' sting victims suffered extreme pain with obvious weal marks visible on the stung area. Although many became somewhat sick and lethargic, there were no deaths in this group during the study. Little did Southcott realise at this time that it would be another eleven years before he would be identifying the jellyfish causing Type 'B' stings, naming it *Chironex fleckeri*,[9] and twenty-two years before he was also to identify the jellyfish causing the Type 'A' stings, naming it *Carukia barnesi.*[10]

Dr Hugo Flecker

Dr Hugo Flecker (*Figure 3.3*) was a radiologist in Cairns, north Queensland for many years. He was a great naturalist and wrote many articles on venomous plants and animals, a subject in which he took a great interest. He was also very interested in the lethal jellyfish in the waters around his area and so on January 20th, 1955 when a 5 year old boy died some 250 kilometres south of Cairns at a town called Cardwell, at Flecker's suggestion the sea in the area was netted.

Three types of jellyfish were caught, one of which was an unidentified, box-shaped jellyfish with groups of tentacles arising from each corner. All three jellyfish were immediately dispatched to Flecker who carefully preserved the unidentified species, before sending it to Dr Ronald Southcott who now lived in Adelaide, South Australia.

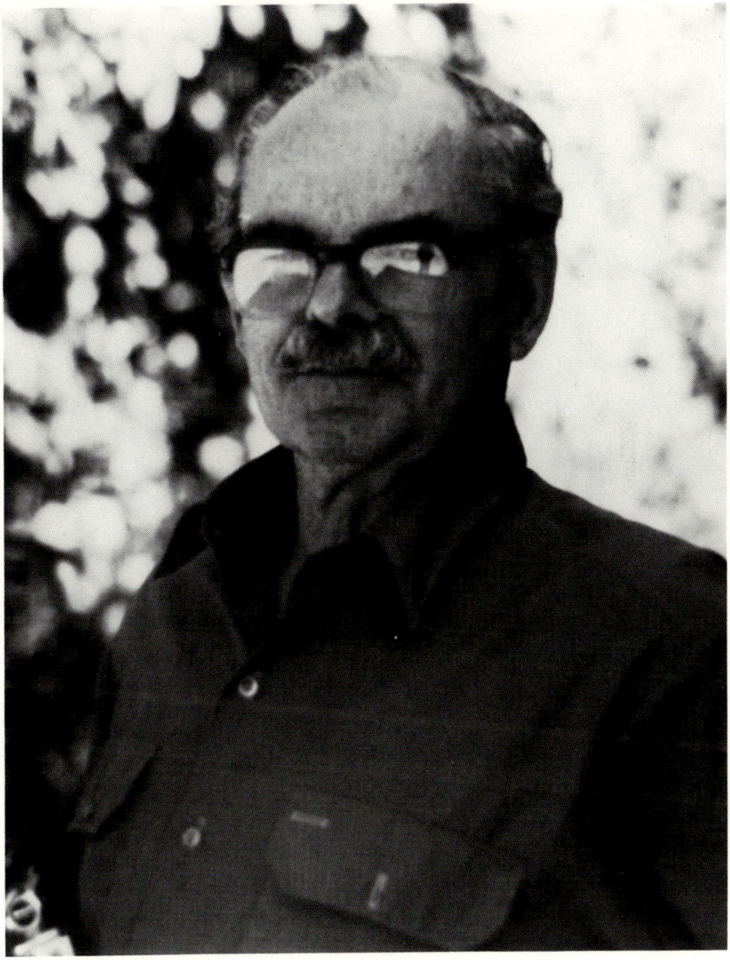

Figure 3.2. *Dr RONALD SOUTHCOTT*

Early researcher into venomous jellyfish in north Australian waters. First identified Chironex fleckeri (known to be the world's most venomous animal) and Carukia barnesi as new Species.

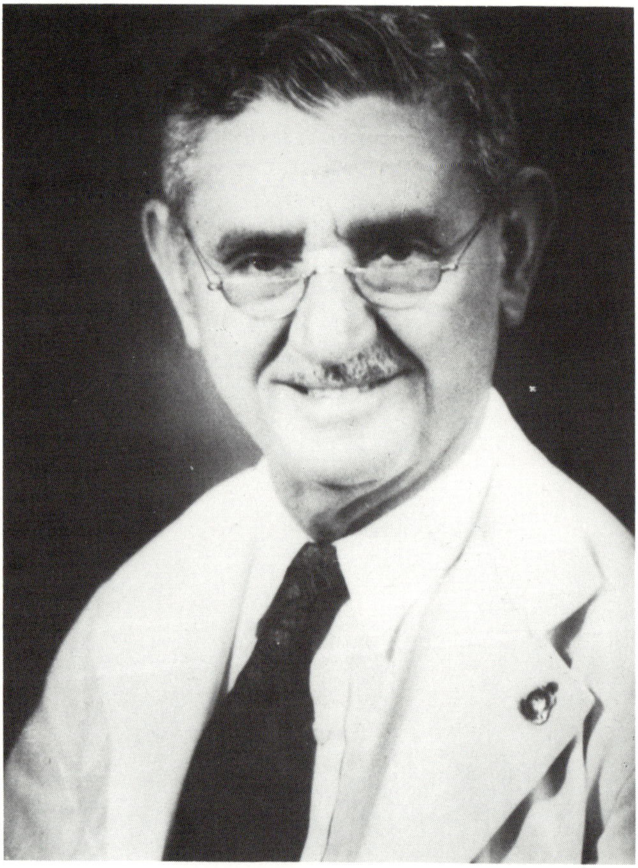

Figure 3.3. Dr HUGO FLECKER (1884–1957)

Former Radiologist of Cairns after whom Chironex fleckeri was named in 1956 as a tribute to his pioneering work in natural history.

This was the first of many similar specimens that were sent to Dr Southcott who had become an expert in Australian jellyfish. On December 29th, 1955 Southcott submitted a paper identifying this new genus and species of lethal jellyfish to the *Australian Journal of Marine and Freshwater Research*, where it was published in 1956.[9] Southcott named the jellyfish *Chironex fleckeri*, the name *Chironex* being derived from the Greek 'cheiro' meaning 'hand', the Latin 'nex' meaning 'murderer', with *fleckeri* obviously named after Flecker who did so much of the original research into this deadly jellyfish.

Flecker was also very interested in Type 'A' stingings and published his article in the *Medical Journal of Australia* where he first named these bizarre variety of systemic symptoms as the 'Irukandji syndrome'.[11] He derived this name from the 'Irukandji', a tribe of aboriginals living in the area around Palm Cove, Cairns where many of the stings occurred. Flecker spent many years trying to identify the marine organism causing this syndrome but unfortunately died in 1957 without success.

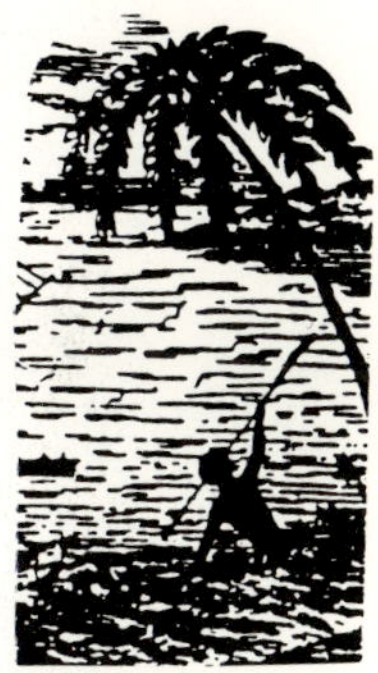

Dr Jack Barnes

After Flecker's death, another Cairns doctor, this time a General Practitioner called Dr Jack Barnes (*Figure 3.4*), was asked to continue the quest to identify the jellyfish responsible for the 'Irukandji syndrome'. Over the next 4 years using detective work rivalled only by Sherlock Holmes, Jack surmised that the organism had to be a very small jellyfish which swam very quickly, and probably close to the surface. After calculating the most likely time and place to catch the animal, as only Jack Barnes could do, he put on his scuba gear and lay on the bottom of the sea bed in shallow water. After many hours his persistence was rewarded when he saw a very small jellyfish swim in front of his mask, which he managed to catch. Later another was caught when a small fish was seen swimming erratically. On close investigation it was found that it was caught in the tentacles of another of these tiny jellyfish.

To discover if these were the jellyfish causing the 'Irukandji syndrome', Jack stung himself, his son Nick, and a surf life saver friend! After the characteristic 30 minute delay all three developed

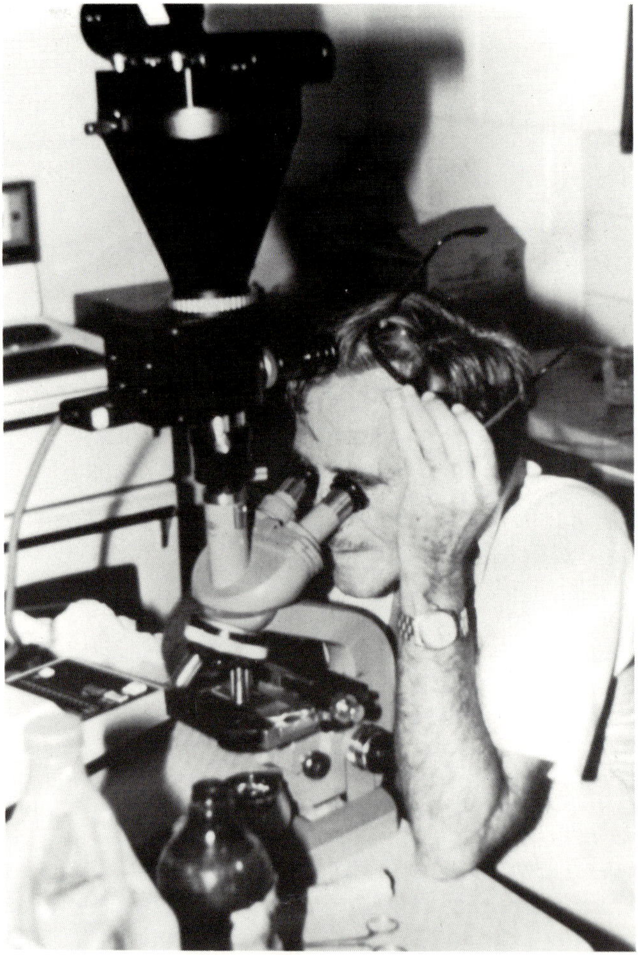

Figure 3.4. Dr JACK BARNES (1922–1985)

General Practitioner in Cairns who first collected Chironex venom from which antivenom was made.

The box jellyfish, Carukia barnesi, (or 'Irukandji') commemorates his name.

the 'Irukandji syndrome' and all had to be admitted to hospital with severe back pain, muscle cramps, nausea, vomiting and headache described in the article in the *Medical Journal of Australia* in 1964.[12]

Ron Southcott again came into the story and another gap in the taxonomy of north Queensland cubozoans was closed. He identified this little box-shaped jellyfish as a new Species, and in 1967 named it *Carukia barnesi.*[10] This name was derived from 'Car' – ex Carybdea, 'ruk' from 'Irukandji', and *barnesi* named after yet another famous north Queensland researcher in the marine field.

Jack Barnes was also very interested in all the large 'box jellyfish' in his area and in 1965 identified another cubozoan. To the untrained eye it looked the same as *Chironex*, although it produced a milder sting pattern and symptoms. His identification of this jellyfish was *Chiropsalmus quadrigatus* and he produced a paper differentiating it from the lethal *Chironex.*[7] However, in 1985 Hartwick and Fenner caught another type of cubozoan in the Philippines, responsible for possibly 20–50 deaths a year, (unpublished report) which seemed to fit more exactly the original description of *Chiropsalmus quadrigatus* Haekel 1862.[13] The taxonomy of these two Species is still a matter for conjecture at this period of time, although research is currently under way. As yet the names, confusing as they are, remain differentiated only by those having to, and are usually referred to as *Chiropsalmus quadrigatus* (Philippines) and *Chiropsalmus quadrigatus* (Australian).

Barnes also believed that there was more than one species of 'Irukandji' and referred to them as 'pseudo-Irukandji'.[14] He was probably correct as Fenner *et al* have recently referenced cases with a more widespread geographical envenomation area than that described for *Carukia barnesi* and described at least one other species of jellyfish producing a similar syndrome.[5]

As the Medical Adviser to the Surf Life Saving Association it was Barnes who first introduced the use of 'pantie-hose' as an effective protective barrier preventing a serious *Chironex* sting. The thickness of the nylon mesh was just sufficient to prevent the tiny stinging cells (nematocysts) on the tentacles being able to penetrate the underlying epidermis and inject their toxic venom.

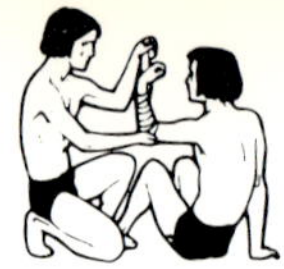

It quickly became a common sight in north Queensland to see Surf Life Savers wearing pantie-hose on patrol, one pair being worn normally to cover the legs and lower abdomen, and the other worn upside down, covering the trunk and arms and with a hole cut for the head. These patrolling members were then able to safely enter the water where they dragged long mesh nets through the shallows to see if *Chironex* were present, thus allowing safe bathing between the patrol flags during times which might have otherwise been possibly unsafe.

In 1964 Barnes also introduced the original first aid treatment for *Chironex* stings, consisting of methylated spirits and tourniquets.[14] It was only in 1975 that further work suggested vinegar and compressive bandages were more effective.[2,15] He also suggested effective medical treatments for severe envenomation by both *Chironex* and 'Irukandji',[16] which still form the basis for current hospital treatments of these marine envenomation cases.

In 1967 Barnes genius led to the development of Commonwealth Serum Laboratories' Box-Jellyfish antivenom.[17] Using a small vacuum flask with an amniotic membrane stretched across the neck, by passing a small electric current through the membrane on which live *Chironex* tentacles had been placed, Barnes was able to induce the stinging cells (nematocysts) to discharge through the membrane, enabling pure venom to be collected. This venom was then injected into sheep to produce an antivenom which was the first really effective treatment for a severe *Chironex* sting. This antivenom still remains a major part of the treatment for a major *Chironex* envenomation,[18,19] although further research is only now showing us ways to improve its effectiveness.[20]

Dr John Williamson

Dr John Williamson (*Figure 3.5*) is also a member of the Medical Advisory Committee to the Queensland Surf Life Saving Association and has provided a significant contribution to our recent knowledge of marine envenomation in Australia. Starting in 1974 as the author of a small booklet called *Some Australian Marine Stings and Envenomations*, John has progressed to produce the third edition called *The Marine Stinger Book* which has now become a reference book worldwide.

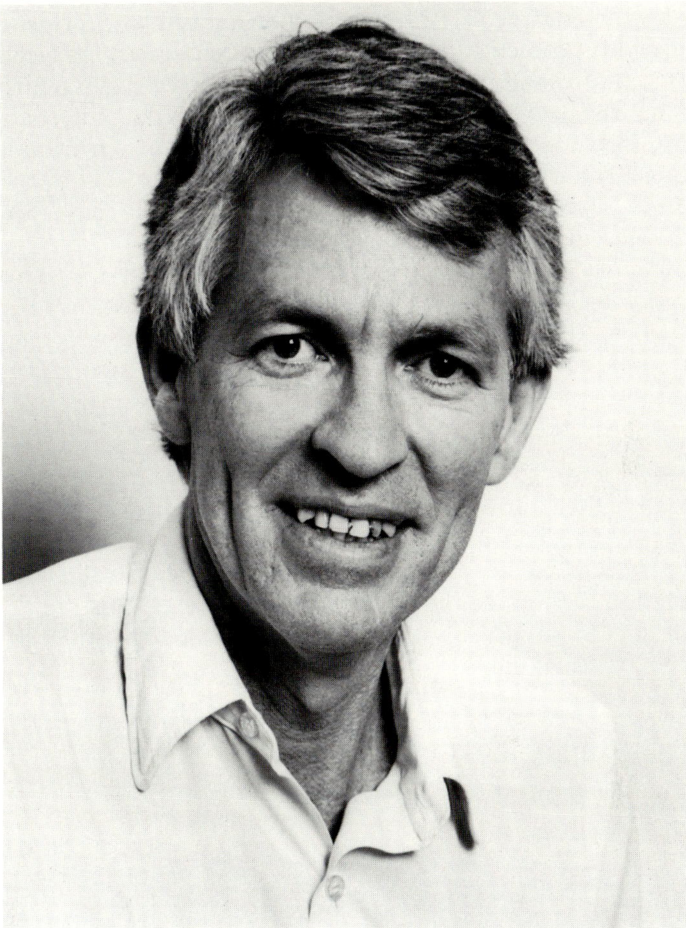

Figure 3.5. Dr JOHN WILLIAMSON

Consultant anaesthetist and Director of the Hyperbaric Medicine Unit Royal Adelaide Hospital, and formerly of Townsville. Responsible for many original papers on marine envenomation.

As an acknowledged leader in this field, John Williamson has also been the author of numerous articles on worldwide marine envenomation problems which have been published in established medical journals and books. He is currently working on the 4th Edition of the *Marine Stinger Book*, collaborating internationally with Professor Joe Burnett of the United States of America, as well as Dr Peter Fenner in Australia.

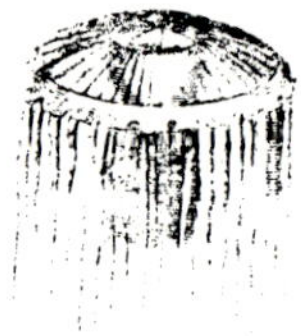

FINALE

We are still at the frontiers of knowledge for research into the causes and treatment of marine envenomation in north Australia. Further knowledge on the treatment of jellyfish stings and envenomation syndromes is continuously being updated, and new species continue to be caught and identified whilst the effects of envenomation are evaluated. I am sure the next 'Historical' book will continue to supply us with more knowledge in this area which is history in the making.

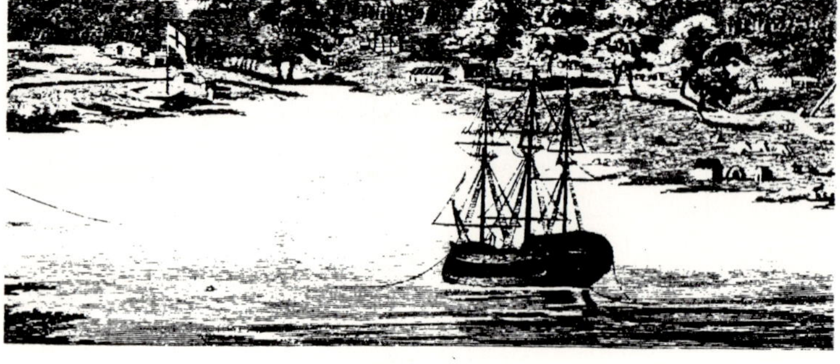

PART II

FEVERS

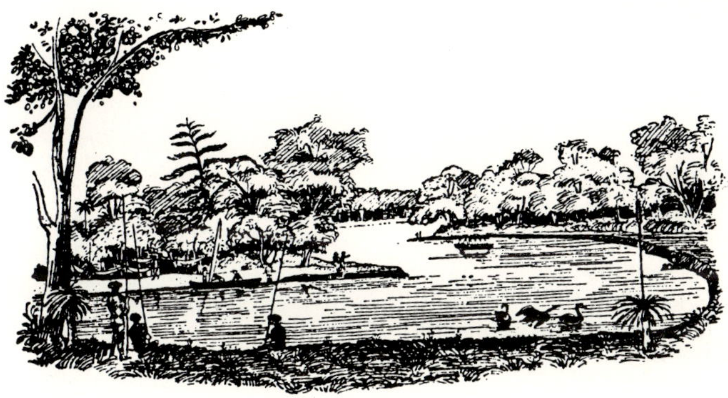

FEVERS AND FRONTIERS 4

CECIL COOK – FRONTIERSMAN OF AUSTRALIAN HEALTH

Ralph Doherty

The North Queensland Medical Conference met in 1954 at Townsville, and held its third meeting at Mackay in 1958. I attended and opened the discussion on one of the invited papers, on tropical medicine in northern Australia delivered by Dr C.E.A. Cook, then a senior medical officer in the Commonwealth Department of Health. It would be hard to claim that I proved a sympathetic discussant. I was there primarily to show the flag for the Queensland Institute of Medical Research, and talked about the work in progress, especially the use we were making of what were then very new virological tools to study problems of infectious disease in north Queensland. I saw the occasion with the arrogance of a 30 year old. Dr Cook clearly spoke from an enormous experience in public health and clinical medicine, and what he and his generation described was important, but it needed to be re-interpreted in 'modern' terms.

The return of the North Queensland Medical Conference to Mackay, 32 years later, and the invitation to present a paper, allows me to look back at that earlier occasion and to some extent atone for my earlier shortcomings. I have come to realise how important was the role that Cecil Cook played in Australian public health, and how little recognition he has received within the medical profession. His retirement from the Commonwealth Health Service in 1962 was the subject of a ministerial press release,[1] but his death in 1987 did not receive the recognition of even the standard *Medical Journal of Australia* obituary. In addition, recently two historians, Ms Suzanne

Saunders and Dr Tony Austin, of the University of the Northern Territory, have focussed attention on the role he played in evolving national policy in Aboriginal welfare, and it seems timely to bring their work to medical notice.

Cecil Evelyn Aufrere Cook was born in England in 1898, and Austin describes[2] –

> *Cook migrated with his family to Australia when he was just three and he spent his youth in Barcaldine in central west Queensland where his father was a general practitioner: it was there, he explained, that he developed what would become a life long interest in the medical problems of the Australian frontier.*

He graduated MB.ChM. in 1920 and proceeded to London to take the DTM&H in 1923, a qualification to which he was to add in later years the Sydney DPH and MD, and the Fellowships of the Royal Colleges of General Practitioners and Medical Administrators. He did well in London and was awarded the Wandsworth Research Fellowship from the School and held it from 1923 to 1925. He consulted Cumpston the Commonwealth Director-General and chose to study leprosy in northern Australia, but interpreted that brief broadly. His own summary stated[1] –

> *During the tenure of this Fellowship conducted research into the Epidemiology, treatment and control of leprosy in Great Britain, Norway, Western Australia, Northern Territory, Queensland and New South Wales.*
>
> *In pursuance of research into epidemiology of leprosy in Australia under Wandsworth Research Fellowship, made a survey of north Western Australia from Onslow to Wyndham in 1924. Attention was directed to –*
>
> *(a) the incidence and epidemiology of leprosy in the white and native populations.*
> *(b) incidence of other tropical diseases in the native population.*
> *(c) recommendations to Western Australian Department of Health, on provision of medical service and methods of disease control in north Western Australia.*
>
> *Similar medical survey of North Australia was made in 1925. Recommendations were submitted to Commonwealth Department of Health and these formed the basis of the national medical services subsequently established in the Northern Territory and north Western Australia.*

His monograph on that study, *The Epidemiology of Leprosy in Australia*, was published by the Commonwealth in 1927.[3] It was, and is, a major contribution to our knowledge of this important disease and will be discussed further below.

He spent 1926 as a medical officer at the Australian Institute of Tropical Medicine in Townsville, and reorganised the hookworm campaign in the Cairns area. Then in 1927, at the age of 29, he was appointed Chief Medical Officer and Chief Protector of Aborigines for the Northern Territory. He held these positions for 12 years. it is recorded that some loss of vision in one eye from a childhood accident meant that he was not accepted as a permanent officer of the public service and was officially classed as 'temporary' for the whole period. It is this period of his life and work, as it applied to his Aboriginal responsibilities, that has come under close scrutiny by Drs Saunders and Austin.[2,4,5]

Cook's own summary of what he achieved in the Northern Territory is impressive. In an application for a subsequent post, he wrote[1] –

> *Enunciated the following principles as the basis of any measures to correct the social and economic problems in the Territory affecting the health administration –*
>
> *(a) Correction of the gross disproportion of male to female population in rural districts.*
>
> *(b) Control and eradication of endemic communicable disease particularly from the native population.*
>
> *(c) The elevation of the native population to the white standard of living.*
>
> *The application of these principles was stated to require –*
>
> *(a) Provision of a medical service competent to treat any condition, readily accessible to any resident of the Territory at any time at a cost well within the capacity of the patient to pay.*
>
> *(b) The organisation of a health service fully informed in the epidemiology of the diseases concerned and devoted to the detection and removal of sources of infection and the correction of environmental influences permitting transmission.*
>
> *(c) Complete medical control of the native population living tribally, on missions or in employment with a view to the detection and cure of disease and to prevent dissemination between the races.*

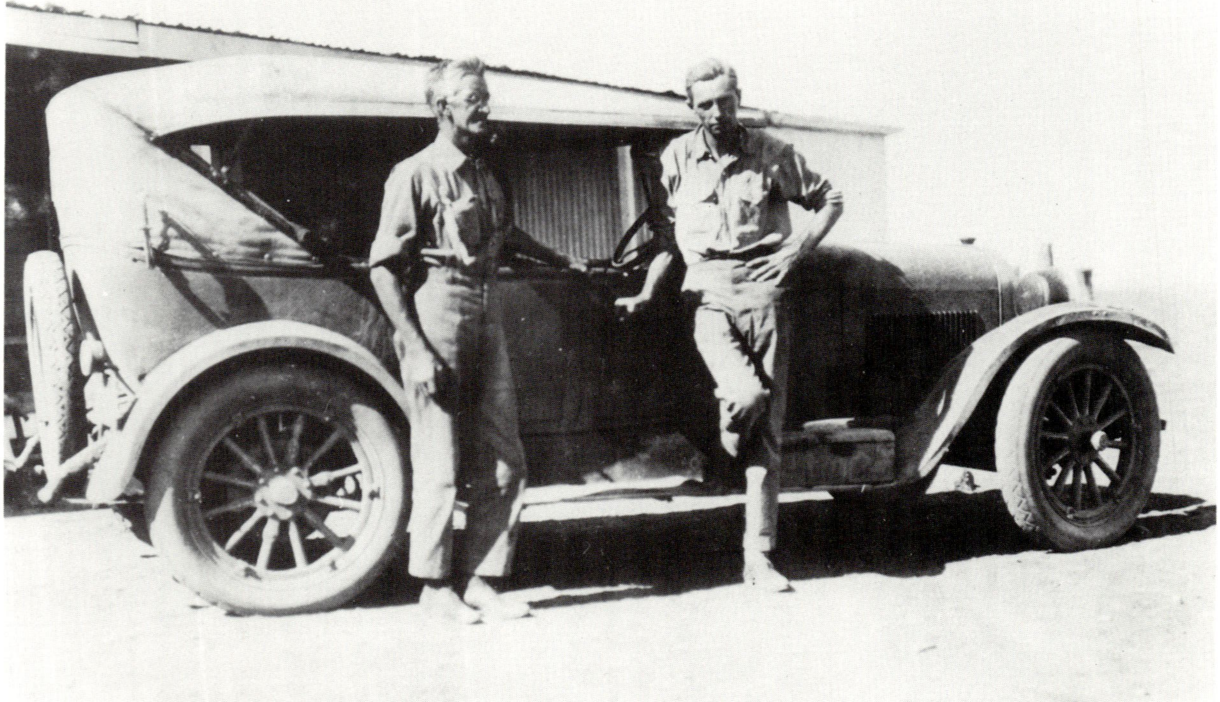

Figure 4.1. *Dr Cecil Cook (on the right) and colleague in the field.*

For these purposes established Northern Territory Medical Service with full time medical officers and trained nurses. Established Medical Benefit Fund permitting free medical, surgical and hospital treatment and ambulance transport (road or air) for the payment of a nominal weekly subscription. Developed system of medical case records to permit study of disease and acclimatisation in the white population. Began routine medical inspection of school children.

Maternity ward provided at Darwin Hospital. Tuberculosis Clinic, Venereal Diseases Clinic, Infant Health and Maternal Welfare Clinics set up. District nurse appointed as a home visitor. Nurses Board set up and the training of local girls in nursing commenced at the Darwin Hospital, for the purpose of relieving trained nursing shortage and providing avocations for Territory girls who, after marriage could serve as nurses in the areas of their residence. Medical Board set up.

Regular and frequent medical inspection of natives was inaugurated. Identity card system was developed as basis of the native census and medical records kept. Leprosarium established, Channel Island.

Regular examination of pearling crews. Endemic diseases ordinance permitting the examination and control of persons entering the Territory and likely to be carriers of tropical disease. Mass vaccination of pearling crews and natives on the northern coast likely to come in contact with them.

Establishment of medical aid posts in remote districts by the training of police and other persons in first aid and sanitation. These were followed in certain areas by the establishment of hospitals staffed by trained nurses and supplemented later by the appointment of medical officers.

Application of the policy of elevating half-castes to white standard including public school education, employment as white apprentices and on marriage, provision of homes designed to white standards.

Control of missions to provide for the hygienic development of the native race, the education of the native to public school standard and provision of medical service to effect the prompt detection and treatment of disease. Improvement of transport and communication by requiring as a condition of licences to employ aboriginals, the provision of wireless communication and landing ground permitting access to small aircraft. Flying Doctor Service.

Legislation for improvement of water supplies. Control of the sale of food. Notification of disease.

Organisation of air quarantine. New hospital, Darwin, Katherine, Tennant Creek, Alice Springs.

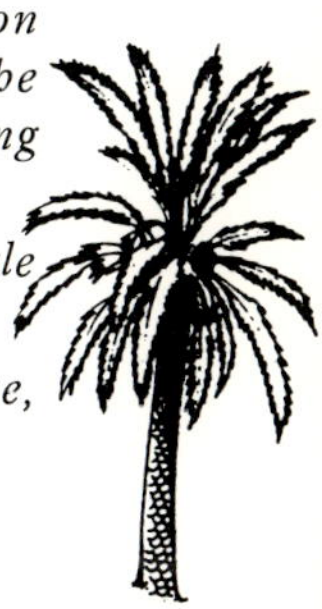

His work achieved recognition from his medical peers, as shown by the award to him of the Cilento Medal of the Commonwealth Department of Health, as well as his appointment later in his career as a Companion of the Order of the British Empire. It has also been seen as important by non-medical historians. Lockwood, in referring to his appointment, commented[6] –

> *... he was to contribute more to taking the Damned out of Darwin than most men before him. He is remembered with affection by survivors from his generation ...*

uncommon praise in the turbulent tale Lockwood tells of Northern Territory politics. Cook certainly comes out in that account in a much more favourable light than, for example, the eminent veterinarian-academic J.A. Gilruth, who served as Administrator of the Territory during World War I. But even in Lockwood's brief and sympathetic treatment Cook comes over as sometimes impetuous and authoritarian. He is quoted as believing that all Aborigines should be medically examined once a year, and 'bang-tail mustered, stripped compulsorily, and examined for V.D., T.B., leprosy, and hookworm'. Recruitment of medical staff was always a problem, and Lockwood reports how Australia's first flying doctor was induced to join the Territory service. In Cook's words –

> *We were desperate for doctors so we got him drunk and sent for his luggage. When he sobered up the Koolinda had sailed.*

Which provides an easy transition back to the historical publications mentioned above. Saunders and Austin are critical of Cook and his work in a number of respects, but also emphasise the difficulties he faced. Austin's particular concern was with the policies and practices adopted in the Northern Territory towards 'mixed-blood' Aborigines, in which he gives considerable attention to Cook's role. He was seen as having the eugenicist biases of his time, such as concern for 'purity of the race'. Austin develops this theme at some length.[2] For example he writes –

> *Cook trained and matured during that period of American and European intellectual ferment dubbed by Michael Roe 'the onslaught of vitalism'. It is clear that he was heavily influenced by that ferment and carried with him to Darwin a progressivist selection of the views of psychologists, anthropologists, geneticists and eugenicists about the racial/hygienic fate of Australian society.*

And later –

> *The crusade-like paternalism of the progressives is nowhere more apparent than in Cook's solutions for the half-caste 'problem'. The nationalist concern for racial well-being, translated into the White Australia Policy, was perhaps the most vital driving force in Cook's policy-making: it undoubtedly over-rode his concern for the half-caste people themselves.*

But he was seen as concerned for the welfare of those for whom he was responsible, bureaucratically efficient in carrying out his duties (indeed Austin heads one chapter 'The eager young bureaucrat graduate, Chief Protector Cecil Cook'), handicapped by Canberra tardiness and political timidity, heckled constantly by both local and southern pressure groups: ahead of his time in many ways but the subject of vitriolic criticism. Some of Austin's statements deserve to be quoted[2] –

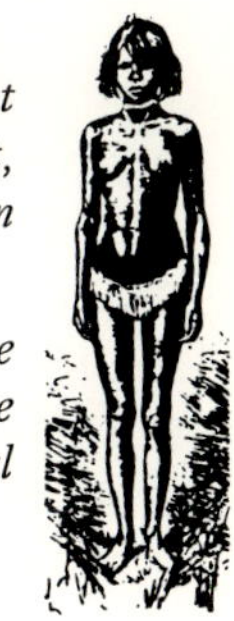

> *For all his attitudinal faults, and whatever we may conclude about the kind of welfare policy he was sent to formulate and implement, he brought with him more bureaucratic care than had ever been experienced by Northern Territory half-castes.*
>
> *He did not bring to the job a set of ready made answers to the problems of Aboriginal welfare ... He insisted from the outset, the Commonwealth should determine a definite policy in the general area of Aboriginal welfare.*

And perhaps as a harbinger of things to come –

> *Cook himself displayed from the outset a condescending disdain for the 'clacking of geese', as he described the lobbying of welfare groups.*

Saunders has documented one particularly difficult interaction, with an intermittently employed pharmacy attendant and hostel supervisor who matured into the famous novelist Xavier Herbert. She records[4] that 'Herbert had first met Cook on his initial visit to the Northern Territory in 1927', just a few months after Cook's own arrival. 'Of similar ages, Herbert being four years the junior, and with mutual interests, they struck up a friendship', and for a short period Herbert was employed at the Darwin Hospital. He found more remunerative and exciting employment on the pearling luggers and 'by August 1930, he was in a position to finance his trip and, taking his fledgling and ultimately unpublished novel *Black Velvet* with him, he set sail for England'. Herbert returned to Darwin in 1935 and again found employment in Cook's area of authority, this time in charge of the Kahlin Compound, the Darwin hostel for Aborigines. Saunders records[4] –

> *From October 1935 until June the following year Herbert became passionately involved in the running of the Compound. 'I am engrossed', he told Dibley, 'in the stupendous task of reconstructing this hideous dump and resurrecting the lost souls that inhabit it.' To this end he improved the hygiene of the compound, fought for better quality food, encouraged a semblance of routine and productivity and, by endeavouring to settle disputes internally rather than in the police courts, to engender a sense of self-worth among the inmates of the institution. He was unable to effect any major material improvements and he accused Cook of refusing to make the necessary money available. Later, in a more conciliatory frame of mind, he admitted that Cook had always been obstructed in his work by 'stinginess from above him and stupidity below' and that government policy was responsible for lack of funds.*

This uneasy balance did not last. 'In a bid to attract increased funds to the Compound and to expose the alleged poor administration of Aboriginal affairs in Darwin, Herbert invited Lancaster, a visiting Commonwealth accountant, to inspect the Compound in Cook's absence ... the plan backfired ... Lancaster condemned the policy, the facilities and the administration of both the Aboriginal Compound and the Halfcaste Home ... Herbert was forced to defend himself and his management of Kahlin ... Cook, who was to have been the victim of Herbert's ploy, was not spared and on his return found himself engaged in voluminous correspondence refuting Lancaster's allegations. All pretence of friendship and support between Cook and Herbert evaporated ... '

Saunders follows the story through, and sees Herbert as increasingly antagonistic to Cook and influencing southern anthropological circles especially through A.P. Elkin, who in turn contributed to the political and administrative decisions that were to lead to Cook's departure. But perhaps Herbert's most waspish reaction to Cook and his whole era of public health and medical practice was reserved for his books. Saunders suggests that Cook was the model for Dr Aintee in Herbert's first major novel *Capricornia*. She writes[4] –

> *Few characters are well developed in 'Capricornia' but, in Aintee, we get a glimpse of a man with a certain amount of wit and good humour who is well liked by his social equals and accorded a somewhat fearful respect by his inferiors. Although the actions of Europeans are described with mockery and derision and the plight of the Aboriginal people exposed with brutal frankness, Dr Aintee is not held personally responsible for the state of poverty and degradation in which the Aborigines live ...*
>
> *Herbert did not allow Cook to escape so lightly a second time around. Dr Cobbity, Dr Aintee's corresponding number in 'Poor Fellow My Country', a character which again 'grew out of' Cook, is portrayed as a mean-spirited but arrogant man who, despite his grandiose ideas, had little understanding of the Aboriginal people and even less sympathy for their condition. And yet, even here, the respect Herbert had for Cook could not be entirely subjugated; while his subordinates and the inmates of the compound mutter darkly about his bloody-mindedness, his power and authority are acknowledged and his medical expertise recognised.*

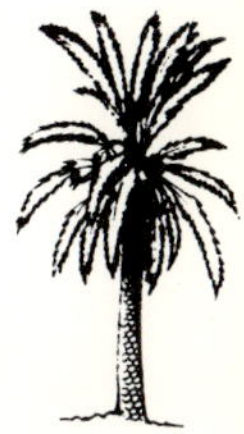

Saunders has also looked disapprovingly at government policies for the isolation of leprosy patients.[5] She saw Cook, and Cilento (who also appears in the history of the North Queensland Medical Conference as delivering one of the major addresses at the first meeting in Townsville in 1954), as contributing to the persistence in Australia of restrictive policies being abandoned elsewhere in the world. The evidence for that view needs sifting. Cook had taken up his early research on leprosy fully conscious of the conflicting pressures and indeed showing sympathy for those who were the victims both of leprosy and of the policies being pursued. He wrote[3] –

> *Here ... on the one hand, is a country where the study of the histories of individual cases appears to exclude contagion as a factor in the spread of the disease, and yet, on the other hand, where sufferers are seized and forcibly isolated on a distant island, in strange, cheerless company, denied in their extremity the society and care of their loved ones, deprived of all there is of interest in their lives, doomed to end their lonely days of misery in exile because their fellow-citizens fear to associate with them.*

But after what must be seen as a careful and laborious investigation he came to see contagion as the only basis of both transmission and control. He was impressed by the outcome of control measures in New South Wales, where 'compulsory notification and isolation at State lazarets has been the law and the practice for over three decades' and 'leprosy may now be considered to be completely under control', an outcome he ascribed to 'the thorough and efficient measures taken for its eradication by Ashburton Thompson'. The facts that Queensland had similarly stringent legislation but an increasing prevalence of leprosy were attributed to administrative failures, inadequate surveillance of suspects, inadequate investigation of contact histories, and inadequate control of discharged lepers. At the conclusion of the study, much of which was a laborious tracking of every recorded case, he supported a policy of isolation which bore most heavily on Aborigines. The conclusions to the report include 'the following suggestions'[3] –

> (i) *Compulsory notification and isolation to continue.*
>
> (ii) *Thorough inquiry into each new case at time of detection, directed towards discovering probable origin.*
>
> (iii) *Institution of regular periodic clinical and bacteriological re-examination of intimate contacts ... .*
>
> (iv) *Such suspects as are not deemed sufficiently definite for committal to the lazaret should be regularly re-examined ... .*
>
> (v) *The criterion for isolation should be different in the white and aboriginal races.*

Cook was after 1950 a senior member of the National Health and Medical Research Tropical Medicine Committee, which had the prime role of advising on national leprosy policy, and which fought hard and ultimately successfully to have isolation requirements relaxed. But that was after the sulphones and other drugs had become available, much more effective than the chaulmoogra and hydnocarpus that he used in the 1930s.

Austin has given a somewhat sad account of the end of Cook's service in Darwin.[2] He had become unpopular, it is suggested, in the south 'for being too conservative in the general area of Aboriginal affairs' and in the north because his 'policies ... were too radical in the more specific area of Half-caste advancement'. The Commonwealth government moved, at last, to changes in Aboriginal policy, changes very similar to what Cook had been urging for years. But as part of those changes, and it is suggested in response to criticisms of Cook and to the anti-Cook lobbying of Herbert and others, it was proposed to separate the positions of Chief Medical Officer and of Chief Protector of Aborigines. Cook strongly disagreed, believing that the two were inextricably related in the Territory, and refused to apply for either of the advertised positions.

> *The Commonwealth Government's desire to dissipate southern perceptions about its own culpability in the area of Aboriginal affairs ... did indeed require a scapegoat and it had to be Cook.*

Cook, Austin suggests, 'had reached a point of intolerable frustration with Canberra's inaction, of anger about his mooted dumping and he maintained a genuine mission with regard to northern health'.

Austin reaches a balanced set of conclusions about Cook's contribution to Aboriginal welfare in the Northern Territory[2] –

> *... he brought a will to actively engage in the development of new initiatives designed to elevate the status of Half-castes in order to engineer their eradication ... In his breeding program and in his advocacy of sterilising Half-caste 'mental defectives', he proved a proponent of some of the worst excesses of progressivism ... On the other hand, Cook also brought to the Territory the most recent anthropological and psychological evidence showing Half-castes not to be as inferior as popular prejudice assumed and the weight of earlier scientific evidence had seemed to demonstrate ... Accordingly, he was, in the Northern Territory, a man ahead of his time, tempering some of the excesses of neglect in education, housing and employment that had earlier characterised a decade and a half of Commonwealth rule.*

So in 1939 he left the Territory and returned to the east, as medical officer at the School of Public Health and Tropical Medicine, the direct successor of the Australian Institute of Tropical Medicine at which he had been based 13 years before.

The subsequent story can be summarised briefly.[1] It is hoped that his biographers will provide a fuller account at some future time. Cook served with distinction in the Army Medical Services from 1940 to 1945: as RMO 2 Armoured Regiment and Lecturer in Military Hygiene, Army School of Hygiene, Sydney in 1940–1; in what was then Ceylon as Pathologist to the 2/12 AGH, AIF, in 1941–3; and then in Papua-New Guinea as Deputy Assistant Director of Hygiene, 2 Aust Corps & NG Forces and Assistant Director of Hygiene, Adv

Land Headquarters. His *curriculum vitae* lists several research interests from that war experience, with special studies of the control of cholera, rabies and filariasis in Ceylon and of the epidemiology and control of malaria, dysentery and scrub typhus in New Guinea.

He returned to civilian life and became Commissioner of Public Health for the State of Western Australia from 1946 to 1949. His own summary of that period, in his typical telegraphic sytle, reads[1] –

> *Gave attention to re-activating local health authorities and health administration – appointment of joint health inspectors to appropriate groups.*
>
> *Established clinic for the diagnosis of tuberculosis by mass X-ray.*
>
> *School of Nursing for the improved training of nurses to staff country hospitals.*
>
> *Measures for improving sanitation and medical service in the north-west.*
>
> *Special attention to the reduction of infant mortality, including provision of laboratory and X-ray facilities at King Edward Maternity Hospital and legal requirements for autopsy after foetal death.*
>
> *Set up a Committee of Advice on infant mortality – comprising obstetricians, paediatricians, physicians.*
>
> *Established State Health Council to facilitate the better integration of the practising medical profession into health administration and prevention of disease.*

He then returned to the Commonwealth Department of Health in Canberra, as Senior Medical Officer to 1958 and then as Director, Division of Public Health until his retirement in 1962. In his Canberra period he was closely involved with the National Health and Medical Research Council, especially its public health wing. He served on and for much of the period chaired the Public Health Committee, one of the Council's three main arms, from 1950 to 1962. After his retirement he lived in Queensland, at Burleigh Heads, until a motor accident forced him to go into a nursing home near family in Sydney. He died in 1987.

The career and achievements of Cecil Cook, and the ways in which they have been perceived and evaluated, raise a number of points for discussion. There are complex political and social questions involved in all aspects of public health, never more clearly so than in those involving the Aboriginal component of the Australian community. Cook's work in the Northern Territory came within what we might define as the 'tropical medicine' era of Aboriginal health, when attention was focussed on a number of infectious or parasitic diseases such as leprosy, hookworm and yaws, which were either uncommon or unknown in the white community. That era was to continue until perhaps the mid-1960s, when the counting of Aborigines in the national census led to more accurate health statistics, the recognition of the deplorable infant mortality on Aboriginal settlements and to a consequent surge of national concern. Times have changed very quickly. The initial interventionist response, to put more money and white professionals into programs of health care and public health activities, has been caught up in and modified by a number of major influences, including the development of Aboriginal health services administered by Aborigines, itself part of a more assertive assumption by Aborigines of responsibility for their own problems, and the recognition of primary health care as the path to the WHO objective of 'health for all by the year 2000'.

We are creatures of our own particular time, and may all find it hard to justify our actions and our words according to the world view and the language of a later generation. Perhaps what is valid in the historians' criticism of Cook's performance in the Territory in the 1930s should more probably be directed at Australian society as a whole, and he himself be seen as what Austin called him, a man ahead of his time.

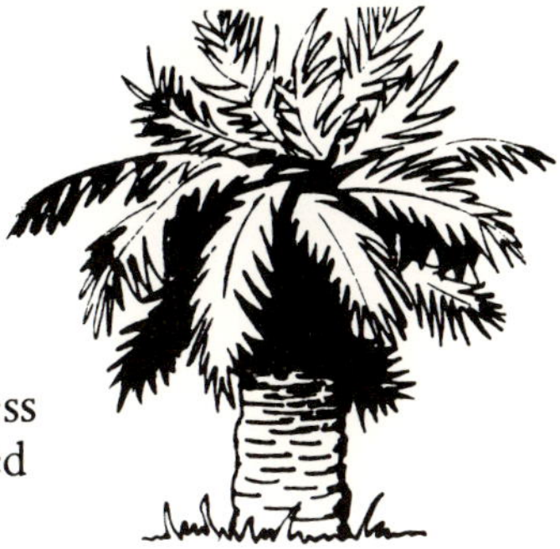

Acknowledgements

I thank Ms Suzanne Saunders and Dr Tony Austin for allowing me to have access to and to quote from their material, published and unpublished, on Dr Cecil Cook.

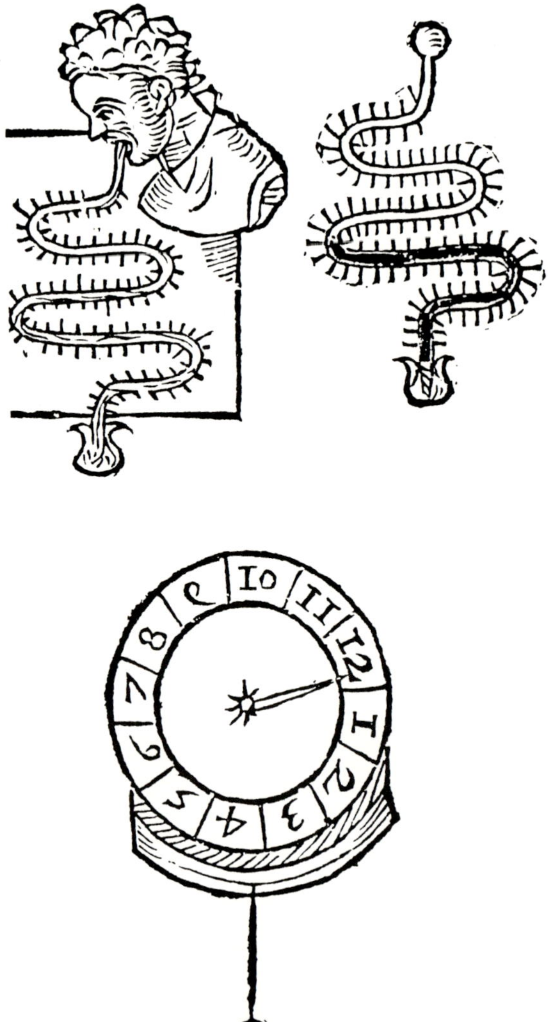

Figure 5.1. Examples of early thermometry – Santorio's thermometer of 1612.

FEVERS AND FRONTIERS 5

THE MEASURE OF NATURE'S INSTRUMENT

An Historical Review of Clinical Thermometry

Mervyn Cobcroft

Why! the Fever itself is Nature's Instrument.

[Thomas Sydenham, 1624–1689][1]

Moses knew. As he harangued the Israelites around about 1260 BC, he clearly identified a relationship between fever and disease –

> *The Lord shall make the pestilence cleave unto thee, until he have consumed thee ... The Lord shall smite thee with a consumption, and with a fever, and with an inflammation, and with an extreme burning ... and they shall pursue thee until thou perish.*[2]

Heat, swelling, pain, redness, and loss of function are literally classic signs of inflammation. Yet fever, its antiquity notwithstanding, remained largely unquantitated until well after other signs, much later recognised, had been elucidated and measured. The stethoscope and pocket watch had evolved to record and monitor heart beat and pulse long before reliable thermometers appeared.

Why?

Several reasons can be advanced. Firstly, instruments such as the microscope and stethoscope revolutionised the concept of disease by establishing the specificity of organs or systems afflicted. Fever, a general phenomenon, did not fit comfortably into this end-organ approach. Searching for the specifics of fevers was singularly unrewarding. There were more spectacular discoveries on which to make reputations. Next, clinicians sensed they could obtain as much or more information by placing a hand upon a fevered brow –

> *... the hand takes account of moisture as well as of actual temperature, convey[ing] more information which the thermometer fails to impart – eg. the 'pungent' dry heat of early pneumonia is most characteristic.*[3]

and, even today, few would deny the value of this hands-on contact. A more obvious factor was the great difficulty in manufacturing and calibrating thermometers. The difference between normal and elevated body temperature is small, a variation which near equated the degree of accuracy of early thermometers. Certainly, those early instruments gave no hint of the normal positional (i.e. armpit, mouth etc), diurnal or ovulatory variations of body temperatures. In fact, normal body temperature was long regarded as being rigidly fixed. Next, these instruments by comparison with today's examples were large and fragile making transportation difficult. A physician could not throw a thermometer into his bag like a stethoscope, so few bothered to carry them. The cost of replacing broken thermometers was enormous. The *Lancet* of 1895 estimated the financial loss through such wastage would provide London hospitals with two extra beds a year, a potent argument against their widespread use. As well, thermometers suffered what today would be called an 'image problem'. By contrast, the stethoscope was a showy invention which looked suitably impressive and took time and skill to master. Not so the humble thermometer. It is no accident that doctors (and others) today drape stethoscopes around their shoulders, not poke thermometers out of pockets, as symbolic clan badges. Everybody wanted a hand in the development of the stethoscope and instrument catalogues were full of illustrations of 'Dr A's new, improved model'. There was little kudos to be had from the pedestrian recorder of temperature.[4,5]

Lastly, there was a fundamental question of philosophy (of which the pioneers were blissfully ignorant and to which we came only with the considerable benefit of hindsight). Temperature, the property of heat or cold, is a sensation perceived by us as individuals. We award it degrees by subjective comparison. Our experience tells us that steam is hotter than ice. The pioneer thermometrists were thus trying to quantitate a subjective experience. It is analogous to trying to measure the greenness of green or to describe the colour to the blind. These thermometrists did not understand what they were measuring. The result was a confusion of temperature scales of varying degrees of rationality. Of course, we now know that temperature is a function of mean molecular kinetic energy. From this it follows that when there is no molecular kinesis we have reached an absolute – not relative – zero, below which it is impossible and illogical to enquire. This absolute zero is the ideal starting point to construct a 'logical' temperature scale which would avoid the idiosyncrasies of our existing ones. The familiar melting point of ice would not now be blessed with 273 Kelvin (eccentric), or 0° Celsius (passable) or 32° Fahrenheit (irrational). We are the victims of history in the same way that electricity erroneously is said to flow from positive to negative.[6,7]

The development of the clinical thermometer can be conveniently if somewhat arbitrarily divided into 4 phases which will now be considered in turn.

Phase One: Construction

The Italian Galileo Galilei [1564–1642] is traditionally credited with inventing the first thermometer in 1592. His instrument consisted of a slender glass tube expanding into a thin walled, air filled bulb at its upper end. The open lower end dipped into either alcohol or water, which liquid partially filled that tube. The air in the bulb expanded or contracted according to the external temperature causing a corresponding shift in the fluid height: the colder, the higher it went up the stem. Galileo does not seem to have provided a scale. The principle underlying the functioning of the thermometer later became known as Charles' Law [1787]. Galileo's instrument was fundamentally flawed for, being open to the atmosphere, the fluid column was also subjected to atmospheric pressure in accordance with Boyle's Law, documented in 1662.[8,9]

The honour of being the first to employ thermometry in physiology and to provide an external scale (i.e. not physically incorporated into the glass) goes to a colleague of Galileo's. Santorio in his 1612 *Commentaries on the Medical Art of Galen* boasted –

> *In a marvellous way, I am accustomed to measure with a certain glass instrument, the cold and hot temperatures of the air and of all parts of the body, and so exactly.*[3]

Santorio's thermometer was basically a modification of Galileo's. (*Figure 5.1*) The glass column was lengthened and convoluted and the scale of 110 points provided externally along the convolutions. (Note it was the length of air within the tube which was measured not the fluid, the reverse of what we use today.) Santorio calibrated his scale at one end by placing the bulb in melting snow and, at the other, by the heat of a candle flame. In measuring his subjects, Santorio had them hold the bulb within their mouths for a standard period of ten beats of a pendulum.[10] Later he would use this pendulum to time how long it took the air to expand to a predetermined mark: the hotter a subject was, the quicker the time. Thus Santorio's time scale is probably one of the most unusual fever measures ever devised. The same atmospheric pressure variations dogged this instrument. It was also fragile, cumbersome, and lacked portability. Despite Santorio's boast, there were only limited sites where the body could safely accommodate the delicate glass bulb.[4]

Although we have been using the term 'thermometer' to describe these early devices, the word did not appear until 1624 in the French book *Mathematical Pastimes.*[11] French physician, Jean Rey, became the first person to measure the expansion of a liquid rather than air. His thermometer however was still an open system with an external scale.[9]

The close of this initial fabrication phase came with the work and encouragement of Ferdinand II, the Grand Duke of Tuscany. Ferdinand eliminated the failings of the open system by having his contrivances hermetically sealed thus disposing of atmospheric influences. The Grand Duke also established the *Accademia del Cimeno* in Florence in 1657 with the object of standardizing the collection of meteorological data from throughout the region. To do this, the *Accademia* employed skilled glass blowers and other instrument makers to construct identical pieces of apparatus including thermometers for distribution to the various data collecting stations. These artisans were among the first to utilize mercury in their thermometers but they preferred alcohol as it had a greater coefficient of expansion.[9,11]

The thermometer now was in the form in which we recognise it today. Development then passed to the second phase.

Phase Two. Calibration

What Galileo was to the thermometer construction, another giant of science, Sir Isaac Newton [English, 1642–1727] was to calibration. To Newton we owe the concept of reproducible fixed points on thermometer scales. It is true that Santorio had upper and lower limits on his scale but he failed to appreciate that ice melts at a constant temperature and that the recorded temperature of a candle flame varies with how far the bulb is held away and with the uneven distribution of heat within flames themselves. Newton however was not the first to suggest fixed and reproducible points. Carlo Renaldini of Padua had done so in 1694 but his work remained unknown and unappreciated. Interestingly enough, Renaldini chose the freezing and boiling points of water as his markers.[11]

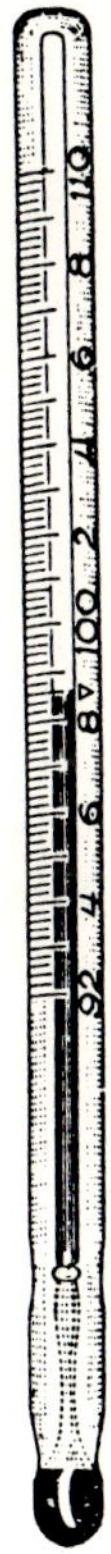

In 1701, Newton chose as his reproducible fixed points those of melting ice (0°) and, with what can only be considerable zenophobia, the axillary temperature of a healthy Englishman. To this upper point, he gave the number 12. This was no random choice on Newton's part for he was obsessed with what he perceived to be the orderliness of Nature. Twelve can be fractioned into half; a third; a quarter; a sixth; two-thirds; three-quarters; five-sixths; five-, seven- and eleven-twelfths to give whole numbers: 'equal parts of heat' as he styled them. Water boiled at 34°. Newton would no doubt have been devastated to learn that an Englishman's armpit was not as good as his word!

Gabriel Daniel Fahrenheit [Germano-Dutch, 1686–1736] came to thermometry with obvious zeal —

> ***When I read that water boils at a definite degree of heat, I immediately felt a great desire to make myself a thermometer so that I might examine with my eyes this beautiful phenomenon of nature and be convinced of the truth of the experiment.***[11]

Fahrenheit adopted Newton's fixed points and in the process adapted them significantly. He found Newton's twelve 'equal degrees' too coarse a measure. At first he doubled twelve to 24, then again to 48, and finally to 96. Fahrenheit was also the first to search for an absolute zero. The most intense cold he could artificially obtain was 'produced by a mixture of water, ice, sal-ammoniac, and even common salt'.[11] This he called 0°. (We now know this temperature can vary according to the quantities employed.) On this scale, water froze at 32° and boiled at 212°. Shortly after his death, these two points were permanently declared as the official markers [1740]. It was found necessary to adjust normal body temperature to 98.6°F!

Andrew Celsius [Swedish, 1701–1744] proposed a scale of one hundred divisions using the markers but with freezing point 100° and boiling 0°! Sensibly another Swede, Linnaeus [Carl von Linne, 1707–1778] persuaded him to reverse this. The centigrade scale was also independently defined by Christin of Lyons the following year. The ninth General Conference on Weights and Measures officially named this scale for Celsius in 1948.[12]

The Celsius and Fahrenheit scales were destined to be the most popular clinically although a rather confused Réaumer scale (0° to 80°) dating from 1740 did find some limited currency in continental Europe.[9]

With the fixity of these markers came a disturbing reality. Thermometers exposed to exactly similar conditions rarely agreed. In clinical settings where temperature differences were never large to begin with, the result was unacceptable. What was the point of one instrument reading 'normal' while another showed 'fever'? Such inaccuracy did nothing towards the acceptance of thermometry.

The fault lay with their manufacture, in all manner of things: the indicator fluid, stem lumens, scale positioning, and even the very glass itself. Several different indicator fluids had been tried such as plain water and linseed oil but eventually it was a contest between alcohol and mercury. Alcohol, which had to be coloured to make it visible against glass, expanded well when heated but not by constant amounts. If a temperature rise of Δt caused an incremental volume expansion of ΔV, there was no guarantee that a $2\Delta t$ rise would be matched by a $2\Delta V$ increase (i.e. alcohol has a variable volume co-efficient of expansion). Mercury on the other hand is far more constant but the incremental volume increase is small. To relate this three-dimensional ΔV change accurately on a linear (one-dimensional), equally-divided scale (Δh) requires one fundamental assumption, namely that the cross-sectional area of the stem lumen (A) remain a constant. Stated mathematically, Δt temperature increase produces ΔV volume change which equals A X Δh. If A is constant, then Δt is proportional to Δh.

Immediately obvious are the practical problems this created –

- To produce lumens of uniform cross-sectional area is technically difficult and was beyond the ability of early glass workers. Consequently, equi-distant scales were inaccurate.

- Alcohol by its variable expansion gave inaccurate readings on equi-distant linear scales, especially over large temperature ranges.

- Mercury in wide lumened stems lends itself greatly to parallax errors.

- Reducing the cross-section area (A) of the lumen increases the length component (Δh) for each degree of temperature change. This reduces parallex but at the expense of increasing the difficulty in reading the instrument and, more importantly, of the effects of any variation in lumen diameter. From the formula $\Delta V = A \times \Delta h$, because A is determined by the square of the radius (r), even tiny variations in the radius when the overall cross-sectional area is small produce enormous changes in Δh which is not so when r is larger. To be accurate, narrow bores demand uniformity.

Thermometers were originally provided with external scales which were engraved on a variety of materials such as strips of bone, ivory, or sometimes paper. The first problem was to correctly position these against the fixed marker points. One can imagine many a scalded finger from the boiling water so I suppose iced water found more uses than just plain calibration. Once aligned the scale had to be glued, wired, or otherwise firmly fitted to the stem. There would always have been the possibility of the scale working loose or falling off thus creating more measurement failures. An external scale also meant the

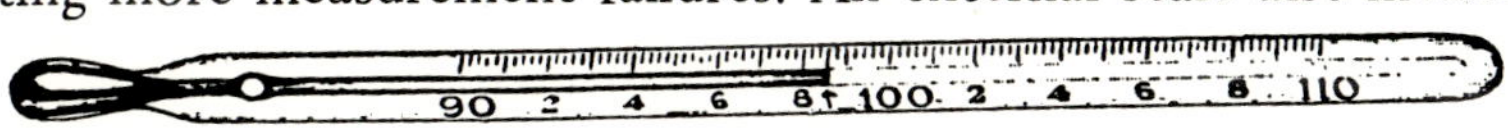

indicator fluid was somewhat physically remote from its measurement point again leading to parallax errors. Surely these objections would disappear if the scale were actually incorporated in the glass itself? One of the first to try direct etching on thermometer stems was Crichton of Paris at the end of the eighteenth century.[4] Unfortunately this did not work very well. Glass is a complex material –

> *... an amorphous, artificial, non-crystalline substance, usually transparent, plastic when molten, ductile when cooling, and glyptic when cold.*[13]

It is also marginally fluid despite its solid appearance and brittle nature. This fluidicity was a particular feature of older glass mixtures as the gravitational ripples on old stained-glass windows testify. Creepage also affected newly made glass so that any thermometer etched straight after manufacture would end up with a great deal of scalar distortion after the passage of a few months. Like good wines, the better thermometers were laid down to mature. Another suggestion was that thermometers be checked regularly for accuracy every year or so at places like Kew Observatory in London or the Thermometric Bureau at New Haven, USA. Good in theory but totally impractical even today let alone the nineteenth century!

Glass also expands when heated, again more so with older styles, so that the scale markings were further apart under hot conditions. Another cause of inaccuracy![4] Because glass is a poor conductor of heat, the glass of the bulb had to be thin enough to allow sufficient heat to expand the indicator fluid. Of course, this thinning contributed markedly to the fragility of the instrument. Even so, it took over five minutes to reach the final temperature reading.

Thus was the sorry state at the end of the second period in the 1850s. But technology was soon to bring a new enthusiasm and new enthusiasts.

Phase Three: Clinical Confidence

Undoubtedly, the greatest clinical thermometrist of all times was Carl Reinhold August Wunderlich [German, 1815–1877] who, after exhaustive clinical investigation, published his monumental *The Behaviour of Body Temperature in Disease* in Leipzig in 1868. This was soon translated into English and re-issued by the New Sydenham Society in 1871. The book revolutionized attitudes towards clinical temperature recording by showing how changes in body temperature related to the progress of diseases. A good example was Wunderlich's demonstration of the crisis and lysis of broncho-pneumonia (*Figure 5.2*) in pre-antibiotic days.[3] It was said of Wunderlich that 'he found fever a disease and left it a symptom'.[14]

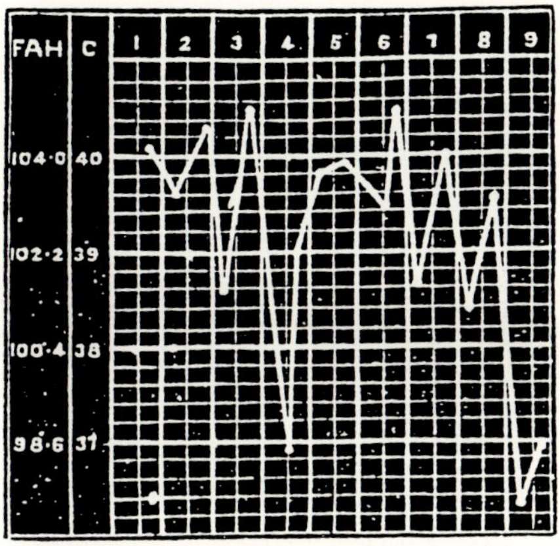

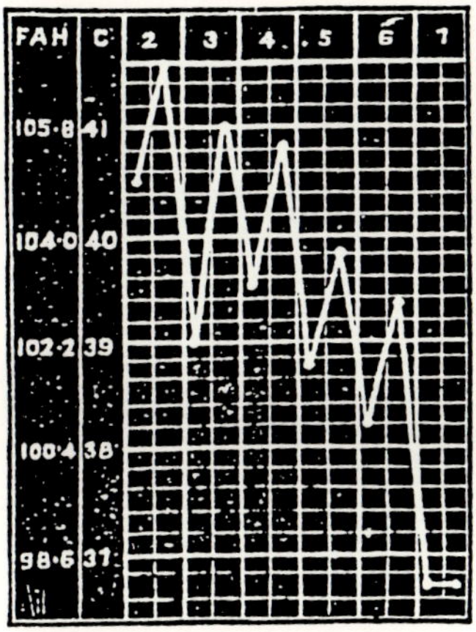

Figure 5.2

Crisis. Case of lobar pneumonia. *(After Wunderlich)*

Lysis. Case of broncho-pneumonia. *(After Wunderlich)*

Others took up and extended thermometry. Sir Thomas Clifford Allbutt [English, 1836–1925] was another champion; his 1870 paper *Medical Thermometry* of 1870 did much to stimulate world-wide interest as did his practical supervision of thermometer manufacture.[14] Allbutt also devised an instrument ('thermopile') for simultaneously measuring temperatures at the surface and in deeper tissues, an important milestone in the physiological understanding of temperature regulation [1868].[4] House surgeon, J.W. Stickler, of the Presbyterian Hospital, New York began the recording of daily temperatures on all patients,not just those with febrile conditions:

> *... the thermometer should be always in the surgeon's hand, and a regular record be kept by the nurse ...*

was the counsel of a standard textbook of 1878.[15] William Carter in Liverpool investigated temperature patterns in normal subjects (nurses on shift duty) and discovered –

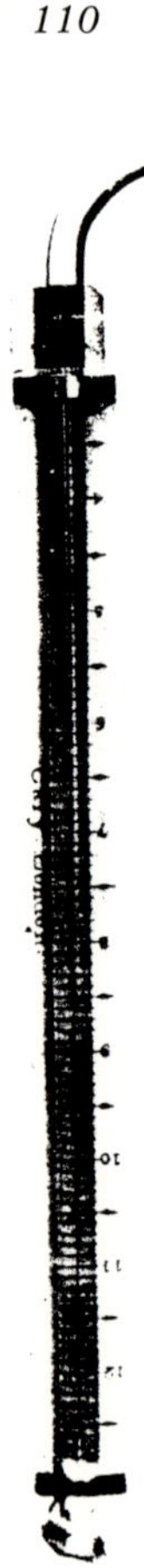

> *... that a daily depression of temperature takes place in the healthy during nights and early morning; that such a change of habit as turns night into day so far as employment is concerned does not permanently affect the character of this depression ...* [It] *is not markedly affected by food.*[4]

What wrought this change in attitude? Simply, reliable and accurate thermometers. Which is where technology triumphed. The second half of the nineteenth century was a period of enormous technical inventiveness in the glass industry with England and Bohemia leading the field in the middle of the century, France slightly later, and the great industrial power of America gradually making itself felt.[13] Machines took over from the eyes, hands, and lungs of man. Machines could draw out hollow tubes of glass to create thermometer stems with the finest, most uniform lumens – far beyond the capabilities of the most capable, steady glass blowers. These precise narrow bores were a great advance: thermometers could be constructed to cover only the narrow clinical range, mercury expansion freed from parallax, and the cumulative effect of the uneven expansion of alcohol minimized. Such instruments were smaller and more compact making them easier to transport and less subject to breakage. Experiment and experience led to new glass varieties culminating in Frederick Otto Schoot of Jena introducing a new stable glass, 'Jena Normal', in 1891.[4] At last the major physical imperfections of earlier thermometers had been defeated.

Figure 5.3
An example of an early clinical mercury thermometer, designed to be read by a doctor or nurse standing behind the patient. Circa 1800.

Concurrently there was a whole succession of minor changes, all of which improved the clinical usefulness of the thermometers. One of these was the invention of the index or self-registering thermometer. Until then the physician or nurse who wanted to take a patient's temperature had to wait the five or so minutes while the indicator gained its maximum extent and then read the instrument *in situ.* If there were a whole ward of temperatures to be taken, this became an irritating waste of time. And if the thermometer had to be removed to examine in a better light, that maximum reading was immediately lost. Some early instruments had been bent almost to right-angles to facilitate on-site inspection. (*Figure 5.3*)

In an attempt to overcome these inconveniences, Francois Walfardin, a French civil servant, placed a small length of air almost at the outer extremity of the mercury column within the stem [1855]. In theory, once the mercury had reached its maximum expansion and the thermometer was removed for reading, the mercury distal to the bubble remained for a much longer time at the correct point while the proximal thread quickly contracted back towards the bulb, the air acting as an expandable buffer zone. Unfortunately this bubble sometimes disappeared into the bulb as the instrument cooled, more so if this happened quickly. At other times, the air became fragmented and the instrument would never work properly again. The problem of fabricating a reliable self-registering thermometer was solved by placing the now-familiar constriction in the lumen just distal to the bulb, which innovation appeared for the first time at the 'Great Exhibition of the Works of Industry of all Nations' in the Crystal Palace, London, 1851.[16]

The principle is simple: the surface tension of a liquid bears an inverse relation to spherical diameter; this increased tension at the constriction is sufficient to hold back the contraction of the indicator fluid within the stem but not the vigorous expansion generated within the bulb nor the centrifical forces produced by shaking to reset the instrument.[4]

Other refinements included placing the scale within the glass itself so that it would not be worn away by constant cleaning and bacteria not lurk within the etched grooves on the surface [Hicks, 1895]; shaping the glass of the stem to magnify the narrow lumen and scale [Hicks, 1895 from an idea suggested by Gall]; flattening the back to prevent rolling off surfaces [Arnold and Sons, 1896]; and dulling or silvering the bulb to increase heat uptake and to reduce equilibration time below one minute [Hawksley, Truax, Fannin and Co., 1890s]. Small, pocket-sized, padded containers also made their appearance which allowed breakage-free transport, a most important consideration in the rough days of the horse and buggy.[4] (*Figure 5.4*)

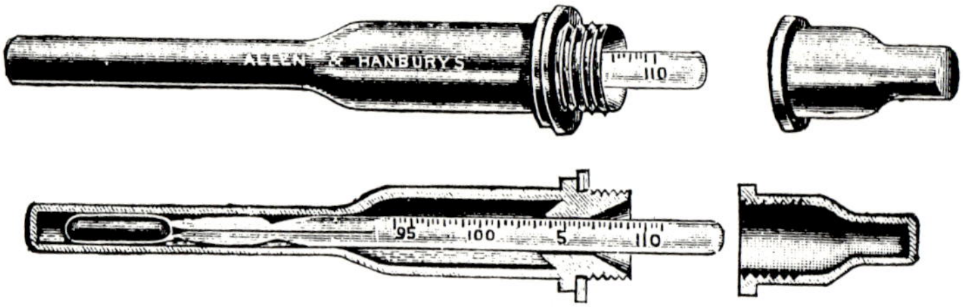

Figure 5.4. Clinical mercury thermometer in a Thorne's silver-plated antiseptic case. Circa 1902. ('Price 3 shillings and six pence')

To some extent we are still in this phase of clinical confidence. The standard glass thermometer is entrenched in clinical practice and 'TPR' (temperature, pulse, and respiration) are still the backbone of clinical observation. But newer and radically different methods of taking temperatures lead us to the fourth phase of our journey.

Phase Four: Couples, Crystals, and Computers

So far, consideration has only been given to liquid-in-glass thermometers which work on the thermoexpansive principle. But other physical properties influenced by heat are making steady inroads into the thermometric landscape including thermoresistance, thermoelectricity, and thermomagnetism.[17]

Sir Humphry Davy [English, 1788–1829] demonstrated that electrical resistance in metals was temperature dependent [1821]. Using this property, Sir William Siemens [English (born Germany), 1823–1883] constructed a platinum resistance thermometer in 1871. Such resistance thermometers function over enormous temperature ranges (–260° to 600°C) and are incredibly accurate (10^{-4} deg C) which, of course, far exceeds clinical requirements. Measurements are made using a modified Wheatstone bridge.[6,9,18] Devices of this type were used experimentally to determine heat distribution in the inflammatory process in the 1880s 'with the greatest exactitude'.[19]

Resistance thermometers are not now put to bed-side use; while extremely accurate, they are slow to respond and bulky.[6] Of far greater importance are the thermoresistance semiconductors ('thermistors'). These devices are part of the electronic revolution which started in 1947 with the American Bell Laboratories' germanium transistor, soon to be replaced by silicon in 1955.[20] Semiconductors are more heat sensitive than metals. They have the advantage of being cheap, fast responding, and very compact, making them ideal for use in miniature probes in such places as the pulmonary arteries and the brain. Unfortunately they are not as resilient as thermocouples and can exhibit hysteresis if subjected to large temperature fluctuations.[6]

Thermocouples work by a phenomenon first described by Thomas Seebeck [German, 1770–1831] in 1821: an electric current is generated in a circuit of two dissimilar metals such as copper and iron where the junctions between the two are at different temperatures.[9] Thermocouples did not find much clinical use until the post-World War Two electronic revolution provided suitable circuitry to remove some complex practical problems (such as keeping the reference junction at a constant reading).[6] Thermocouples have the same advantages as thermistors but are longer lasting. The probes can be made very small indeed for deep body positioning. Both can provide continuous read-outs much employed in operating theatres and intensive care units.[21] They can readily be incorporated into computer-run monitoring systems.

Until the last few years, the liquid-in-glass thermometers have held their own in ward and office use but their day is almost done, victims of the integrated circuit and liquid crystals. They are rapidly being replaced by disposable and digital thermometers. Disposable thermometers are easy to manufacture, cheap, unbreakable, accurate to 0.1°C, and overcome any worry of disease (AIDS, hepatitis, etc) transmission.[21] They are either made of materials which melt at specific temperatures or liquid crystals.[12] Liquid crystals, first made commercially available in 1975 by the British,[22] are substances that flow like liquids but exhibit solid-like molecular alignment at specific temperatures. These changeable molecular arrangements are accompanied by pronounced colour shifts which are a most useful temperature indicator.[12] One of the neatest adaptations of liquid crystal technology is the self-adhesive, flexible strip thermometer – a single-use device which can easily be fixed to the skin over any body contour. (*Figure 5.5*)

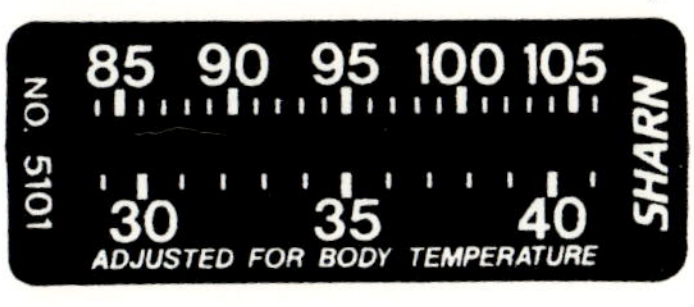

***Figure 5.5.* Disposable strip thermometer for clinical use. 1990.**

Strip thermometers find use in short-term continuous monitoring such as during surgery. Other liquid crystals will align themselves in electric fields and, when placed against polarizing film, block out light. This feature is a basis of one type of digital display, notably that employed in digital timepieces.[20] Another type of digital display employs light-emitting diodes (LED) invented by Holonyak in USA in 1960.[22] These technologies combined with integrated circuitry have resulted in electronic thermometers now marketed by numerous medical equipment suppliers. Electronic thermometers have all the advantages of their disposable cousins: robustness, accuracy (0.1°C), speed (45–60 second read-outs), economy, ease of use, cross-infection prevention (disposable sheaths), and adaptability to many sites (rectal, axillary, oral).[23]

Although I tend to agree, perhaps I would not be as extravagant as Charles W. Ingraham's utterance in 1895 –

> *Not a day passes but that the fever-thermometer gives additional evidence of its being one of the most accurate and scientific diagnostic instruments ... Though the thermometer is but a piece of glass containing mercury, yet it diffuses information that sways the opinions of physicians in council, it indicates the best course of treatment to pursue, it decides doubtful points, and brings order and method out of confusion and uncertainty. In the practice of every physician, many lives are annually saved by what the fever thermometer had detected and brought forth for consideration. Fatal complications are averted and unfavorable changes, particularly in the course of acute disease, are by its use detected sufficiently early to allow of prompt treatment. We cannot but wonder how our ancestors could have intelligently practised medicine and surgery without the aid of the thermometer.*[4]

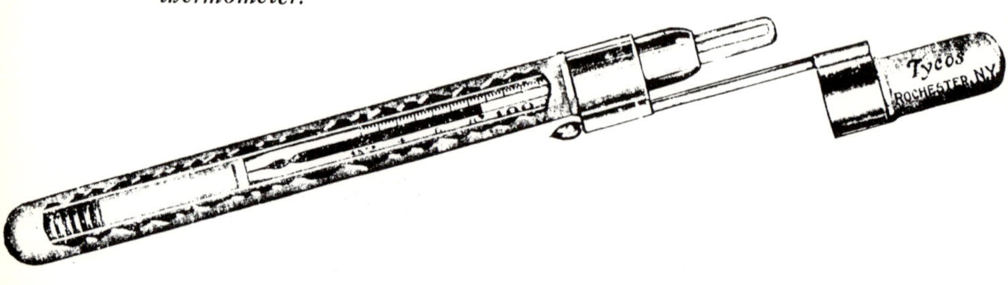

PART III

FRONTIERS OF THE HEALTH PROFESSIONS

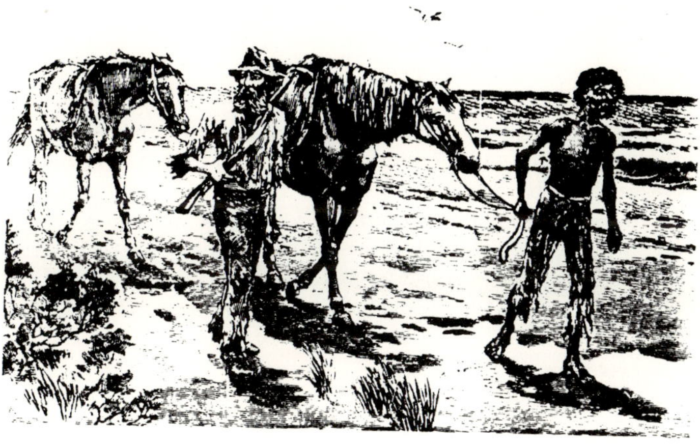

AUSTRALIAN
COLLEGE OF
NATURAL
MEDICINE

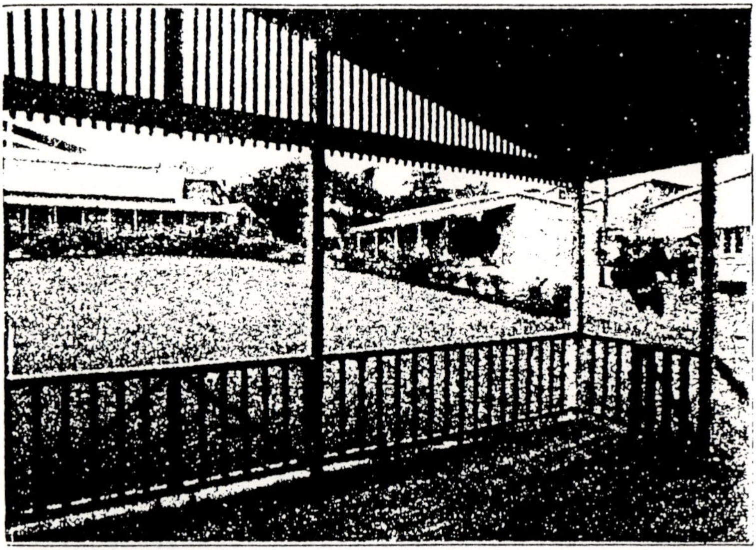

HANDBOOK
1990

362 Water Street, Fortitude Valley, Brisbane, Australia. 4006. Phone: (07) 257 1883 Fax: 257 1889

* Incorporating: **Acupuncture Colleges Australia (Brisbane),**
Australian College of Natural Therapies, College of Classical Homeopathy &
Brisbane College of Traditional Acupuncture and Natural Therapies

Figure 6.1. 1990 Handbook, Australian College of Natural Medicine

FEVERS AND FRONTIERS 6

COMPLEMENTARY MEDICINE: A NEW FRONTIER

John Thearle

By the dawn of the twentieth century scientific medicine in Australia, as in other parts of the western world, dominated all other healing systems, due to the general public's faith in its methods and also because of the official registration of medical practitioners. Registration had the effect of placing the three traditional branches of the profession (physicians, surgeons and apothecaries) under one legal umbrella. While this contained the practices of other, unconventional healers, they were not banished from treating patients. The state may proscribe but it cannot prevent a citizen's beliefs and practices.[1] The establishment of the Commonwealth Department of Health in 1921[2] was followed by a major upheaval in the health care system, including improving quarantine procedures, the investigation and prevention of disease, health education and setting up hospital health benefit schemes.

Once again Australian health care is undergoing structural changes as a result of challenges from within and outside the scientific, or conventional, system. Technological and scientific advances have led to the reconstruction of hospital-based medicine which has been at the core of medical training. Specialisation has flourished, divided into areas primarily by age, for instance, adolescent medicine and geriatrics. Within the traditional specialist sphere new technology has brought further subdivision. For example, in recent decades various types of specialist and organ transplant surgeons have emerged. Ironically, even general practice has now become a speciality!

However, of particular importance has been the challenge from complementary or alternative medicine, brought about not only by consumer demand. Orthodox practitioners are either referring patients to alternative practitioners or using alternative therapy themselves, especially for chronic conditions not curable by scientific methods. The dramatic rise in alternative medicine is the result of better organised practitioners and the establishment of schools. The advertisements and medical and lay press reports in Figures 6.1 to 6.4 bear this out. The reasons for this rise will be examined and the history of these alternative methods investigated.

Alternative Health Services

See Also –

Acupuncture
Biorhythm Services
Chiropractors
Herbalists
Homoeopaths
Hypnotherapy
Masseurs &/or Masseuses
Naturopaths
Osteopaths
Relaxation Therapy
Yoga

[Address and telephone numbers for 34 practitioners or clinics listed under this heading]

Figure 6.2. Alternative Health Services advertisement in Brisbane Yellow Pages, 1990. Telecom Australia.

The 1960s witnessed an upsurge in the use of alternative, unconventional therapy in health care and treatment of disease. People, especially the young, were searching for new values, were concerned about the environment, were seeking pure and natural foods and occasionally new medical discoveries seemed to turn into life-threatening manipulation.[3] In 1977 Ivan Illich, a priest, published a controversial book entitled *Medical Nemesis* which criticised modern scientific medicine and stated that the medical establishment had become a major threat to health.[4] Illich identified iatrogenesis at three levels: clinical, social and structural or cultural. Clinical iatrogenesis comprised illnesses which would not have come about unless sound treatment had been applied. Social iatrogenesis related to the medicalisation of life. Structural iatrogenesis was the paralysis of health responses to suffering.[5]

Resorting to alternative medicine has increased in Australia as well as elsewhere in the world where official health care is based on scientific medicine. Government concern at this increase was voiced in August 1974 when the Commonwealth Minister of Health, Dr D.N. Everingham, set up a Committee of Inquiry into Chiropractic, Osteopathy and Naturopathy, with Homeopathy added later. Professor E.C. Webb was Chairman of the committee and the other three members were two eminent scientists and a medical practitioner with expertise in health administration. The committee, which was unanimous in its deliberations, issued its report, known as *The Webb Report,* in 1977.[6]

Assessing the use of alternative medicine, the Australian Health Survey 1977–8 found that over a four week period as many as 356,000 people visited an alternative medical therapist. This number corresponded closely with those who sought advice or help from a chemist, a community nurse or a dentist.[7] Unsubstantiated figures for 1983 provided by the Australian Natural Therapists' Association (ANTA) implied that in that year therapists gave over eight million consultations.[8] Detailed costs are not available but, using an average fee of $19 per consultation as a conservative estimate, it would appear that $150 million was spent by patients for consultations alone during that year. In addition there would have been a considerable, but unascertainable, sum spent on proprietary drugs, herbals and vitamins. When compared with the cost of the national health system which subsidises orthodox medicine, this shows a significant amount is spent on alternative methods.

In Australia in 1987–8, the Health Insurance Commission paid $3,096 million for medical benefits under the Medicare system introduced in February 1984 by the Commonwealth Government. For the same period the Pharmaceutical Benefits Scheme paid $1,047.6 million for drugs issued under the provisions of the *National Health Act*.[9]

The Victorian Government directed its Social Development Commission in 1984 to enquire into the safety of herbal medicines and megavitamin use. The commission also investigated the range of alternative therapies. This survey of users and providers of alternative

Medicare

therapy included the attitudes of general practitioners and provided hitherto unavailable information on alternative medicine in Australia. In summary, following interviews with 1202 adults, 22 percent admitted using alternative medicine in the previous five years, 12.5 percent had sought alternative advice for their children, 17 percent had visited an orthodox medical practitioner who used alternative medicine and, significantly, 83 percent believed that alternative practitioners should be allowed to practise alongside orthodox doctors and other health professionals. Following a study of general practitioners, over two thirds of the 179 surveyed considered the methods of manipulation, acupuncture and hypnotherapy were effective, 69 percent thought mineral/vitamin therapy ineffective, while 55 percent were dubious about homeopathy. It was also evident that doctors themselves were using alternative therapies and 67 percent had referred patients for acupuncture treatment. Only 15 percent had used chiropractors or osteopaths. The usual reasons for such referrals were either inadequate training in these areas or lack of improvement in the patient's condition.[10] Both the increased use of alternative treatment and a desire shown by medical practitioners for more information and training in alternative techniques have been reported in similar investigations carried out in the United Kingdom and in Holland.[11,12,13,14,15]

The resurgence of this competition for orthodox medicine, which is largely subsidised by the government and private health insurance, seems to indicate that there is 'something to offer' in compensation for the financial burdens adherents of alternative therapy have. The evolution of these alternatives, some of which have roots in antiquity, needs to be examined in perspective rather than simply dismissed as quackery. Their continued existence suggests that they have stood the test of time, in some cases for thousands of years, while the scientific medicine of the last two centuries is still in its infancy, relatively speaking.

A large variety of complementary medicine is available in Australia. To discuss all of them is beyond the scope of this review. Manipulative therapy (chiropractic and osteopathy), naturopathy, homeopathy and acupuncture are relatively well established in western cultures and form the major component of alternative medicine. These are the healing practices which will be discussed.

'YIN AND YANG WITH ACUPUNCTURE'
Australian Dr Weekly, 9 March 1990

'ACUPUNCTURE ACCEPTED'
Australian Dr Weekly, 6 April 1990

'CONGRESS ON OLD AND NEWMEDICINE'
Australian Dr Weekly, 6 April 1990 [World Congress, Perth, September 1990]

'CHIROPRACTORS GAIN WIDER SUPPORT'
Australian Dr Weekly, 13 April 1990

'EXAMINING THE MYSTERY OF HOMEOPATHY'
Australian Dr Weekly, 13 April 1990

'CHIROPRACTIC IS ON THE WAY UP'
Australian Dr Weekly, 27 April 1990

Figure 6.3. Medical press headlines for articles on complementary medicine.

Terminology and Principles of Scientific and Complementary Medicine

The terms *scientific, conventional* and *orthodox medicine* are used for an aggregate of diagnostic and therapeutic concepts and practices which attempt to adhere to modern scientific principles. Where they are not adhered to an alternative system may be said to be in use. It is impossible to define with exactness the whole range of therapies which fit into this category. Nevertheless, it seems reasonable to group them together under the term *complementary medicine.* This is preferable to *alternative medicine* as the therapies never entirely replace conventional medicine, while the terms *fringe, unorthodox* or *unconventional* may appear hostile.

Complementary medicine attempts to recruit the self-healing capacity of the body and uses all the symptoms as guides to the source of the patient's upset or imbalance. Symptoms are assessed against the individual's personality and the individual as well as the symptoms are treated. Health is broadly defined as going beyond a state of complete physical and mental well-being, with poor vitality and low resistance being regarded as states of health. Complementary medicine improves health and well-being by using preventive methods. It is most at home treating psychogenic and chronic diseases where resistance and the health of the patient are important in recovery. The goal is self-healing and, if practised competently, should be harmless and non-toxic. Diagnosis is not invasive and essentially consists of sensitive observation of areas and functions of the body and the patient's feelings, habits and life style. Faculties beyond normal explanation also play a part in diagnosis and are today regarded as some kind of physical phenomenon below the threshold of normal perception and beyond that of current scientific explanation.

Holistic Medicine

Although orthodox medicine has always claimed to treat the whole individual, holistic medicine is a movement within the medical profession which is evolving in response to the need to find new ways of dealing with stress-related and degenerative health problems. It is also a reaction against increasing specialisation. In practice, holistic medicine uses conventional and complementary treatments simultaneously and is concerned with the long-term development of each patient rather than his or her short-term response to each incidence of disease. Recognising the possible emotional roots of a disease, it also brings the family into the process of healing.

Complementary Medicine and its Place in the History of Medicine

In pre-history primitive society's medical practices were based on magico-religious concepts and work on the principle that both illness and its relief derived from a deity, evil spirits or another person. The medicine man or physician-priest possessed superior knowledge with far reaching powers in many areas, including medicine, although this was restricted to internal diseases which he treated with secret formulae and rites. Ordinary therapists existed such as bone-setters, healers of wounds and herbalists; they dealt with conditions which had an obvious cause but they were never free from the supernatural.[16]

It is recorded that, although the Babylonians (*c.* 2000–3000 BC) and the Egyptians (*c.* 1000 BC) practised magico-religious medicine, they were also practitioners who employed surgical techniques and used herbs and their hands for therapy.

With the advent of Greek civilisation (*c.* 600–500 BC) man's view of his place in the world (cosmology) changed. The Greeks asked what, not who, was the cause of phenomena and events. The Hippocratic school of medicine, the forerunner of western medicine, based its enquiries on reason rather than religion, and attributed disease to natural phenomena. Health was highly valued. The ill, unless restored, were misfits in society. Hippocratic therapy included surgical procedures as well as aligning fractures and skeletal derangements.

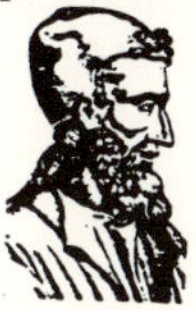

The Graeco-Roman physician Galen (130–200 AD) achieved medical fame by synthesising all existing medical knowledge and establishing a medical tradition that was to last for the next one thousand years. Galen retained the Hippocratic belief in humoral pathology, that health was achieved by restoring equilibrium to the fluid essences (humours) of the body. He maintained good health, always precarious, was susceptible to the constant changes of six 'non-neutrals': the air; food and drink; motion and rest; sleep and waking, inanition and repletion. Treatment was usually by diet and drugs, usually a polypharmacy of plant and animal tissues (Galenicals).

When the Roman Empire declined, the centre of culture moved to Byzantium. Greek medicine continued to be practised but magico-religious elements reappeared and alternative medicine flourished. In Europe priests assumed responsibility for caring for the sick until about the year 1200 when the Italian School of Medicine was established at Salerno and medicine moved from the control of the clergy to the laity.

Eventually, during the Renaissance, scientific enquiry spread to the study of anatomy which led in turn to surgical advances, while improved technology and clinical observation at this time allowed greater understanding of disease. Although physicians acquired a greater status, the barber-surgeon practised as a craftsman and the tradesman apothecary compounded drugs, while quacks practised without restriction. Manipulation and surgery of the vertebrae was denounced, yet Ambrose Paré (*c*.1517–1590), the great French surgeon of the Renaissance known as the father of modern surgery, advocated using other types of healing including massage and alignment of the spinal vertebrae.[17]

During the next four hundred years scientific enquiry continued apace and the boundaries of medical knowledge of disease and its treatment were constantly widening. By the end of the nineteenth century these advances had laid down the theory of scientific medicine as practised today. Medical education improved and registration established the profession by distinguishing between trained and untrained practitioners.

It is evident from this brief summary that complementary methods which have the same roots as scientific medicine, have been placed outside current legitimised medicine. Interesting paradoxes have occurred. The herbalist has been ousted by the pharmaceutical chemist who has refined herbal cures and isolated new drugs. Many of the traditional treatments of non-technological cultures have been incorporated into modern medicine. At the same time scientific medicine has moved away from the personal contact of the manipulative and hands on therapies of earlier times.

BRITISH MEDICAL JOURNAL VOLUME 287 30 JULY 1983 337

YOUNG DOCTORS' VIEWS ON ALTERNATIVE MEDICINE

DAVID TAYLOR REILLY

"... what is taken for today's unorthodoxy is probably going to be tomorrow's convention."

PRINCE CHARLES, PRESIDENT OF THE BMA.

Figure 6.4. Headline from the British Medical Journal, 30 July 1983

MANIPULATIVE THERAPY

Historical development

For a scientific appraisal of manipulative therapy it is appropriate to consider osteopathy and chiropractic together as they have common roots which can be traced back to the bone-setters of the eighteenth and, particularly, the nineteenth centuries. These bone-setters used empirical methods and developed great skills and reputations as healers when their results contrasted, often more than favourably, with those of orthodox medicine based on scientific theory. For joint displacements their methods were gentler and surer than the barbaric contraptions used in treatment by orthodox surgeons of the time. For example, in 1869 Dr Theodor Billroth, an orthodox practitioner, recommended the use of multiplying pulleys for treating dislocations (*Figure 6.5*).

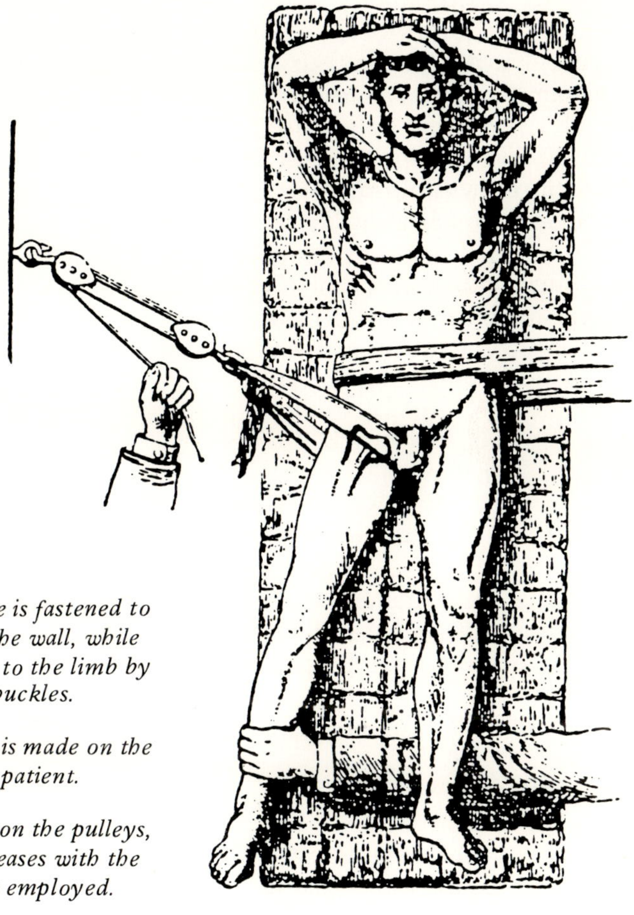

One end of the rope is fastened to a strong hook on the wall, while the other is applied to the limb by straps and buckles.

Counter-extension is made on the body of the patient.

An assistant draws on the pulleys, whose power increases with the number of pulleys employed.

Figure 6.5.

Nineteenth century apparatus for treating hip dislocation.

Although some nineteenth century orthodox medical practitioners used joint and spinal manipulation, it was the osteopaths and chiropractors who developed manipulative therapy further.

Osteopathy

The osteopathic school of therapy was founded by a self-educated American, Andrew Taylor Still (1829–1917). His concept, which was the fruit of divine revelation, was that correction of alignment of the spine would relieve obstruction to spinal arteries and nerves and allow essential substances to restore health. Spinal manipulation was his panacea for all illness. His system was in direct competition with orthodox medicine. Since Still's first School of Osteopathy was founded in 1892 at Kirksville, Missouri, many schools have flourished in North America. Although his basic tenet, the need for spinal adjustment for health, has remained, the osteopathic concept has been broadened to the need for total adjustment of health to be carried out at three levels: structural (osteopathic manipulation), biochemical (by natural or pharmaceutical means) and psychological techniques.[19]

Osteopathy in Australia

In 1977 the Webb Committee of Inquiry into Alternative Medicine found the osteopathic situation confused.[20] Osteopaths were small in number and mostly self-taught, although a few medical practitioners had trained at the London College of Osteopathy and used manipulation as a therapeutic supplement. The majority of manipulators, who used osteopathic techniques and often preceded therapy with local massage and palpation for diagnosis, called themselves chiropractors and were mainly trained in Australia.

Chiropractic

The system of chiropractic was founded by Daniel David Palmer, a Canadian grocer and fish pedlar, who emigrated to the United States when he was twenty years old. After excursions into osteopathy, phrenology and spiritualism, he embarked on a quest for the cause of human disease. This was allegedly found by him in 1895 when he cured two patients, one with deafness and the other with heart disease, by replacing vertebrae manually. His principle was that subluxation of the vertebrae or incomplete dislocation caused 95 percent of all diseases.[21] He maintained they elongate the pathway of the nerve, modify impulses and cause functions to be performed abnormally. It followed that treatment of all diseases could be effected exclusively by manipulation of the vertebrae to re-align joints.

Palmer founded the Palmer School of Chiropractic in 1895 which was successively run by his son and eventually his grandson who changed its name to Palmer College. This success spawned other colleges and converts to the system. One of these was an Oklahoma lawyer, William Carver, who established a chiropractic school in Oklahoma City. However, he taught that chiropractic should employ other forms of treatment and this caused a schism, resulting in two schools of chiropractic thought. Those who follow Palmer call themselves 'straights'. Carver's adherents are referred to as 'mixers' because they apply other types of treatment such as massage, heat, herbs or tablets in addition to chiropractic adjustment. This approach has brought chiropractic much closer to the naturopathic tradition.

Chiropractic in Australia

It is difficult to give an accurate statistical account of chiropractic practice because the area is bedevilled by the fact that many healers perform manipulation and some call themselves chiropractor along with other titles. In 1977 the Webb Report listed 866 members of associations which admitted chiropractors and, although allowance was made for overlapping membership, non-association chiropractors were not taken into account.[22] Following the recommendations of the Webb Report, all Australian states had set up registration boards by late 1979 to oversee the practice and educational standards of osteopaths and chiropractors. This had the effect of raising the status and rewards for these practitioners as well as eliminating the unqualified and incompetent.

NATUROPATHY

Naturopathy is in essence the oldest alternative system, going back to pre-history. It espouses the belief of Hippocrates of *vis mediatrix naturae*, that is that nature has a reactive and curative power. It is therefore a system of treating ailments which recognises that healing depends upon the vital and curative force within the human organism. Its preventive approach is that the body can be maintained and strengthened by using natural foods, herbs and mineral supplements, water both internally and externally, exercise, sunlight, fresh air, purging and freedom from worry. The curative approach accepts disease as an entity to be treated by herbs and minerals.

Two major stimuli have renewed interest in naturopathy, the heroic nature of eighteenth and nineteenth century orthodox medicine and, since the 1950s, the unwanted side effects of new pharmaceutical drugs.

Naturopathy in Australia

A characteristic of Australian naturopathy is its wide and varying range of aids to diagnosis and treatment. Therapy includes dietary advice, manipulation, remedies of a herbal, mineral or homeopathic nature, zone therapy, acupuncture and colonic irrigation.

HOMEOPATHY

Homeopathy was founded in 1811 by a German medical practitioner, Samuel Hahnemann (1755–1843). Its origins lay in the doctrines of the seventeenth century physician, Paracelsus, whose 'doctrine of signatures' held that diseases or sympoms are curable by those particular drugs which produce similar effects on the body. Hahnemann's own aphorism was *similia similibus curantur* (like is cured by like). In contrast, conventional medicine generally prescribes allopathically, *contraria contrariis*, which means that treatment is based on principles other than symptom similarity. In allopathic medicine this principle of opposing disease or palliate symptoms has changed as it has evolved. For example, in the eighteenth and nineteenth centuries leeching attempted to remove congestion, cooling was used to treat fevers and sedatives were given in excited states. Now, following acceptance of Pasteur's Germ Theory, antiseptics and antibiotics are used to treat infection.[23]

In homeopathy the desired effect of drugs is heightened by giving them in infinitesimally small doses (potentisation) by dilution of soluble drugs or by trituration, the grinding up of insoluble drugs with an inert substance. Also, chronic diseases are regarded as a manifestation of suppressed itch or *psora*. Hahnemann made two major contributions to modern medicine. He modified the practice of using massive doses of drugs to the limit of their toxicity and he strongly advocated using a single drug rather than complex mixtures (polypharmacy).

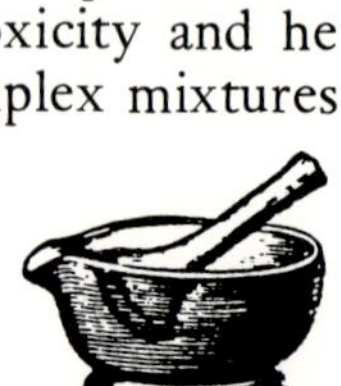

Homeopathy in Australia

Following the empirical success of homeopathic physicians at the time of a cholera epidemic in the 1830s and royal patronage at that time, homeopathy established itself in Great Britain. A small number of British homeopaths came and practised in Australia in the mid 1860s. Their remedies did not inspire the same distaste as did those of orthodox medicine and the herbalist. As a result its popularity rose, posing a threat to orthodox medicine in the latter part of the century. Modern pharmaceuticals in the early twentieth century and a series of *Poisons Acts* limited to registered medical practitioners the use of preparations employed by homeopaths and others. Nevertheless, homeopathy has continued to be practised, even by a few orthodox practitioners. The principles continue to be 'like cures like', the high potency of the microdose and a programme of individualised treatment. Although the Webb Committee found that homeopathy could not be supported by any scientific evidence, it continues to be popular and enjoys royal patronage with members of the British Royal Family using and promoting homeopathic methods.

ACUPUNCTURE

Acupuncture is part of traditional Chinese medicine which also uses herbs, diet and exercise in the treatment of disease. Its theory dates back to between 770 and 476 BC and the ancient text,

> *Nei Ching* (the Yellow Emperor's classic of internal medicine).

Acupuncture's popularity has waxed and waned over the centuries. However, in China today it is used alongside western medicine according to the doctor's judgement of which is more suitable for the individual patient.

Acupuncture is a term coined by French Jesuit missionaries working in China in the seventeenth century and is derived from *acus*, a needle puncture, and means to pierce. Acupuncture cannot be easily assessed in western terms because of the different philosophy of Chinese medicine. Life is activated by *chi* or the vital life force (energy) which pervades all things. As long as *chi* flows freely throughout the body, health is maintained. The principal premise is that health is achieved by balancing the opposing forces of *yin* and *yang* (*Figure 6.6*). When either predominates, health disorders result. Chinese medical

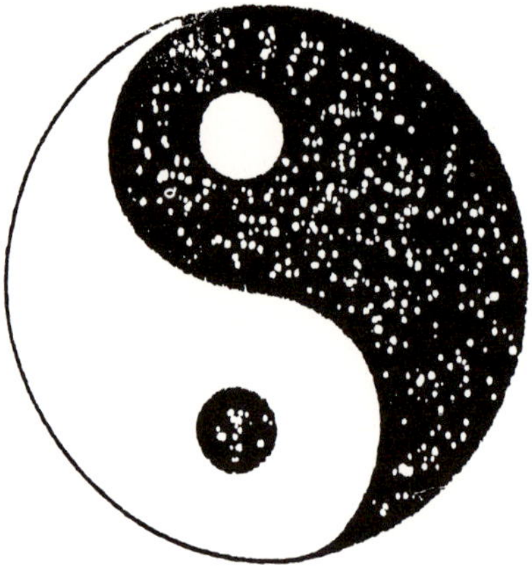

Figure 6.6

The Tai Chi t'u', the Chinese symbol representing the balance of Yin and Yang.

philosophy also regards man as a whole being of an indivisible combination of mind, body and spirit where it is impossible to treat one aspect without affecting the others. The patient's *chi* is manipulated at certain points along a series of body networks or meridians. These meridians connect with inner organs by channels through which energy can pass and achieve balance.

Acupuncture plays an important part in therapy. Once diagnosis has been made, treatment aims to stimulate or gather energy by inserting needles along predetermined meridians. Some conditions require the use of *moxa* which involves burning a cone of herbs, traditionally dried mugwort leaves, over the acupuncture point before inserting the needle. This moxibustion tones and supplements the energy. The acupuncture needles are made of stainless steel varying in length from 12 cm to 37 cm and usually penetrate only a few millimetres beneath the skin.

針灸

Acupuncture in Australia

Many Chinese who came to Australia during the gold rushes of the mid 1850s used acupuncture but it roused little interest in Europeans until the late 1960s, after the Cultural Revolution in China. At that time foreigners visiting China observed the apparent success of acupuncture used in the treatment of many conditions, including major surgery on conscious patients.

After a fact finding visit to China by senior medical experts under the auspices of the National Health and Medical Research Council (NHMRC) in 1973 and the report issued the following year, qualified support was given for clinical trials of acupuncture used for certain conditions including pain alleviation, dental and obstetrical analgesia, sciatica, joint pain, deafness and drugs including alcohol withdrawal.[24] The report recommended the use of acupuncture be restricted initially to registered medical and dental practitioners although, if trials were successful, acupuncture might be undertaken by nursing and paramedical personnel under medical supervision.

Enthusiasm for and interest in acupuncture (and traditional Chinese medicine) has grown since the 1960s. An Acupuncture College was founded in 1969, an Acupuncture Association in 1972 and in 1973 the Australian Acupuncture Society was formed for medical practitioners as well as an Acupuncture Ethics and Standards Organisation (AESO). In 1978 private insurance funds gave rebates for services from accredited members of the AESO and, from the late 1980s, Medicare rebates were introduced for acupuncture therapy provided by registered medical practitioners.

RELATIONSHIP BETWEEN OSTEOPATHY, CHIROPRACTIC AND ORTHODOX MEDICINE

Competition is strong in the area of manipulation.[25] For osteopathy and chiropractic it is the exclusive therapy. Orthodox medicine and physiotherapy, which follows the medical model, use manipulation along with other forms of therapy, but it tends to be palliative rather than curative and is limited by a number of contra-indications to its use. The differences are based on theory rather than the technique itself. Both use X-rays as a major diagnostic tool but, in examining them the chiropractor may see subluxations whereas the orthopaedic surgeon does not. Physiotherapists emphasise mobilisation, which is the gentle coercing of a movement by limited passive oscillations performed within or at the limits of muscle range. While some physiotherapists use manipulation, they also use hot and cold towels, rubbing and warming instruments, vibrators and pulsating devices.

The main area of contention has been medico-political. It was felt that chiropractic theory did not stand up to scientific clinical scrutiny and research, whilst physiotherapy, which had been outside the conventional medical framework, had been incorporated into the orthodox system by the 1960s. Following the Webb Report in 1977, which rejected chiropractic and osteopathy as an alternative health system but saw them instead as specialists in spinal manipulation,[26] chiropractic was legitimised.

ASSESSMENT OF COMPLEMENTARY MEDICINE

In assessing complementary medicine the greatest concern is over the use of methods which have not been proved to bring reliable improvement in the patient's condition, using criteria normally adopted for scientific clinical trials. Many therapies in complementary medicine have not been proved to be totally safe from toxic or long-term side effects, for instance, the use of herbals.[27] Physical methods using massage may cause damage to bruised or previously injured tissues. Another danger is the use of complementary methods by people who lack medical qualifications or adequate training where incorrect diagnosis may endanger life. In spite of the need for minimum standards for complementary therapy, progress in registering practitioners has been slow in Australia. It is feared that legalising some therapies may have the unwanted effect of implying acceptance of all of them.

Attempts at research into complementary medicine have been thwarted by government and commerce refusing to invest money. Nevertheless, following a challenge by Prince Charles, when he was President of the British Medical Association in 1983, to re-examine the basic assumptions of scientific medicine and be more open-minded about alternatives, some research has been undertaken. A research council for complementary medicine has been established in the United Kingdom to study suitable research methods.[28]

Complementary medicine itself is beset with difficulties caused by its theory, the importance of the individual practitioner in the therapeutic results and the singularity of each patient and his problems. It seems unlikely, therefore, that any serious appraisal will be forthcoming for a long time. The case may just rest with –

Let the best man win!

as suggested in 1981 by the Editor of *Lancet.*[29]

CONCLUSION

An attempt has been made to place complementary medicine in a contemporary context. The popular and medical press bear witness to an undoubted increase in its use. The difficulty in assessing it, the fears of orthodox medicine about its safety, especially in the hands of unscrupulous healers, and the possible harmful interaction between homeopathic, naturopathic and pharmaceutical drugs, all provide grounds for concern. Nevertheless, complementary medicine should be considered as a new frontier which has to be challenged, in some cases to be tamed and accepted. In others, rejection may be the order of the day.

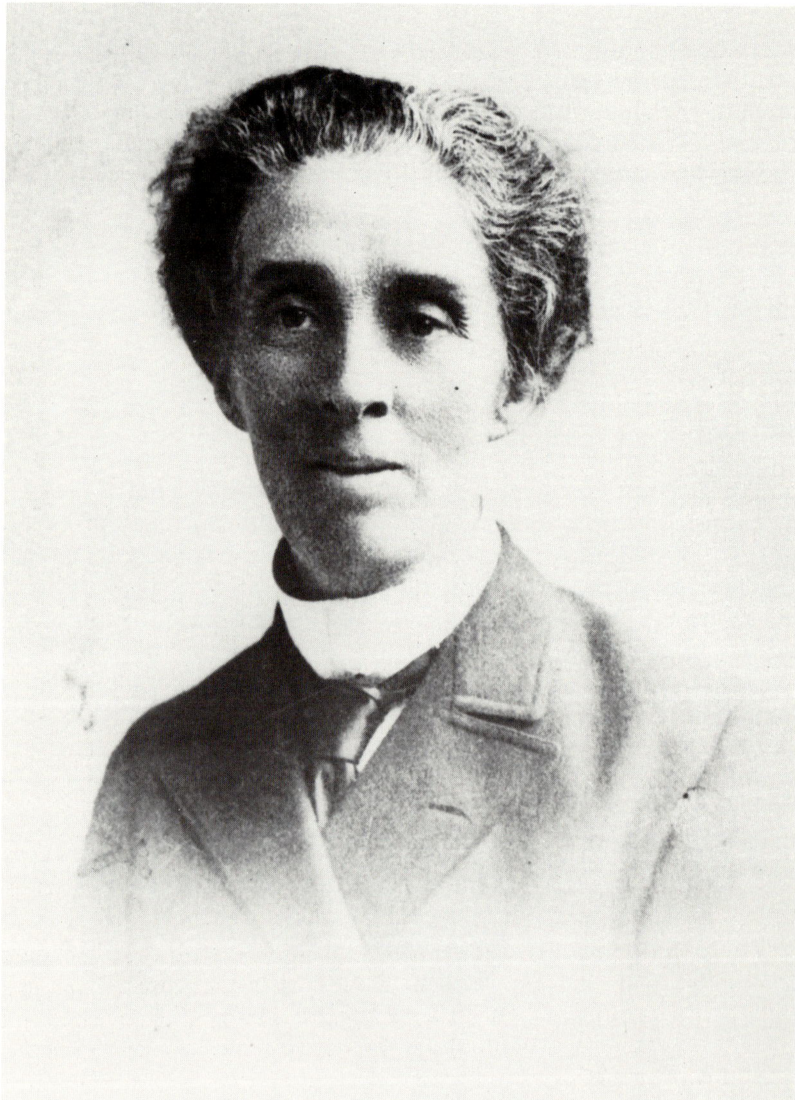

Figure 7.1. Dr Lilian Violet Cooper, LRCP&S (Edin.), LFPS (Glasg.) 1890, the first medical woman to practise in Queensland. Photo by permission of the John Oxley Library, Brisbane)

FEVERS AND FRONTIERS 7

FEMININE FRONTIERS

Queensland's Early Medical Women

Lesley Williams

On 7th February 1990, Australia Post issued a stamp to commemorate one hundred years of medical women in Australia. Constance Stone, having been refused entry to the medical course at Melbourne University left Australia in 1884 to study at the Women's Medical College of Philadelphia.[1] She obtained a Doctorate in Medicine in 1885 and then proceeded to Trinity College, University of Toronto – where she successfully gained the degree of MD ChM in 1888. Finally in order to make her case for applying for registration in Australia as watertight as possible she went to London where the following year she obtained the Licentiate of the Society of Apothecaries, the first London instituion to open its doors to women.

For a short time Dr Stone worked in London with Dr Elizabeth Garrett Anderson before returning to Australia where she was registered in Melbourne on 7th February 1890. She opened her own general practice which she ran with great success until her untimely death in 1903.

Queensland's First Medical Woman

Just one year after Constance Stone began her Australian medical career, there arrived in Brisbane, Dr Lilian Violet Cooper who had graduated LRCP & S (Edinburgh) and LFPS (Glasgow), 1890. (*Figure 7.1*) She trained at the London School of Medicine for Women and the Royal Free Hospital and had sailed from London on 10th April 1891 on RMS *Lusitania,*[2] arriving in Sydney on 25th May. The Sydney-Brisbane journey was made on the AUSN ship *Aramac* which berthed in Brisbane on 29th May.[3] As Lilian Cooper had a contract to work with Dr Booth in Cordelia Street, South Brisbane, she lost no time in finding a cottage in Russell Street and in applying for registration and this was granted on 4th June 1891 – Medical Practitioner No. 489.

Her arrival in Brisbane apparently made no impact with the local press; the passenger list did not mark her out as anyone different from the other young women on board. She travelled as 'Miss Cooper'.

Thus began practice in Brisbane, Queensland's first female medical practitioner.

The assistantship was far from satisfactory through no fault of hers, and after six months she was able to cancel her contract with Dr Booth.

On 24th, 26th, 29th and 31st December 1891, there appeared in the *Courier Mail* under 'Professional Notices' the following paragraph (*Figure 7.2*) –

Professional Notices

DR. LILIAN COOPER, L.R.C.P. and L.R.C.S., Edin., L.F.P. and S., Glasg., having resigned her assistantship to Dr Booth, has COMMENCED PRACTICE in Brisbane. Consulting Rooms, 5 George-street Mansions. Hours, 11 to 3 p.m. Private Residence, Russell-street, S.B.Hours, 8.30 to 10 a.m. and 6 to 8p.m. Dr Cooper has made a special study of the Diseases of Women and Children.

Figure 7.2. The Courier Mail 24th December 1891.

In the beginning few patients crossed her threshold; the public, many women included, were not sure they liked the idea of a lady doctor. Her male colleagues certainly did not want her; it is said they refused to give anaesthetics for her operations; they refused to see patients referred by her; there was no social or professional contact. However, they did not count on her indomitable spirit, her resilience, her determination, her dignity and professionalism. She was tall and rather daunting in appearance, but children, in particular, saw beyond the forbidding brusqueness, and found a kind, sympathetic gentleness and it is not surprising that in 1896 she became Honorary Medical Officer of the Hospital for Sick Children.

Gradually her practice built up. She applied in 1891 for membership of the Queensland Medical Society and it took two years before this was granted. In 1897, she moved her rooms to 106 George Street next to the Government Printing Office and her practice was flourishing. Many Brisbane women consulted her and brought their children to her for treatment and she was meticulous in her attention to their problems. When the Lady Lamington Hospital opened in 1900, she was appointed Honorary Medical Officer there as well. Thus began her care of the women and children of Queensland that lasted until her death. In 1906, she became Honorary Surgeon at the Mater Misericordiae Hospital when it was established at North Quay – an association with the Mater that lasted until her retirement. She also served on the first Mater Public Hospital Board.[4]

In 1911–1912 Dr Cooper visited the Mayo Clinic and the Johns Hopkins Hospital in the United States, and in Durham, England, she was successful in obtaining an M.D.

She served with distinction during World War I, with the Scottish Women's Hospitals in the front line in Serbia. Her companion Mary Josephine Bedford who had accompanied her from England and was heavily involved in charity work in Brisbane, was in charge of the Ambulance Unit. They were awarded the 4th and 5th Order of St. Sava respectively by the King of Serbia.

When the Royal Australasian College of Surgeons was founded in 1928, Dr Lilian Cooper became a Foundation Fellow.

All Queensland women, not only medical women, owe Dr Lilian Violet Cooper a deep debt of gratitude. She was the first. On her shoulders was laid a huge responsibility. Her dedication to the task of caring for the sick and needy, her expertise as a physician and as a surgeon were subjected to very close scrutiny by some of her male colleagues and members of the public. She was not found wanting. (It is said she met some of their patronising comments with a suitable flow of language.) Had she failed, the cause of the Australian-born girls who in the 1890s were still fighting for equality of opportunity in the medical world would have been impeded.

In 1926, the two friends had moved into a beautiful home, *Old St Mary's* in Main Street, Kangaroo Point. It had been built about 1860 by the first Rector of the first Anglican Church[5] in the area, Rev. J. Robert Moffatt.

After the death of Lilian Cooper on 18th August 1947, Miss Bedford approached the Sisters of Charity and offered the home as a hospice for the incurable and terminally ill. This was Lilian Cooper's expressed wish and today Mt Olivet Hospital which rose from the site of *Old St Mary's*, perpetuates the memory of her life and work. Mt Olivet is her lasting memorial and the Lilian Cooper Nursing Home perpetuates her name.

The First Queensland-born Medical Woman

While Lilian Cooper was fighting her battles, a young Ipswich girl, Eleanor Constance Greenham, (*Figure 7.3*) daughter of John and Eleanor Greenham of Limestone Street, was attending the Brisbane Girls' Grammar School and when the Ipswich Girls' Grammar School opened its doors on 1st February 1892,[6] she was the first girl enrolled by Headmistress, Fanny Hunt (the first woman to graduate B.Sc. from Sydney University). In her Senior year Eleanor Greenham won the Botany medal and prizes for History, Geography, Latin, Euclid and Science. The following year, she remained at school doing advanced work prior to enrolling in the Faculty of Arts at Sydney University in 1895. She transferred to Medicine and graduated MB ChM in 1901, thus becoming the first Queensland-born woman to graduate in Medicine.

UNIVERSITY OF SYDNEY

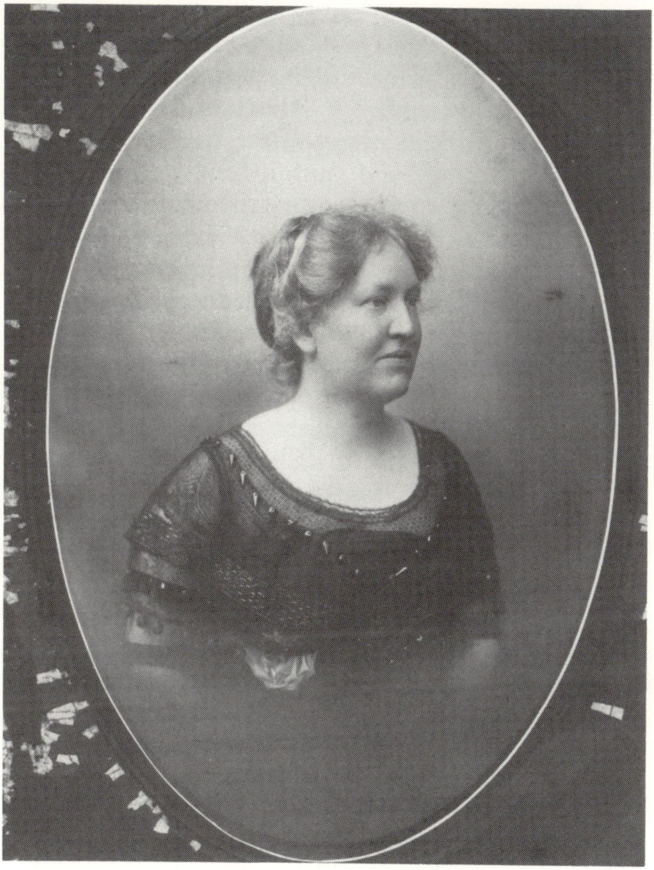

Figure 7.3. Dr Eleanor Constance Greenham (1874–1957), the first Queensland-born medical woman. Photo, courtesy of Mr Keith Greenham.

Dr Greenham was registered – No. 711 on 2nd May 1901 and immediately received an appointment as resident medical officer at the Lady Bowen Hospital on Wickham Terrace, Brisbane. She was thus the first female to receive a resident hospital position. From the beginning, she received great encouragement from Lilian Cooper and they became firm friends.

Dr Greenham was intent on general practice and in 1903 she took rooms in City Chambers at the corner of Edward and Queen Streets, Brisbane, where Wallace Bishop's shop trades today. For a time, she too found business very slow but she had a bright sunny personality and her optimism was firm. Gradually she built up a successful practice among the business women of Brisbane. Her records show that her patients came from all over North Brisbane as well as from the city itself.

Late in 1907 she moved to Association Chambers, 284 Edward Street, next door to the site where the foundation stone of the new YMCA building had recently been laid. She occupied the first floor with her surgery, waiting room and office in the front of the building and her private living quarters across the passage at the rear. The household chores were taken care of by a faithful housekeeper, Miss Drysdale and when she retired, by Miss Murphy. Dr Greenham was one of the first women to own a car; in 1907, she drove a Darracq and after a few years changed to a Hupmobile with a self-starter. Indeed, she became a major shareholder in Evers Motors of Petrie Bight, the Hupmobile agents.[7]

A few years prior to her death in 1957, Eleanor Greenham moved to Merthyr Road, New Farm. Her nephew, Keith Greenham, remembers her well —

> ... *a large lady fond of flowing floral garments.*

He lunched with her every Thursday when attending the University of Queensland, then at George Street. He said she always claimed she was a pioneer, never a traditionalist. She was an excellent pianist and played for relaxation. She never married, but took great interest in her nephews and nieces and became Director of Greenhams Ltd of Ipswich, owners of much of the central business district in that city. She was generous in her support of the family and paid the university fees of at least one of her nephews.

Eleanor Constance Greenham was well-loved and respected by her many patients and friends. Her great-niece Dr Wendy Greenham, Casualty Registrar at Toowoomba General Hospital, is carrying on the tradition of the first Queensland-born medical woman.

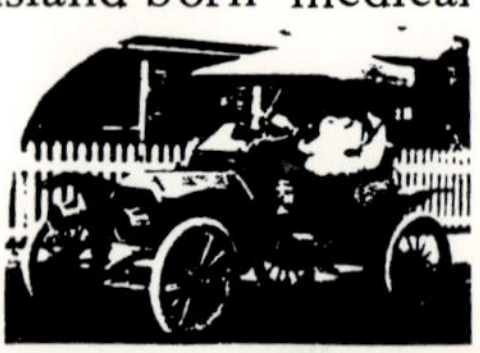

Queensland's First Medical Sisters

A short time after Dr Lilian Cooper opened her own practice in the *Mansions,* in December 1891, there arrived in Brisbane on *The Scottish Lassie*[8] Dr John Ure, a widower, with his young family of three daughters and four sons. From Dr Herbert Churchill he bought an elegant two-storied colonial house named *Blackall* (*Figure 7.4*) at 63–65 George Street, Brisbane, next to the Shakespeare Hotel (later the Hotel Cecil) and diagonally opposite the *Mansions,* in the Margaret Street–Mary Street block. George Street in those days had many similar homes. About the end of 1906, Lilian Cooper and Miss Bedford bought *Auckland House* just two doors from the Ures and on the corner of George and Mary Streets.

Lilian Cooper and the Ures were good friends, and doubtless, she took an interest in and encouraged the girls, all of whom attended

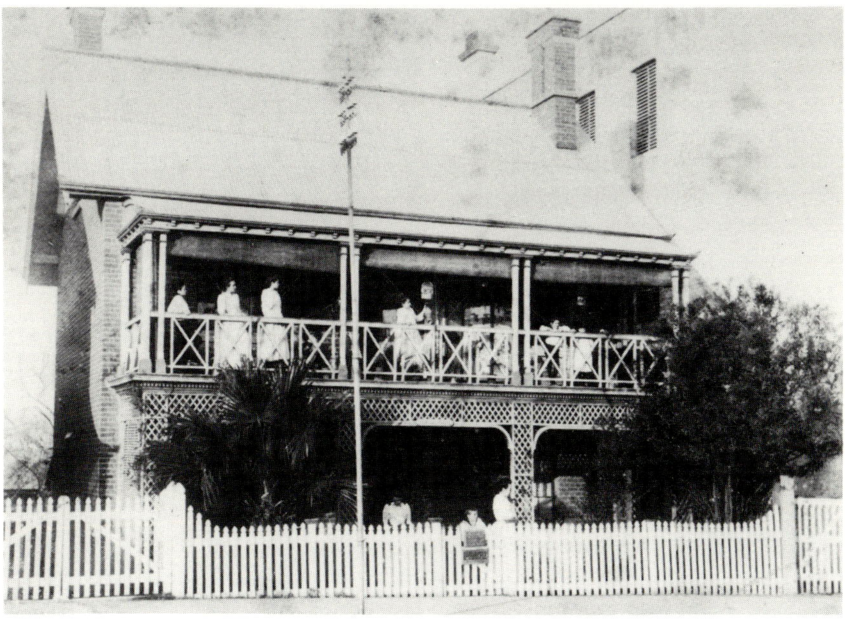

Figure 7.4. ***Blackall House, at 63-65 George Street, Brisbane, home of Dr Edith and Dr Lulu Ure. Photograph, courtesy of Dr Noel Ure.***

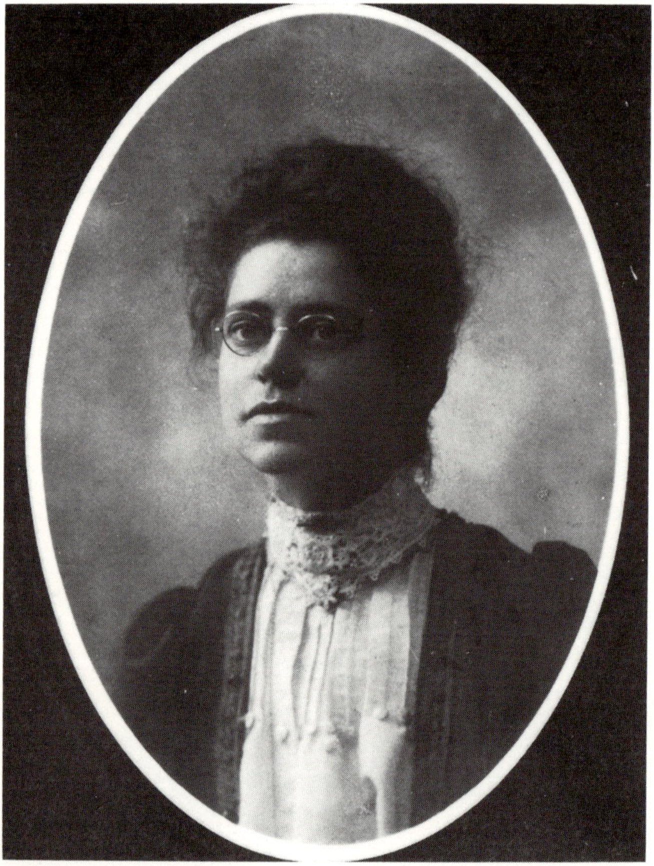

Figure 7.5. DR EDITH URE
Photograph, courtesy of Dr Noel Ure

the Brisbane Girls' Grammar School. Edith, the eldest of the family, (*Figure 7.5*) having passed the Senior Examination, enrolled at Sydney University in Medicine and graduated in 1902. On her return to Brisbane, she was registered on 3rd April 1902 and immediately joined her father in his medical practice. He described himself as —

... medical practitioner and accoucheur.

Sarah Louisa, known as 'Lulu' (*Figure 7.6*) followed Edith to the Women's College and the Medical Faculty of Sydney University. In 1904, John Ure died and Edith carried on the practice alone. Over a period the Sydney women medical students suffered a number of failures (including Alice Pritchard, already an Arts graduate, who failed her 4th year four times, but later practised in Queensland). Lulu failed her finals but was successful the following year and became Queensland's 811th medical practitioner on 2nd February, 1905.

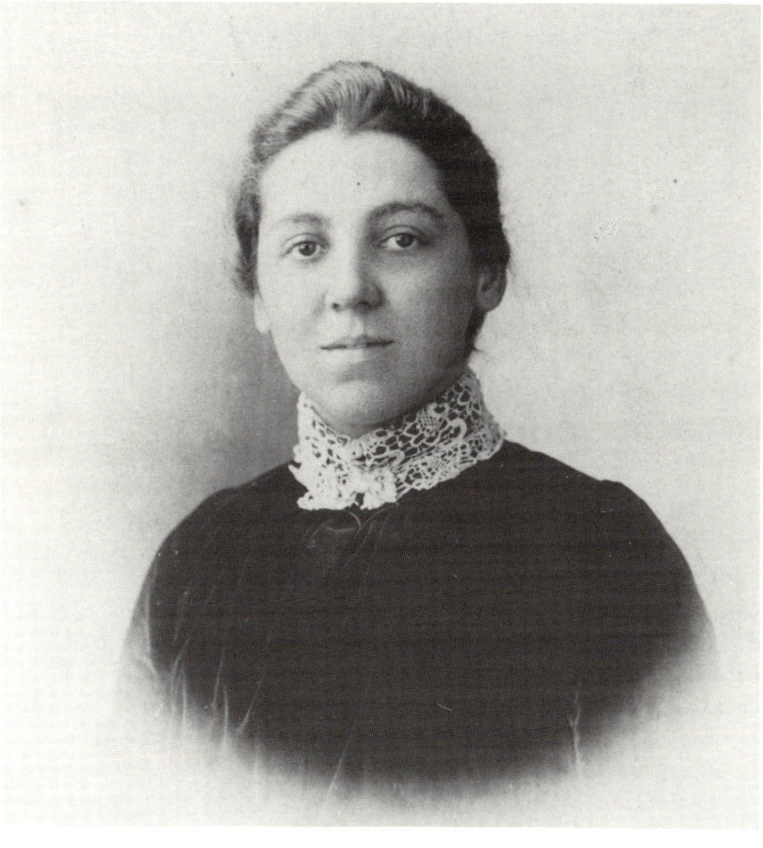

Figure 7.6. DR SARAH LOUISA LOCHHEAD (née URE)
Photograph, by permission of the John Oxley Library, Brisbane.

Prior to Lulu Ure's graduation, the small community of women doctors in Queensland had risen to five with the arrival of Dr Lucy Gullett from Sydney in July 1902 and Dr Effie Stilwell from Melbourne just one month later. They were the first of the influx of medical women from the South, who, finding it very difficult to obtain hospital positions in their own States, came to Queensland for the necessary training.

Dr Gullett and Ella Greenham had been fellow-students at Sydney University and it is certain they kept in close contact over the years. Lucy Gullett was appointed RMO at the Hospital for Sick Children and Effie Stilwell took Ella Greenham's place at the Lady Bowen Hospital. Both of these women, however, had only a short sojourn in Queensland. Lucy Gullett moved to private practice at Bathurst and later at Pymble. She is remembered as one of the founders of the Rachel Forster Hospital for Women in Sydney. Effie Stilwell went to India as a medical missionary.

When Dr Lulu Ure returned to Brisbane she was appointed Resident Medical Officer at the Brisbane General Hospital and in 1908 she accepted a position at the Lady Bowen Hospital. After a year, she shared the practice with her sister Edith until her marriage and migration to New Zealand. Edith retained the practice until 1915, when, tragically, she developed peritonitis and died on 10th May. Dr Noel Ure who is living in retirement at Bribie Island, is a nephew of Sarah and Edith.

The Builder of a Tuberculosis Sanatorium

When Dr Effie Stilwell resigned as Resident Medical Officer of the Lady Bowen Hospital in August 1903, her place was taken by Dr Helen Shaw (*Figure 7.7*) who had graduated MB BS, Melbourne, in 1901. She was warmly welcomed and encouraged by Dr Lilian Cooper and after her twelve months' residency, she took rooms in the same building as Lilian Cooper at 106 George Street next to the Government Printing Office.

In 1905, Dr Shaw decided to move to Stanthorpe, a town noted for its —

> ***... salubrious climate, its fruit production, its tin sluicing operation and its wealth of minerals.***[9]

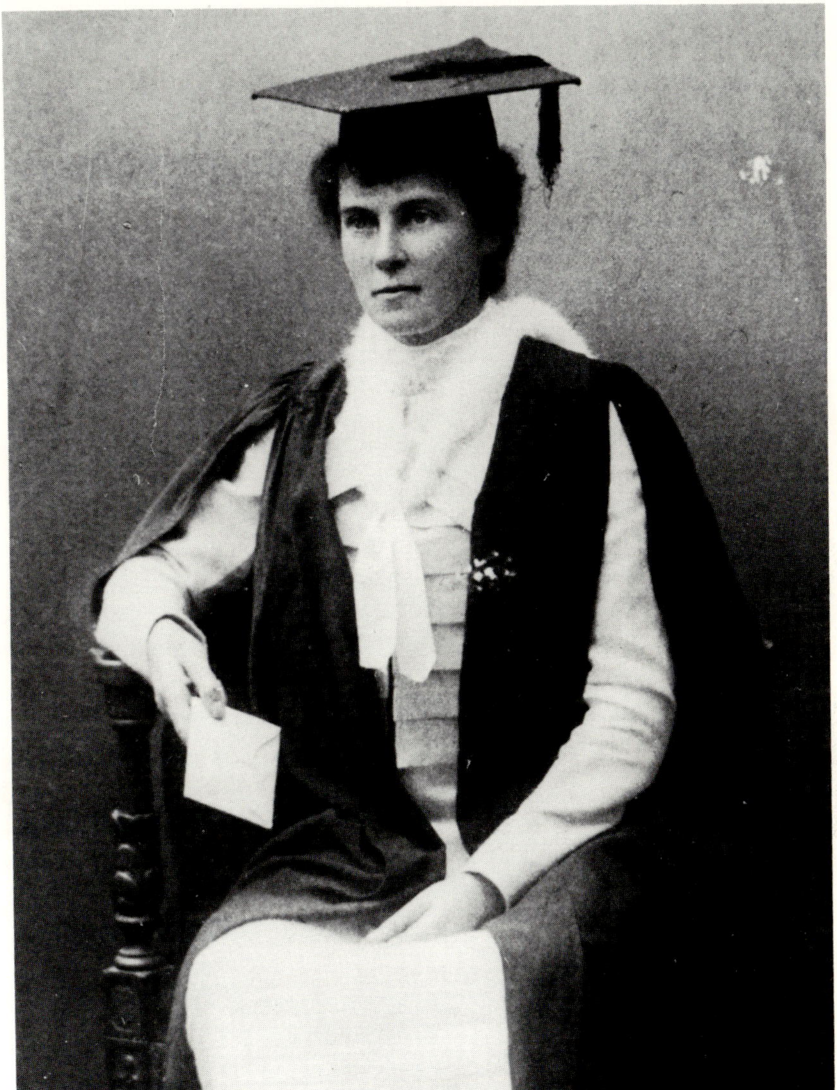

Figure 7.7. DR HELEN SHAW
Photograph reproduced by permission of the John Oxley Library, Brisbane.

The Stanthorpe Border Post of 9th June 1906 reported that at the meeting of the Hospital Board Mr C.P. Sheahan suggested that half the hospital beds should be placed at the disposal of Dr Helen Shaw and that 'the Hospital Board salary at present paid to Dr Orton be shared between them'. This recommendation must really have set the cat among the pigeons and it is not known how cordial was the relationship between Dr Shaw and Dr Orton.

In 1904, tuberculosis was declared a notifiable disease in Queensland, mainly due to the efforts of Dr Jefferis Turner, visiting medical officer to the Diamantina Hospital for Chronic Diseases. For many years southern Queensland had been regarded as the ideal climate for TB sufferers and a State Sanatorium had been opened in 1900 close to Dalby. Mrs Allison, a resident of Sugarloaf near Stanthorpe, financed the building of a Sanatorium at The Three Mile on the Stanthorpe–Sugarloaf road.[10] (*Figure 7.8*) Later the district was known as Kyoomba. *The Stanthorpe Border Post* of 2nd February 1907 reported that Dr Helen Shaw was medical officer in charge. After nine years there, she moved to a private practice at Sherwood Road, Toowong before going to England in 1920. The Commonwealth Government took over the Sanatorium and greatly enlarged it to cater for servicemen who had returned from World War I with tuberculosis.

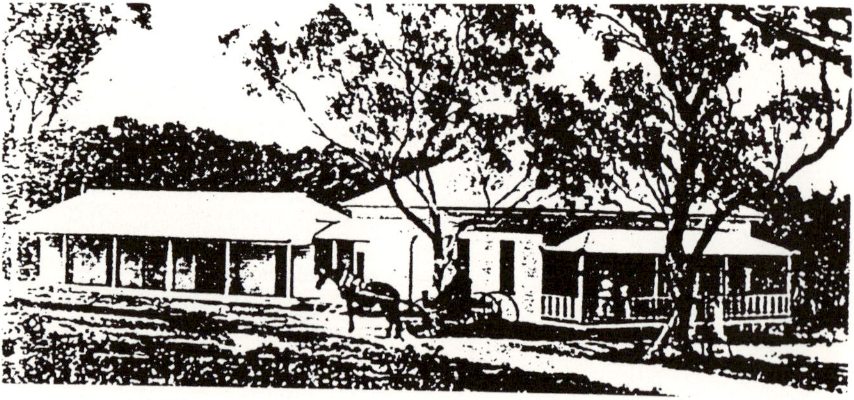

Figure 7.8: Dr Helen Shaw's sanatorium at 'The Three Mile' on the Stanthorpe–Sugarloaf Road.
Photo, courtesy of Stanthorpe and District Historical Society.

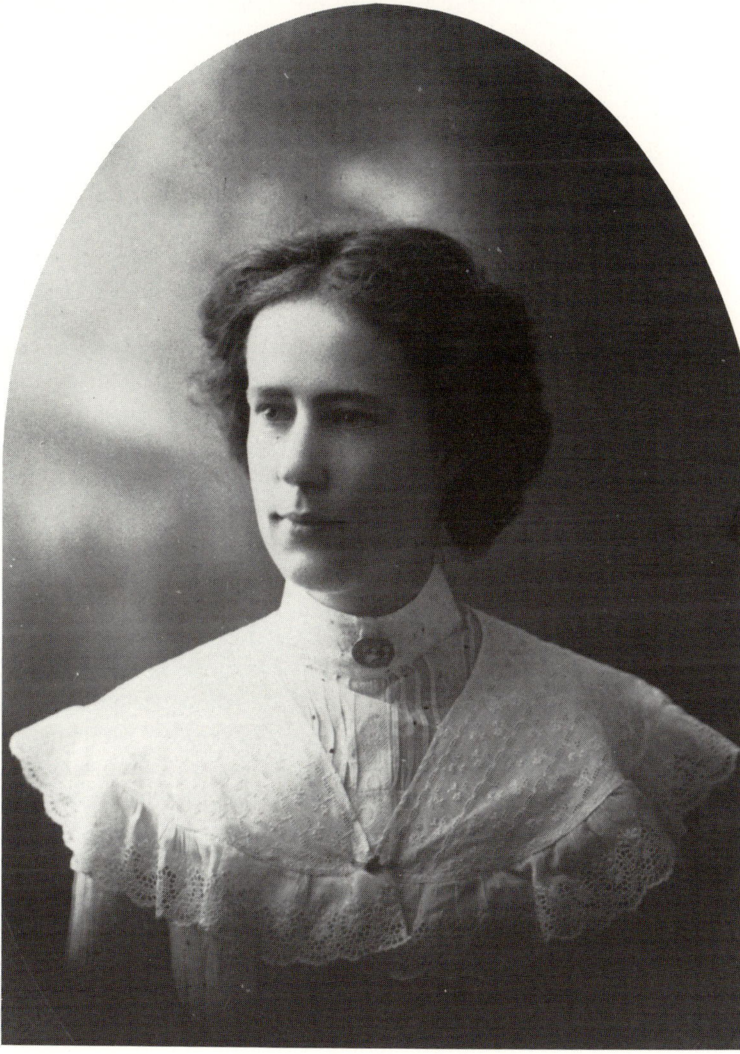

Figure 7.9. DR ELEANOR ELIZABETH BOURNE
Photograph reproduced by permission of the John Oxley Library, Brisbane.

The First Medical Inspector of Schools in Queensland

Just two months after Dr Helen Shaw was registered as Queensland's 766th medical practitioner on 6th August 1903, Dr Eleanor Elizabeth Bourne (*Figure 7.9*) began her professional career in her hometown of Brisbane.

She was born at South Brisbane, the eldest child of John Sumner Pears Bourne and Jane Elizabeth (*née* Hockings). She had a privileged childhood; her father was a clerk in the Lands Office and later became Commissioner; her mother had received a good education for girls of her day at Mrs Unsworth's school, Harris Terrace,[11] George Street, opposite *Blackall*, which was to become the Ure family home. One uncle was Director of Posts and Telegraphs, one the Registrar of Titles and another the Receiver of the Treasury. Her grandfather, Albert John Hockings was Mayor of Brisbane and he also represented South Brisbane in Parliament and was associated with Sir Charles Lilley in drafting the first *Education Act* for Queensland.

Eleanor was educated at the Central School and won a three year Scholarship to the Brisbane Girls' Grammar School. In the 1890s, the general financial depression caused the School to sacrifice some of the advanced subjects due to the shortage of teachers. By arrangement with Mr Roe, Headmaster of the Brisbane Grammar School, girls wishing to learn Latin for the Senior Public Examination of Sydney University were allowed to attend classes with the boys.

At this time the only Scholarships available in Queensland for tertiary education were three Exhibitions of £100 per year for three years, awarded annually. Mrs Bourne was anxious that her elder daughter should have a University education and approached the Chief Justice, Sir Samuel Griffith, who was also Chairman of Trustees of the Grammar Schools to ascertain whether girls were eligible to compete, as previously no girl had thought to apply. Sir Samuel decided that in the text of Conditions for Applicants for Exhibitions, the word 'he' would embrace 'she'.[12] Thus Mrs Bourne had opened up the opportunity for all girls to compete for university scholarships.

Advanced Mathematics was another subject not offered at BGGS and Mr Roe allowed Eleanor to do all her 6th Form subjects with the boys. Not only did she become the first girl to win an Exhibition (1896) but she was also awarded the Botany medal, the Grahame and the John West medals and the Women's

College Bursary. Having graduated MB BS at Sydney University, she returned to Brisbane and was registered on 1st October 1903. She obtained an appointment as Resident Medical Officer at the Brisbane General Hospital – the first woman to be appointed to the medical staff of that hospital. In 1905 she transferred to the Hospital for Sick Children to broaden her experience. Lilian Cooper had paved the way very well for the early medical women in Queensland. They were appointed on their merits as resident medical officers and they measured up.

Eleanor Bourne spent the next few years in private practice at 69 Wickham Terrace, during which time she held honorary posts as Outpatients' Physician at the Children's Hospital, Anaesthetist at the Lady Lamington Hospital and Physician to the Creche and Kindergarten Association.

Dr J.S.C. Elkington, Commissioner of Public Health, had come to Queensland from Tasmania where he had filled the same position and where he was instrumental in setting up the first school health services in Australia. It was obvious to Dr Elkington, following the report of ophthalmologist Dr William Taylor, that children particularly in the west of the State were not performing to their optimum because of various physical conditions, including trachoma, that were treatable and preventable. Dr Eleanor Bourne took up duty on 1st January 1911 as the first Medical Inspector of Schools in Queensland, (*Figure 7.10*) with a salary of £400 per annum. In her first six months on the job she established the procedure for medical inspection of school children and personally examined 3068 pupils,[13] mostly in the Brisbane area. She found that 31% suffered some physical defect that would interfere with their work. She also worked out the procedure for notification of parents and follow-up inspection.

Dr Bourne was assisted in this work by a nurse, Miss Ina Neilson who was appointed on 6th March 1911 at a salary of £104 per annum plus £10 for uniforms. The routine included measurements of height and weight, examinations of general physique, heart, lungs, glands, teeth, throat, spine and limbs. Vision was tested by optotype designed by Dr Gertrude Halley and Dr Hogg of Tasmania, which allowed children as young as 4 years of age to participate

Among the children examined, 61 were found to have heart defects, many of which were unknown to the parents. They had

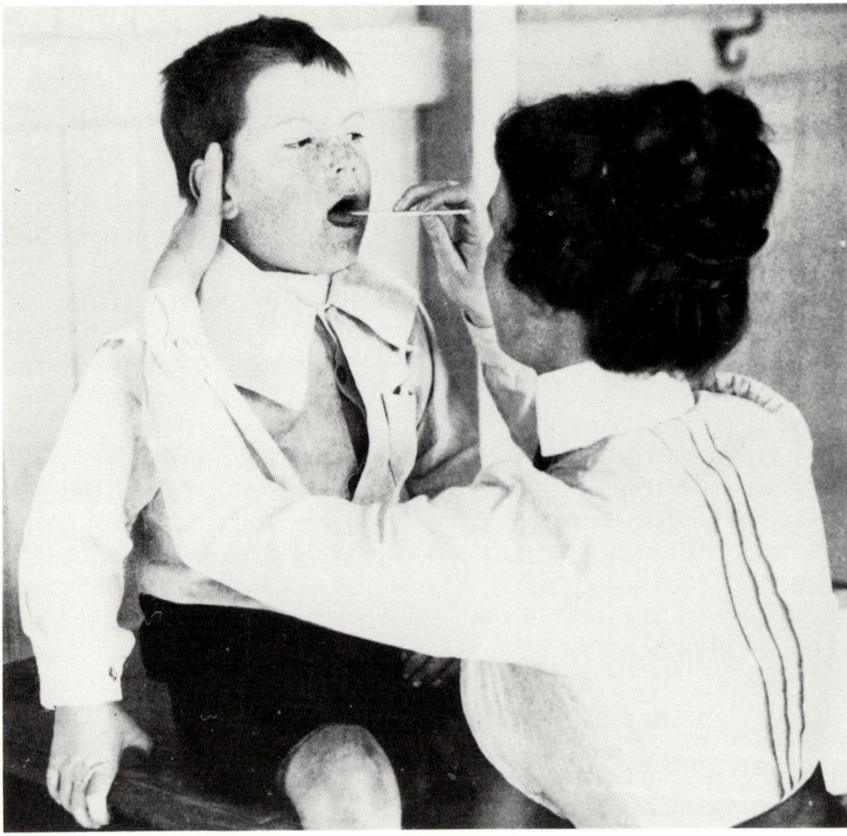

***Figure 7.10.* Dr Bourne in her role as Medical Inspector of Schools for the Education Department of Queensland. Photograph reproduced by permission of the John Oxley Library, Brisbane.**

thought the children simply had 'growing pains'. Three hundred and eighty-one children had defective vision and Dr Bourne considered that 534 were probably anaemic because of their pallor (in summer) and general languor, and 843 had some physical defect. In an effort to identify carriers of scarlet fever, she also scrutinised 2000 other children in five schools where outbreaks had occurred and she excluded 68 who had peeling skin and also their home contacts.

At each school she visited, Dr Bourne lectured to parent groups and had also given a course of lectures on school and personal hygiene to teachers at the Central Technical College and to Teachers' Associations at Ipswich and Toowoomba. She displayed a remarkable energy and an immense capacity for hard work; there was no let-up in the programme she set for herself and her nurse assistant, Miss Neilson. From July to December 1911,[14] she turned her attention to Western Queensland but maintained a watchful eye on schools with diphtheria cases.

The two women went first to Charleville and on to Cunnamulla[15] where they hired a car to go to Thargomindah. They took a Cobb & Co. coach to continue the journey to Augathella but one of the horses broke down and they walked the last two miles before night-fall. They bedded down on a mattress under the stars and continued on early next morning. Their equipment was transported in a large box and when the driver carried it into the schoolroom and dumped it on the table, he announced 'The Doctor's instruments'. A yell arose from the 73 children and it took time to calm them down. The next stop was Eulo, then Blackall, Longreach and Barcaldine.

Dr Bourne examined 1532 children and checked the eyes of 1616. As well as 38 heart defects and 22 cases of deafness, she found 301 children had conjunctival problems. The other cause for concern was the number of children with nits – 56.24% of girls and 6.86% of boys. She drew up a pamphlet detailing treatment, to send home to the parents.

In that year she read two papers, one to the Queensland Branch of the British Medical Association and one to the Public Health Section of the Australasian Medical Congress in Sydney. Her report recommended the appointment of part-time Medical Inspectors, one for Townsville and one for Rockhampton and also the appointment of an ophthalmologist (Dr Douglas Rodger) to tackle the trachoma problem.

In 1912 Dr Bourne concentrated on the schools in the Coastal area of Queensland and investigated the incidence of ankylostomiasis. She and Nurse Neilson travelled 5217 miles and interrupted their itinerary to attend to a large diphtheria outbreak in the Mackay district.[16] Here alone, she examined 2570 children and visited 44 schools.

A conference of medical inspectors was planned for January 1914 in New Zealand and Dr Bourne applied for leave to attend. She was advised that if she took it as recreation leave, the Minister would approve return railway and steamer fares from Australia to New Zealand, but no other expenses. She went!

In October 1913, Dr Elizabeth Sweet, a recent Melbourne graduate joined the staff of the Department and she too carried out a very busy programme of inspection, but with the outbreak of World War I, the work of the School Health Services was curtailed with the enlistment of Dr Rodger and in March 1916, Dr Bourne sailed for London to join the staff of the 500 bed Military Hospital in Endell Street, staffed entirely by women. Dr Flora Murray and Dr Louisa Garrett Anderson were in charge and they were supported by women specialists in all branches. They coped with convoys of wounded soldiers evacuated from the Front. After the Armistice, Eleanor Bourne was appointed Medical Controller in the Northern Command and later in Eastern Command and arranged medical and sanitary supervision of camps and billets of detachments of Queen Mary's Army Auxiliary Corps.[17]

After the War she qualified for the Diploma of Public Health of the Royal College of Physicians London and the Royal College of Surgeons England in 1920, and at this stage decided to remain in England to gain experience in Public Health. She received an appointment as Medical Officer for Maternity and Child Welfare in the city of Carlisle and once again her immense capacity for work was demonstrated. She was in charge of a new maternity hospital servicing a large district; she conducted two antenatal and three infant welfare clinics per week; she supervised the work of midwives and health visitors; she carried out medical inspection of schools, as well as many other duties.

In 1928 Dr Bourne applied for the position of Commonwealth Director of Maternal Hygiene and Children's Welfare in Australia. She was offered the position but refused it when she found that the starting salary offered, was less than that stated in the advertisements! She returned to Brisbane in 1937, having resigned due to ill-health and she lived in retirement at Manly. Shortly before her death on 23rd May 1957, she completed 50 years' membership of the Queensland Branch of the British Medical Association.

Mrs Jane Elizabeth Bourne, mother of Dr Eleanor Bourne, was foundation President of the Standing Committee of Women's College in the University of Queensland and continued in the position until 1922. Eleanor and her sister Florence Ida (Headmistress of Maryborough Girls' Grammar School for 16 years) also supported the Women's College[18] with generous gifts and endowed a room in memory of their mother who contributed so much to the success of their careers.

Eleanor Elizabeth Bourne set a high standard of dedication to her work, far beyond the expectation of the position.[19]

The Southern Influx

While Dr Lulu Ure and Dr Eleanor Bourne were working as resident medical officers in Brisbane hospitals, Sydney women were finding great difficulty in obtaining appointments to the large teaching hospitals.[20] Dr Constance D'Arcy had graduated 6th on the list in 1904 but was refused a position by both the Sydney and Royal Prince Alfred Hospitals, a man of lower grading being appointed. She went to the Adelaide Hospital.

In 1905 Dr Susie O'Reilly passed her finals 4th on the list. She applied to North Shore, Royal Prince Alfred and Sydney Hospitals. In the case of the latter, six positions were available and normally a graduate 4th on the list was assured of a position. The Board decided there was no accommodation for a resident lady doctor and she was passed over, and she too went to Adelaide for her postgraduate hospital appointment. (It is interesting to note that forty years later, 'lack of accommodation' was still the reason given for passing over, for resident positions at the great teaching hospitals in Sydney, five women who had graduated with Honours.)[21]

The following year, Dr Jessie Aspinall applied to the Royal Prince Alfred and began work as a junior resident before ratification by the Conjoint Board (consisting of the Sydney University representatives and the Hospital Board). The Conjoint Board refused to ratify the Hospital Board's decision and Dr Aspinall was dismissed for no other reason than that she was a woman. A furore erupted involving the press, the public and women's groups. Brisbane hospitals were asked for an opinion and the medical superintendent of the Brisbane General Hospital, Dr J.B. McLean, said that during the last couple of years Dr Bourne and Dr Ure had been employed as residents and both women had performed their duties most capably. Dr John Thomson, President of the Medical Board in Queensland said that wherever medical women were practising medicine in Queensland, they were giving the utmost satisfaction.

In the years between 1906 and 1910, a number of women newly graduated from Melbourne and Sydney as well as some who had graduated in Britain, came to Queensland to take hospital appointments. The positions in Brisbane were limited but many country towns had no doctor. In 1907 Mabel Crutchfield was appointed to Boulia[22] hospital, Mary Edelsten to Jundah; Alice Pritchard to St George, Adela Williams[23] to Muttaburra. A Queenslander, Constance Binney was at Longreach, Alice Kirke[24] was practising at Queenton, Charters Towers and Robina Harlin[25] assisted her husband Dr F.W. Harlin at Peak Downs Hospital, Clermont. (*Figure 7.11*)

In the following year, Dr Williams moved to Kingaroy, Mary de Garis took her place at Muttaburra and Laura Weir began a long association with Springsure.

By the year 1911, twenty years after Lilian Cooper arrived in Brisbane, there were twenty-one medical women practising medicine in Queensland, nine in Brisbane and twelve in centres as far removed as Urandangie, Kingsborough and Boulia.

Table showing the total number of Medical Women practising in Queensland in the Fifty Years 1891 – 1941

Year	*In Brisbane*	*Outside Brisbane*	*Total No.*
1891	1	0	1
1901	2	0	2
1911	9	12	21
1921	5	13	18
1931	17	12	29
1941	19	20	39

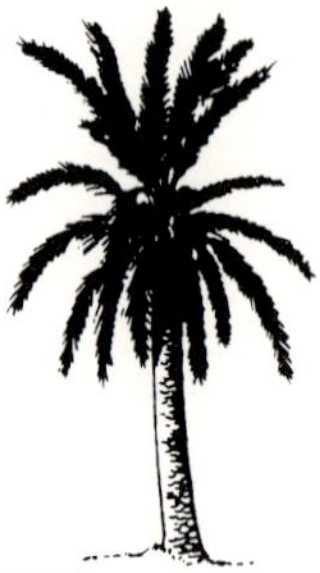

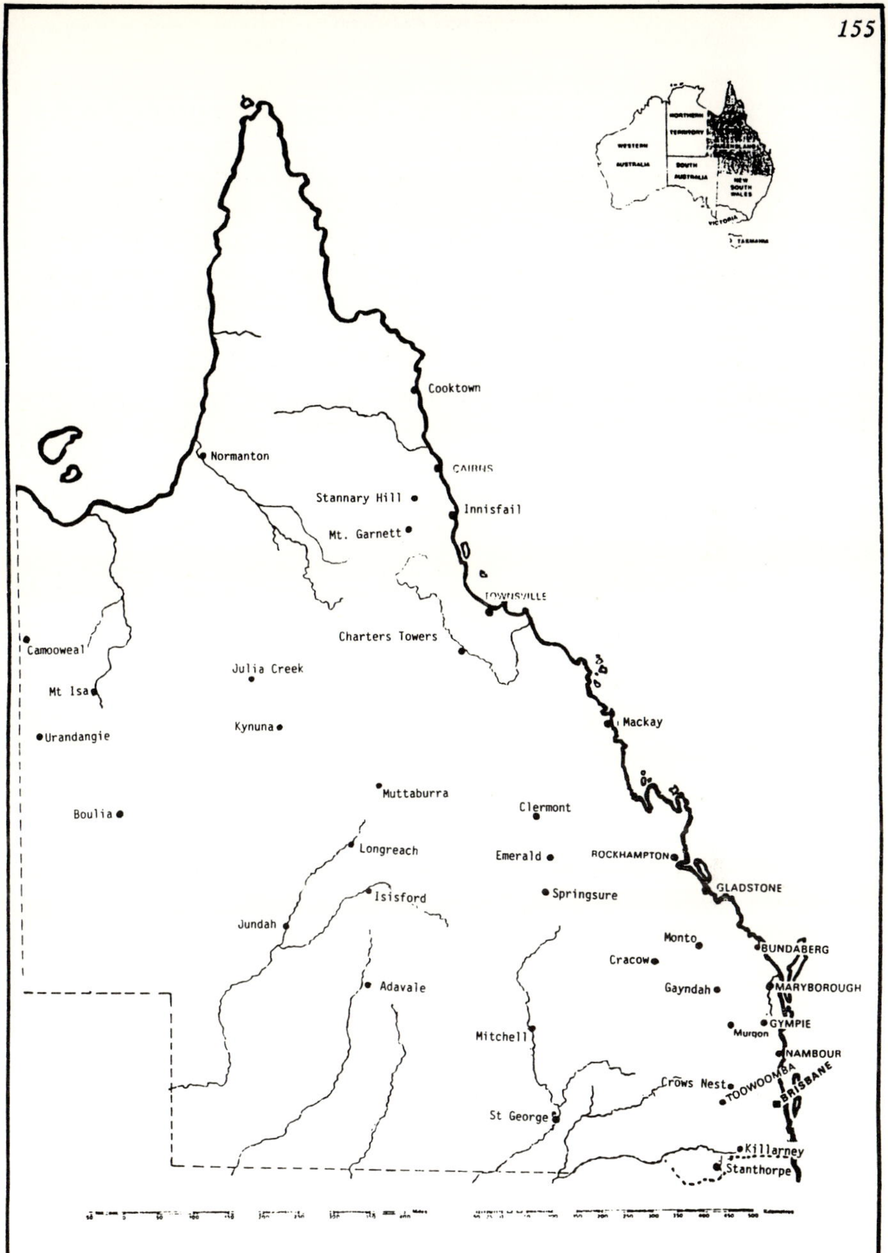

Figure 7.11. Map of Queensland showing centres where the early medical women practised their art.

An Early Queensland Medical Mother

Alice Lavarack,[26] (*Figure 7.12*) born at Wellington Road, Kangaroo Point on 5th February 1883 attended the Brisbane Girls' Grammar School and won a Queen's Scholarship to Melbourne University. She graduated in 1908 and after working for eleven months at Melbourne Hospital, she took up the vacancy at Muttaburra. She was petite and pretty and accustomed to country life as her father, Cecil Wallace Lavarack, owned a property, *Consentes,* near Julia Creek. When called to patients, she rode side-saddle and took a .45 Colt revolver with her but it is doubtful if she ever had to use it.[27]

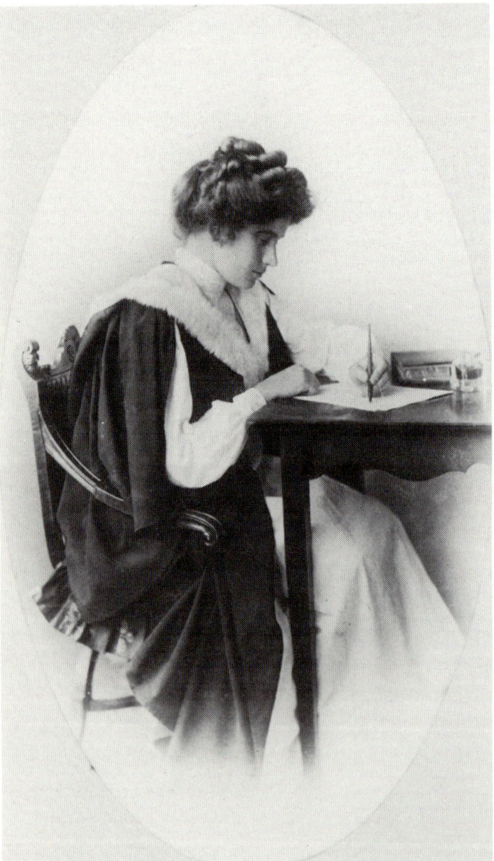

Figure 7.12. Dr Alice Jones (née Lavarack) Photograph courtesy of Mrs J.H. McCrea.

Muttaburra, in those days was a frontier town and Alice kept a stockwhip at the hospital and threatened to use it on some of the difficult inebriated out-patients! At Muttaburra, she met Frank Jones, manager of *Lerida.* They married and bought *Cabanda,* 45 miles from Julia Creek. Alice cared for the health of everyone for miles around, even as far as Dalgonally and she also raised a family of five children during their ten years at *Cabanda.* (*Fig. 7.13*)

In 1923, they moved to *The Summit*, Stanthorpe, where Frank Jones was occupied in the fruit industry. Not long after the birth of their seventh child, Frank Jones died and Alice

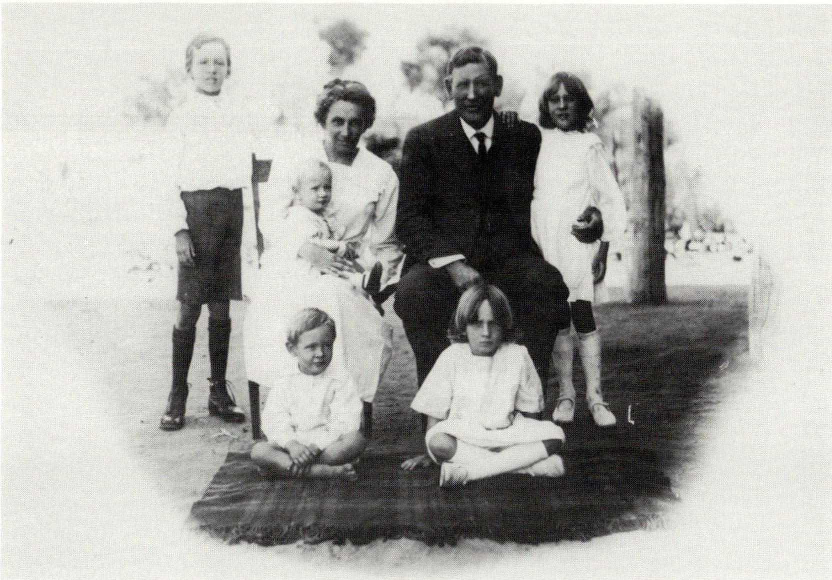

Figure 7.13. Medical mother, Dr Alice Jones with her husband Frank and five of their seven children, at Cabanda, Julia Creek, c. 1922. Photograph courtesy of Mrs J.H. McCrea.

was left to raise her young family single-handed. She resumed active practice and with the beginning of World War II, she moved to Brisbane where she did a refresher course. She received an appointment to the Mater Children's Hospital and she also did many *locums* around Brisbane.

Later Dr Jones took a position at Cracow where she lived in a large house next to the hospital and each week, she took a cab to Theodore for an afternoon surgery. After a few years, she moved to Texas and it was there she suffered a stroke. She recovered under her daughter's care at Wellington Point and then resumed work again, taking hospital rounds for Dr Trevor Allen. She died on 30th June, 1955.

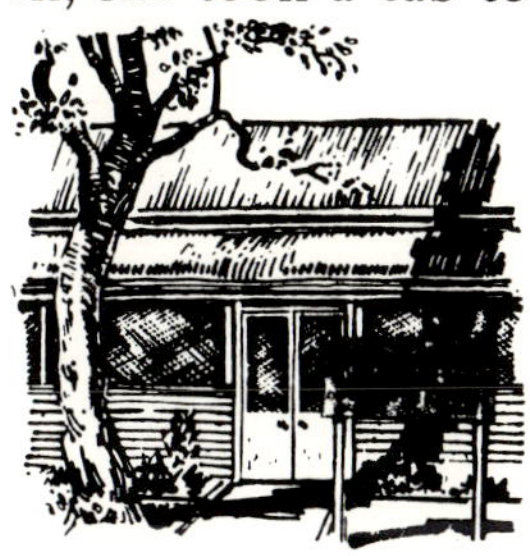

Alice Jones was one of Queensland's earliest medical mothers.

There remains much more to tell of the lives and work of Queensland's early medical women. They were a privileged group in that they came from well-to-do homes with fathers in secure positions often in the Public Service, the Military, in Medicine or in private business. The parents were well educated and were desirous that their daughters also should be educated to their potential. Money was, of course, necessary because, in the case of girls from Queensland where there was no Medical School until 1936, they had to board in Sydney or Melbourne and despite scholarships, this was an expensive exercise.

Although these girls did not have the bitter struggles encountered by Elizabeth Garrett and Sophia Jex-Blake in Britain, they nevertheless met with many difficulties and open opposition from male colleagues and sometimes even the public. For ten years Lilian Cooper stood alone but firm, walked tall and secure in the confidence of her knowledge and expertise. She paved the way well and those who followed her received encouragement and friendship.

Today it is possible for women of ability and limited means and the same dogged determination displayed by Lilian Cooper, Eleanor Greenham and Eleanor Bourne to qualify as medical practitioners. In 1990, there are 557 women undergraduates in the Faculty of Medicine in Queensland out of a total of 1,315 students (42%). They have earned their entrance and attend their classes as is their right. They are accepted by their male *confrères* with never a thought that to share the dissection of a cadaver was once considered indelicate for women. May they spare a thought that this total acceptance was won by the strength of character, the quality of work and the dedication of the early medical women of Queensland.

Acknowledgements

Thanks are due to Lady White for information on her aunt, Dr Lilian Cooper; to Mr K. Greenham, Mrs L. Greenham and Mr R. Greenham for recollections and photographs of their aunt, Dr Eleanor Greenham; to Ms J. Hill, Principal of the Ipswich Girls' Grammar School for access to the School Archives and for early photographs; to Mrs J.H. McCrea for photographs, records and recollections of her mother Dr Alice Jones; to Mrs J. Harslett, Secretary of the Stanthorpe and District Historical Society for information on Dr Helen Shaw and Dr Robina Harlin and to Mrs Riha and Miss D. Byrne of the Oxley Library for their assistance and interest.

FEVERS AND FRONTIERS 8

Yet a Frontier

Contraception in Colonial and Post-Federation Australia

Pamela Chick

Women and men have always wanted to control their fertility. This has been true for thousands of years across diverse cultures, and has been equally true for Australia from colonial times until the present day. But progress has not come easily. The barriers of controversy and moral outrage have had to be overcome, and safe effective contraception developed. Slowly the frontier has been pushed forward but advances have been difficult to achieve. There is still much to do.

Birth Control in the Colonies

From the time of its original colonization, Australia was geographically isolated from the rest of the world. From 1788 it has never been isolated from outside ideas and philosophies; these were eventually brought to the colonies by travellers and immigrants.

The birth control movement was given impetus by Thomas Malthus (1766–1834) with his theories on population –

> *I say that the power of population is infinitely greater than the power in the earth to produce subsistence for man.*

This idea was embraced as one providing a more socially acceptable *raison d'etre* for fertility control than one which merely afforded comfort to the individual who might not want more children. Malthus himself did not favour birth control; he proposed that the control of fertility should be by moral restraint, which entailed delayed marriage and strict pre-marital chastity.[1]

However, more realistic social reformers believed that Malthus' suggestions would not be very popular and felt that birth control would be a far better solution. In 1833, Dr Charles Knowlton's pamphlet, *Fruits of Philosophy*, which advocated birth control by vaginal douching, was published in England. This was later republished by Charles Bradlaugh and Annie Besant in 1877 as a test case against obscenity laws. For their trouble they were very nearly imprisoned. The pamphlet was described as indecent, lewd, filthy and obscene. However, it became available in Australia where it met with some opposition, but Justice Windeyer, in 1888, ruled that it was not obscene. As a result of this court action, publicity for birth control was enormous.[2]

Various methods of birth control were advocated in the 19th century. These included *coitus interruptus* (withdrawal), periodic abstinence for varying periods, condoms, pessaries containing quinine or mercury, sponges soaked in various solutions, douches of lysol and caustic. Strenuous laughing and holding the scrotum to prevent ejaculation were also recommended. Purgatives were widely used in the hope of producing abortions. Women commonly swallowed substances containing arsenic, strychnine and mercury.[3]

Unfortunately much of the advice given was completely wrong and some even increased the risk of pregnancy. Much was useless. Dr James Beaney, of Melbourne, advocated abstinence for three days before and for eight days after the period and cold douching at other times. This advice must have added substantially to the population as he was largely advocating intercourse in the fertile time. Another advocate for birth control was Mrs Brettena (Bessie) Smyth, also of Melbourne, a flamboyant figure who sold medicines, corsets and surgical appliances. She advertised widely and was very critical of all contraceptive methods other than the *Prentif Pessaire* (a cervical cap), which was the one she sold and which had 'never been known to fail where instructions were carried out'.[4]

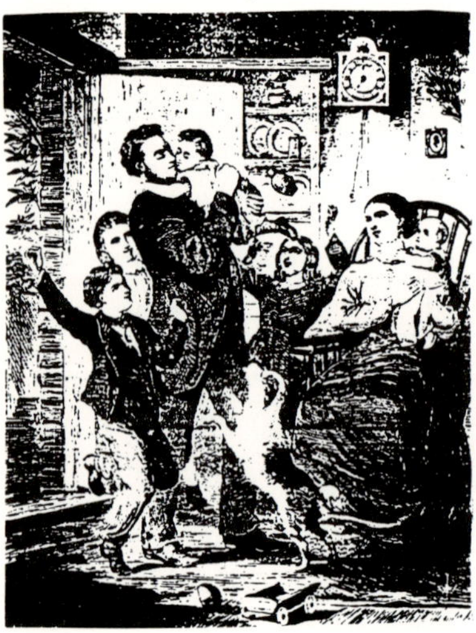

As has occurred throughout history, abortion was practised and advertised in colonial Australia. Doctors played very little part in assisting people with birth control, and the provision of contraceptive advice was considered unethical by the medical profession.[5] In the *Australasian Medical Gazette* of August 20th, 1897, a call was made for the *Indecent Advertisement Act* to be enforced, and for the Medical Board to be given the power to refuse registration to –

> *... those who do not conform their conduct to the honourable rules of life.*[6]

The Early Twentieth Century

It is tempting to believe that control of fertility has only become possible with modern methods of contraception. However, Australians managed to achieve a substantial fall in the birth rate during the Depression years of the 1890s. In all, the birth rate fell by over 30% from 1890 to 1902. (*Figure 8.1*)

This was seen as a cause for concern and 1904 saw the establishment of a Royal Commission on the Decline of the Birth Rate and the Mortality of Infants in New South Wales. The outcome of this was that the Commissioners pronounced that it was the duty of all married women to have as many children as possible, and that to limit child bearing was an extremely selfish act. Contraception was viewed as evil and Part II of the Report which contained details of safe methods of birth control was completely suppressed.[3]

The views of at least some of the medical profession were apparently similar to those of the Commissioners. Dr Sandford Jackson, in a presentation which he made to the Queensland Branch of the British Medical Association said –

> *It is abundantly evident that there is a knowledge of methods of race suicide that is positively amazing. Young people begin their married life with the determination to have no children.*[8]

One wonders if the Commissioners and the medical profession ever thought of the impact their pronouncements might have had at an individual level. The author's own grandmother, who was a young married woman at the time, went on to have thirteen children and 'so many miscarriages that I lost count'. Her last child, the author's mother, was born when she was forty-two years old. One does not

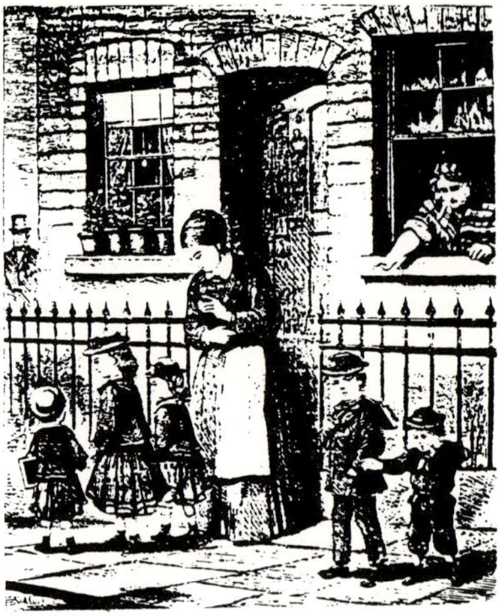

know if she was individually influenced by the Commission's findings; whether it was the pressure of society's mores; or she simply did not have access to contraceptive advice. Perhaps she even really wanted such a large family. However, although she was a devoted and much-loved mother, one certainly gained the impression that she was somewhat relieved when she finally became menopausal!

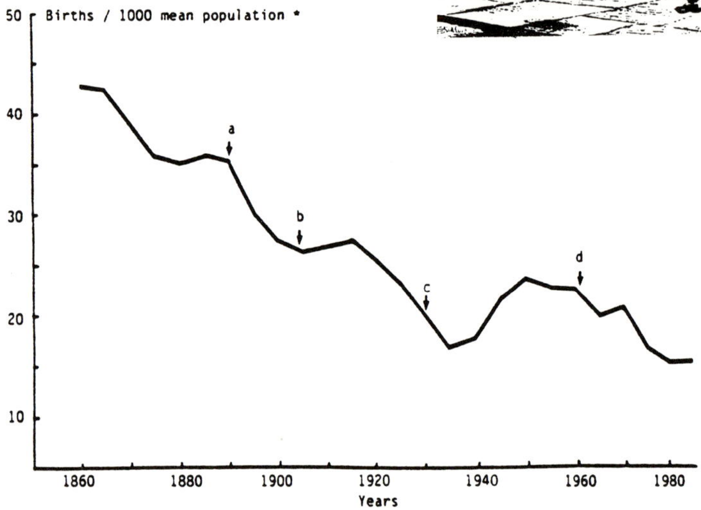

Figure 8.1. Crude Birth Rates, Australia 1860–1988

(a) Depression, 1890
(b) Royal Commission on Decline of the Birth Rate and Mortality of Infants in New South Wales, 1904
(c) Depression, 1930
(d) Introduction of oral contraceptive pill, 1961

*Excludes full blood aborigines before 1966.

Reference: Australian Bureau of Statistics – *Demography,* 1947. Bulletin No. 65; *Demography,* 1971. Bulletin No. 87; *Social Indicators, Australia* 1984. Cat. No. 4101.0; *Births, Australia,* 1988. Cat. No. 3301.0.

Development of the Family Planning Associations in Australia

In spite of official views on the evils of contraception and a belief in the need to populate the country, the demand for birth control continued. Gradually those who believed that it should be available became organized and the birth control movement grew. This movement comprised individuals and organizations who came together and formed the precursors of the Family Planning Association.

By the early 20th century there were a number of people who were advocates for birth control and who sought to further its acceptance. On the 27th April, 1926, the Women's League of New South Wales called a meeting which resulted in the Race Improvement Society. This was incorporated into the Racial Hygiene Centre of New South Wales in 1927 and an office was established at 82 Pitt Street, Sydney. Its aim was to eradicate venereal disease, teach sex education and further the community's knowledge of eugenics. In the 1920s the eugenic movement had some community acceptance although many would now find this philosophy distasteful.

In 1929, the Race Improvement Society became the Racial Hygiene Association, and early patrons and subscribers included prominent citizens of New South Wales. The Advisory Board had members of the judiciary, medical profession and churches well represented on it. The Executive Committee of the Association had women as 14 of its 16 members. This interest in, and control of, the Family Planning Association by women is still largely the case today.

The Racial Hygiene Association provided advice on contraception from its inception, (*Figure 8.2*) but the first clinic did not open until 1933, at 14 Martin Place, Sydney. The Clinic service was promoted in a conservative way, possibly to mollify the community. Dr Katie Ardill-Bryce who was in charge of the clinic was quoted in *The Sun* newspaper (24th November, 1933) as saying that every effort would be made to confine birth control to married women; and that while it would not be practicable to ask every woman to produce her marriage licence, single women – if it were apparent that they were single – might be asked to do so. However, she was courageous enough to say –

> *Even if our service should unwittingly prevent a few illegitimate children from being born, I should not be sorry.*

Racial Hygiene Association of N.S.W.

The lack of preparation for marriage means

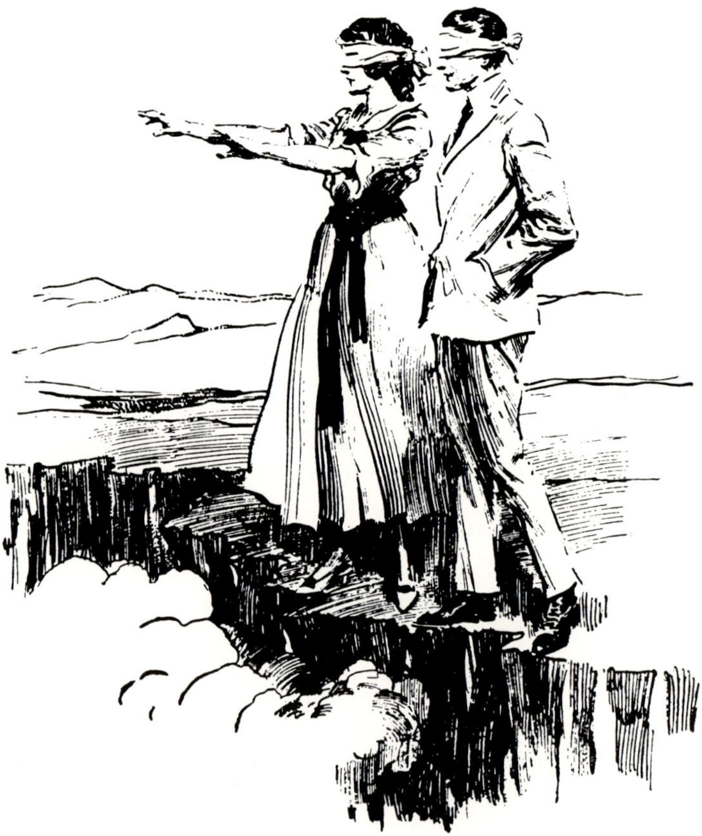

WE SAY

KNOWLEDGE means SAFETY

GIVE THEM LIGHT !

Figure 8.2. Poster, Racial Hygiene Association of New South Wales Annual Report, 1929, in the Mitchell Library, State Library of New South Wales.

It is also stated in the same newspaper article that the Police Commissioner had advised that the Clinic was perfectly legal.

After an enthusiastic and buoyant start the Clinic experienced difficulties during the years of World War Two. The Government grant was withdrawn; there were complaints to the Minister of Health, often by women's organizations themselves; there was a shortage of rubber to make diaphragms although there was enough to provide condoms for the troops! In 1941 there was even a protest against the inclusion of the name of the Clinic in the Sydney telephone directory. In 1943–44 the Clinic was forced to close.

The Racial Hygiene Association struggled on and in 1944–45 rubber again became available for diaphragms the Clinic re-opened. After the war the numbers of women attending expanded rapidly,* and in 1952 the first Branch Clinic was opened in the Sydney suburb of Leichhardt.

In 1960 the Racial Hygiene Association became the Family Planning Association of Australia. In the next decade it took an increasing interest in the part Australia would play in the wider world. In 1969 it became a full member of the International Planned Parenthood Federation (IPPF). Soon after, IPPF provided a small grant to assist in the establishment of individual Family Planning Associations in other States. This money, together with grants from the States, meant that by 1973 every State and Territory had its own Association. In 1974 funding was provided by the Commonwealth Government through a National Family Planning Program. This has continued to the present day, although channels of funding have varied somewhat according to the different policies of the Governments of the time.[9] In Australia these Associations now provide over 240,000 consultations annually.[10]

A further milestone was achieved with the removal in 1972 of the 27½% luxury tax on oral contraceptives.

The Women's Movement and women's issues were intensely topical during the 1970s. Nineteen seventy-five was nominated 'International Women's Year' and during that year a conference on *Women's Health in a Changing Society* showed that family planning, unwanted pregnancies, sexuality and provision of services for these issues was of great concern to women. The Royal Commission

*Oh, how graphic. [Ed.]

on Human Relationships Report in 1977 gave an analysis of sexuality and fertility control. This was the first time that such a comprehensive analysis had been carried out.[9]

However, the Family Planning Associations have not had universal acceptance. As well as those who oppose family planning on moral grounds, it is thought by some members of the medical profession that the Family Planning Associations encroach on traditional general practice.

In attempting to argue the case against family planning, comparisons have been frequently made between costings for family planning services and the Medicare rebate for a standard general practitioner consultation.*

It is erroneous to do this as there is no common basis for direct comparison. A private medical practice is a business enterprise and therefore services which are not chargeable against medical schedules cannot be developed or provided. On the other hand, the functions of a Family Planning Clinic, whilst including scheduled medical services, also include a wider range of paramedical services which are not chargeable against the medical schedules.

To begin with, many of the services are longer than the standard consultation of 25 minutes because of the nature of the clientele. Many women are young (20% under 17 years), some are outside the mainstream of society, and some are migrants needing interpreters. Sexual counselling and the management of complicated cases are also a part of the service. Intra-uterine device insertion and vasectomies also attract a greater-than-standard consultation fee. In addition, postgraduate and undergraduate medical training is carried out in the Clinics and a reduction in the number of patients seen becomes necessary if proper attention is to be given to teaching.

As well as services provided by the medical practitioners, services are also provided by nursing sisters. For example, in Queensland in 1988/89 these included over 17,000 interviews, 5898 pregnancy tests and 37,000 calls for telephone information.[11] Nurses also provide education and information for clients.

The Family Planning Associations provide one focal point for the birth control movement. As such their role is political, which takes administrative time, and therefore money.

*In 1990, a 'Standard Consultation' was defined in the Medicare Rebate Schedule as one lasting 5-25 minutes.

Medicare

CONTRACEPTIVE METHODS

Traditional Methods of Contraception

The first diaphragm was invented in Germany in the 1880s. It became known as the Dutch Cap however because it was so widely used in Holland. There were many variations on this theme, with diaphragms and caps of different shapes and sizes becoming available. (*Figure 8.3*) They were brought into Australia from overseas but in 1923 this ceased because Federal Government customs regulations were introduced making it illegal to import contraceptives. This restriction on the use of caps in Australia persisted until 1935 when Dr Francis Harding brought back a sample of a Racia cap from the United States of America. He managed to hoodwink His Majesty's Customs by presenting it as a type of pessary which could be used to 'support women inside'.[12] The cap was then patented by the Racial Hygiene Association and made in Australia by the Nutex Rubber Company.[4]

The diaphragm was at its most popular in the 1950s but its use declined sharply, particularly among young women, with the introduction of the oral contraceptive pill in 1961.[13] By 1977 it was used by only 1% of married women.[14]

Condom use also declined markedly at that time, although 'rhythm' and 'withdrawal' methods remained at their previous levels.[15] The maintenance of the levels for withdrawal has been due to increasing migration of central Europeans who have traditionally used this method. Its use by Australian-born couples declined with the advent of the contraceptive pill.[16]

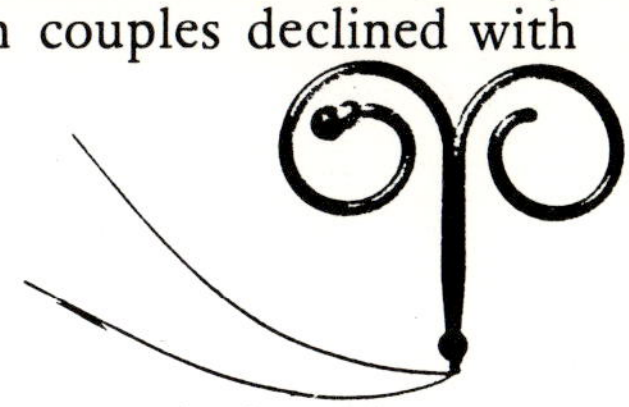

The Intra-Uterine Contraceptive Device

Although not strictly an IUCD, an intra-cervical 'collar stud' device made of a material 'lighter than aluminium' was available in the early 1900s. It was made in four sizes, the largest being for women who had more than seven children. This device was placed in the cervix by the woman herself using an introducer. It was advertised by the No More Worry Company and could be ordered by mail from Brisbane.[4]

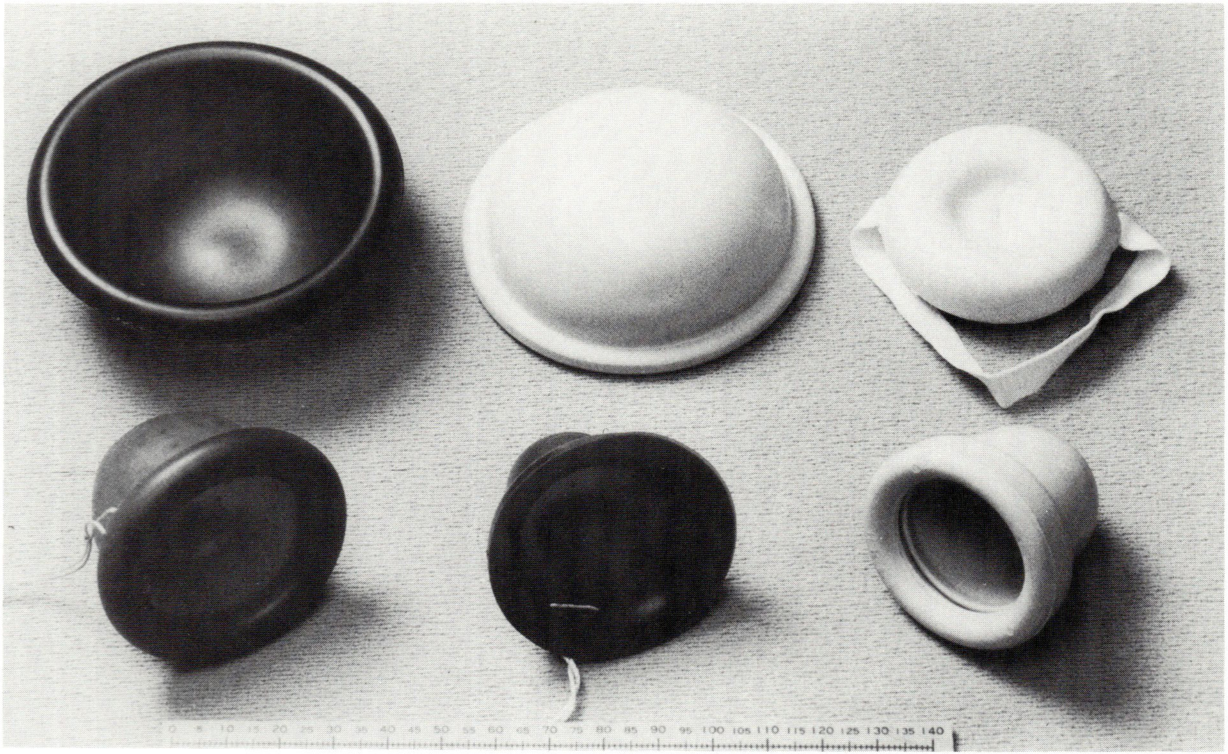

Figure 8.3. *Samples of various diaphragms or 'caps' for contraceptive use.*
From top left (clockwise) – Dumas Cap, Ortho Diaphragm, 'Today' Vaginal Contraceptive Sponge, Cervical Cap, Vimule, Superchex.

Many different types of intra-uterine contraceptive devices (*Figure 8.4*) were being developed and tried throughout the world in the early twentieth century. It is not known to what extent these were used in Australia, except that the Grafenburg Ring was the contraceptive of choice for 6% of women in Melbourne in the 1950s and early 1960s.[15] This device was placed entirely within the uterus.

The inert plastic devices, Lippes Loop, Saf-T-Coil and Dalkon Shield were introduced in the 1960s, and these were the first devices to have a string protruding into the vagina. This allowed for easy removal and checking that the device was in place, but it has been postulated that it also allows the ascension of bacteria from the vagina into the normally sterile uterine cavity.

The next generation of IUCDs, which had a copper wire wound around their stem (Gravigard, Gynae T, Multiload) became available from the mid 1970s. These were also stringed devices but had the advantage of being smaller, with similar 'break–through' pregnancy rates to those of the inert devices. With these smaller devices the side effects of bleeding and pain were considerably reduced.

The 1980s saw the advent of the Nova T which was also a copper bearing device. However, there was a silver core in the copper wire and this, by increasing the active life of the copper, allowed the device to stay in position for longer than the two years that was currently accepted for other copper bearing devices. However in Australia the recommendation remained that all copper bearing devices should be changed every two years and this applied equally to the Nova T, Gravigard, Gynae T and Multiload.

It was initially thought that IUCDs would be very popular; however their use has been limited because of the side effects of increased bleeding and pain in some women, and the higher incidence of pelvic inflammatory disease.

The introduction of IUDs coincided with the era of greater sexual permissiveness, which resulted in an increasing incidence of sexually transmitted diseases. It is probable that most cases of pelvic inflammatory disease in IUD users are primarily sexually acquired. However, the occurrence of pelvic inflammatory disease in association with IUD use which has been well publicised in recent years has reduced their popularity, and litigation[17,18] in other countries has had the effect of further reducing the availability of these devices.

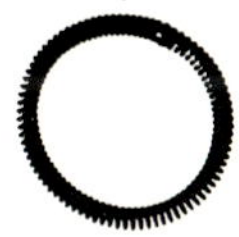

In September 1989, the Commonwealth Department of Community Services and Health advised that it would conduct a review of all IUDs imported into Australia, and requested additional clinical data. As a result of this, only one company, Organon, which distributes the Multiload device and has the major part of the market in Australia, believes that it is commercially viable to continue. Other manufacturers, who have a smaller share of the market, believe that it is not financially worthwhile to use their resources to provide data within the time frame and format required, as well as conducting ongoing monitoring programmes.[18]

The result of this is that the choices for Australian women have been narrowed, and women for whom IUCDs are an excellent method of contraception will be disadvantaged.

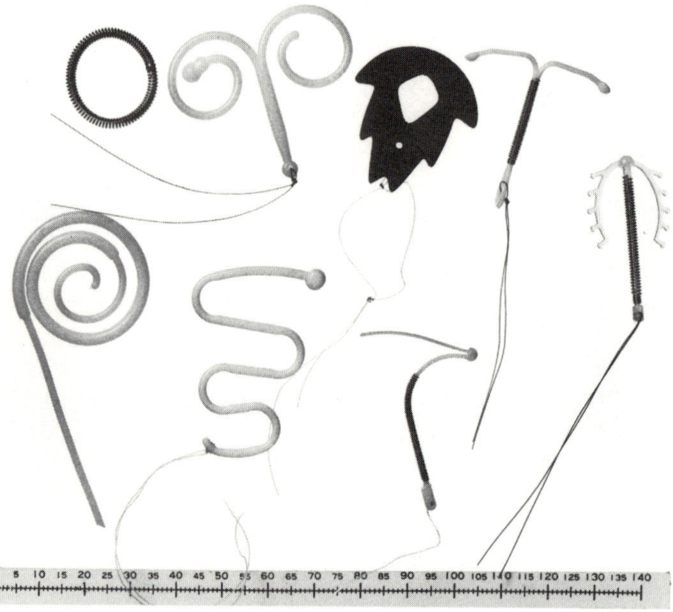

Figure 8.4. Intra-Uterine Contraceptive Devices.
From top left, (clockwise) – Grafenburg Ring, Saf-T-Coil, Anderson's Leaf, Nova T, Multiload-cu 250, Gravigard, Lippes Loop, Gynaecoil.

The Oral Contraceptive Pill

The oral contraceptive pill was introduced into Australia in 1961 and eagerly accepted. In 1966 Australian women had a higher rate of use than any European country and almost twice as high as that in the U.S.A.[4] Its introduction also coincided with the Women's Liberation Movement, and it could be argued that without the Pill's almost 100% guarantee of fertility control this Movement would not have had anywhere near the impact that it did. Once women could control their fertility, they could have sexual freedom, the ability to develop careers around the birth of children and to delay the birth of those children if they wished. This freedom, both sexual and financial, (this latter due to increased access to money which the ability to work has given them) has facilitated power changes in relationships between men and women. Depending on one's point of view, this has had beneficial or disturbing effects.

The oral contraceptives of the 1960s contained about three times the dose of the current 'low dose' ones. In the 1970s the first euphoria of use faded somewhat when the British Committee on the Safety of Drugs warned that there may have been an association between high dose oestrogen pills and blood clotting leading to embolism. As a result of this sales fell dramatically from 1976, but following a switch to the lower oestrogen dose their use soon increased.

Over the years there has been considerable media coverage given to possible adverse effects of the 'Pill'; sadly, insufficient balance has been given to its benefits. Frequently there has been a failure to counterbalance the risks of the 'Pill' against those of childbirth and pregnancy. Consideration also needs to be given to social factors such as the distress and consequences to a woman who finds herself pregnant when she does not wish to be. The reality is that, except for those women over forty who smoke, it is safer to use an oral contraceptive than it is to have a baby.[19] Having a baby is not an incredibly dangerous procedure and we think of it as being a reasonable and safe thing to do; yet it is often not recognized that the use of an oral contraceptive is even safer.

It is interesting to note that people accept that there is an advantage/disadvantage balance for most areas of their lives, be it travelling in a car, playing football or hang-gliding. However, there is often a failure to recognise that the same balance applies in the area of medicine. Many of us have an unrealistic expectation that medicine will provide all benefits and no risks. Of course, one recognizes that in medicine especially, most people expect to have their health improved by what is done, and it is reasonable to hope for and expect this.

Depo Provera (depo medroxy progesterone acetate)

Depo Provera is an injectable, long acting progestogen. It is a very effective contraceptive, and while not suggesting that it is free of all side effects, it does have definite medical and social advantages for some women. It has been available in Australia from the early 1960s and is currently on the NHS, listed as a Specified Purpose drug for breast cancer, endometriosis, endometrial cancer and renal cell cancer. Although approved for contraceptive use in many countries including the United Kingdom, New Zealand and Sweden, it is not approved as a contraceptive in Australia. However, the Australian Drug Evaluation Committee expressed the following view in 1976, since reconfirmed –

> *After discussion it was agreed that the use of the drug as a contraceptive must be regarded as investigational since there are unresolved questions relating to its safety for this indication. The Committee noted however, that the drug is available on the market and though it cannot be promoted as a contraceptive it may be used as such when the doctor being acquainted with the facts considers that it is the most appropriate treatment. This situation allows for responsible use such as that where informed consent is obtained!*

There has been continuing controversy about the use of Depo, largely led by consumer groups. This is often centred around reported use in aboriginal and intellectually disabled groups. However, the very real issue of the need for users to give informed consent has sometimes been obscured by factual inaccuracies and biased criticism of the drug itself. This has led to a general confusion of the issues.

With regard to its safety, Professor Ian Fraser, the Chairman of the Steering Committee, Long Acting Agents for Fertility Regulation, WHO has reviewed the scientific data thoroughly and concludes that –

> ***DMPA does not face any more unresolved issues from the scientific point of view, than oral contraceptives, intra-uterine devices, sterilization, some of the new and future methods of contraception and very many drugs that we use with relative impunity.***

Professor Fraser also asks –

How safe does a drug have to be before it is given marketing approval?

and concludes that –

> ***... it should be as safe as reasonable precaution by all concerned can make it consistent with appropriate therapeutic benefit.***

He believes that Depo Provera certainly meets these criteria.[20]

In spite of continuing consumer group opposition, there are many women who find this the most satisfactory method of contraception and wish to use it. This particularly applies to a number of women who come from New Zealand, where it has been readily available for a number of years, who become somewhat irate when told of its investigational status in Australia.

Meanwhile it continues to be prescribed and its use also has the support of the Royal Australian College of Obstetricians and Gynaecologists –

> *There is no evidence for serious long term complications of treatment but increasing evidence for substantial protection against endometrial cancer, ovarian cancer, pelvic inflammatory disease and endometriosis.*
>
> *It is the belief of the College that Depo Provera offers an additional option in the range of available contraceptive methods in Australia, which may be particularly suited for some individuals. It should only be prescribed with proper counselling of clients to assure awareness of the issues involved, by medical practitioners who understand these issues.*[21]

However the manufacturers, Upjohn, appear to have given up and do not currently have an application for approval before the Australian Drug Evaluation Committee, so there is no prospect of change in the status of Depo Provera in Australia in the near future.

Sterilization

Sterilization operations are now widely performed in Australia and it has been estimated that 60% of couples will choose this as their ultimate method of birth control.[22] In 1988/89 alone nearly 20,000 tubal sterilizations and over 26,000 vasectomies were performed in Australia.[23]

There has been a big increase in both male and female sterilization since the early 1970s where only 3.6% of women and 0.2% of men had chosen sterilization.[24] In the Royal Commission into Decline of the Birth Rate in 1904, there is reference to operations which would have produced sterilization in women, but these were ostensibly done because of pathology. While operations primarily for sterilization were performed in the first half of the century, the numbers were small and there was concern about its legality and morality.

However, there are no laws which specifically mention sterilization in any State in Australia and one wonders if queries about legality may not have masked basically moral concerns. Although the law has not changed, with changing moral views the incidence of sterilization has increased dramatically. Earlier moral attitudes were reflected in the views of the AMA (NSW Branch), when as recently as 1962, it was stated that –

> *Except for therapeutic reasons, no member should perform an operation for sterilization of a male or female. Not only is it ethically wrong to do so, but it is legally wrong even if consent has been given.*[4]

Legal concerns have been whether the operation can be said to be performed for the benefit of the man or woman. Whereas, in female sterilization, the benefit for the woman is direct, there has been controversy over whether a vasectomy is for the benefit of the man or of his partner. However, vasectomies are performed openly and attract a Medicare rebate. No one has ever been prosecuted for having one, or for performing one with reasonable care.

The legality of sterilization is a matter for each State, but it is now generally believed that sterilization is not against the law.[25] Nevertheless there is still uncertainty in people's minds and as a result of this some do not consider sterilization as an option, when it may well have been suitable for them.

Recent Contraceptives

Contraceptives which are not available in Australia, although they are being used in comparable countries include –

- oral contraceptives with new progestogens
- the contraceptive sponge
- RU486
- long acting progestogen implants
- medicated IUCDs containing progestogen.

Many of these methods have been used for a number of years in overseas countries with apparent advantage and yet are denied to Australian women. One of the reasons for this is that Australia is a small market and for the drug companies the effort and expense of obtaining approval to introduce new products, compared with expected profit, is not financially worthwhile. And it is believed that the time and money taken to negotiate the bureaucratic processes does discourage them from marketing their products here. While it is agreed that all care must be taken before approving new products, it is felt that there should be a review of the administrative processes. One way in which this could be done is the development of collaborative procedures with other countries with the aim of reducing the time and expense taken for approval, without compromising safety.

However, bureaucratic processes are not the only barriers to either the introduction of, or the ability to trial, new contraceptives. The introduction of RU486, a pill which in association with prostaglandins is apparently effective in providing a safe early abortion is violently opposed by some churches and anti-abortion groups. They believe it would lead to an increase in the nation's abortion rate. As a result of this small but vocal minority the manufacturers, Roussel-Uclaf, have not applied to the Australian Drug Evaluation Committee to market the drug in Australia, and have no plans to do so in the near future.

THE FUTURE

Men and women have searched for ways to control their fertility for thousands of years[26] and the progress towards safe and effective contraception in this century has been quite remarkable. As yet no perfect contraceptive exists, but many are very good indeed when used appropriately.

Contraception is very much an individual matter with medical, social, moral and psychological factors all contributing to the choice. Perhaps it is because so many factors are involved that the issues around contraception become confused. There is a need for intellectual honesty and informed debate between people of different views, but this is not happening often enough. In spite of the fact that modern contraception is safer than pregnancy and childbirth in the vast majority of cases it is still under frequent attack. There is a tendency for side effects and possible problems to be given prominence in the media, whereas beneficial effects are either not mentioned at all, or relegated to a small article towards the back pages of a newspaper. Sadly such adverse publicity has an effect. It is particularly distressing to see a woman, distraught with an unwanted pregnancy, who had abandoned safe and effective contraception because of a completely false perception of danger.

There also must be a recognition of one's true motive in either promoting or opposing a method of contraception. It is not reasonable to attack a contraceptive inappropriately on medical grounds when one's true motive for wishing to see it discontinued is based on a moral belief that contraception is wrong, any more than it is proper for someone who believes wholeheartedly in contraception to ignore possible side effects.

Controversy is valuable however, even though it is sometimes seen as being only negative and disruptive. Because so many social and moral issues are involved with contraception, it is an essential part of pushing the frontier forwards. Discussion and controversy allow society to test its values and arrive at a position on these. What must be guarded against however is the tyranny of a minority view over the majority. Contraception is a personal matter and while the majority have no right to insist that the minority act in the same way they do, neither can the minority be allowed to dictate society's values.

Today, in Australia, there are many barriers to be overcome. We have come a long way but there is still a long way to go. Contraceptive choice is very limited compared with many comparable countries, and worse still the options here are decreasing. Increasing litigation, a small market for manufacturers, bureaucratic processes and a small vocal minority are all responsible for this. If further losses are to be contained and new gains made, the belief in the right to safe and effective contraception, and the will to fight for it, must be maintained.

Acknowledgements

I thank Dr Stefania Siedlecky and Ms Diana Wyndham for making available information from the manuscript of their book *Populate and Perish. Australian Women's Fight for Birth Control*, to be published by Allen & Unwin. I also thank Mrs Marjorie Millburn, Administrator, Family Planning Association of Queensland who, for many years, has maintained a file on items of historical interest and kindly made that available.

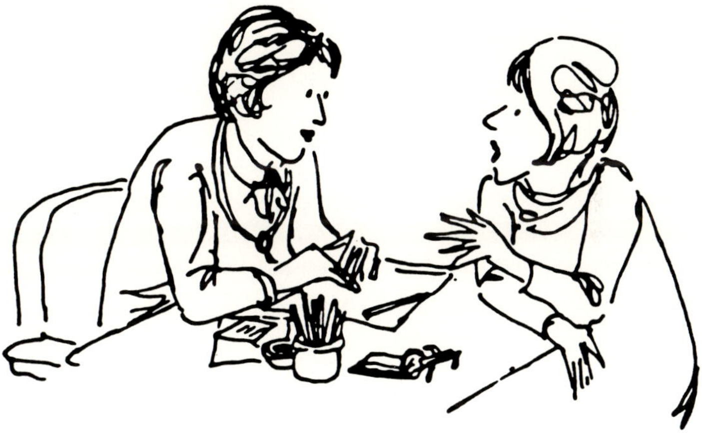

I'd like a spontaneous romantic form of contraception that enhances libido and interpersonal communication.

Reprinted with the permission of the artist, Merri Collier (From Healthbright 1986, 6(1):16)

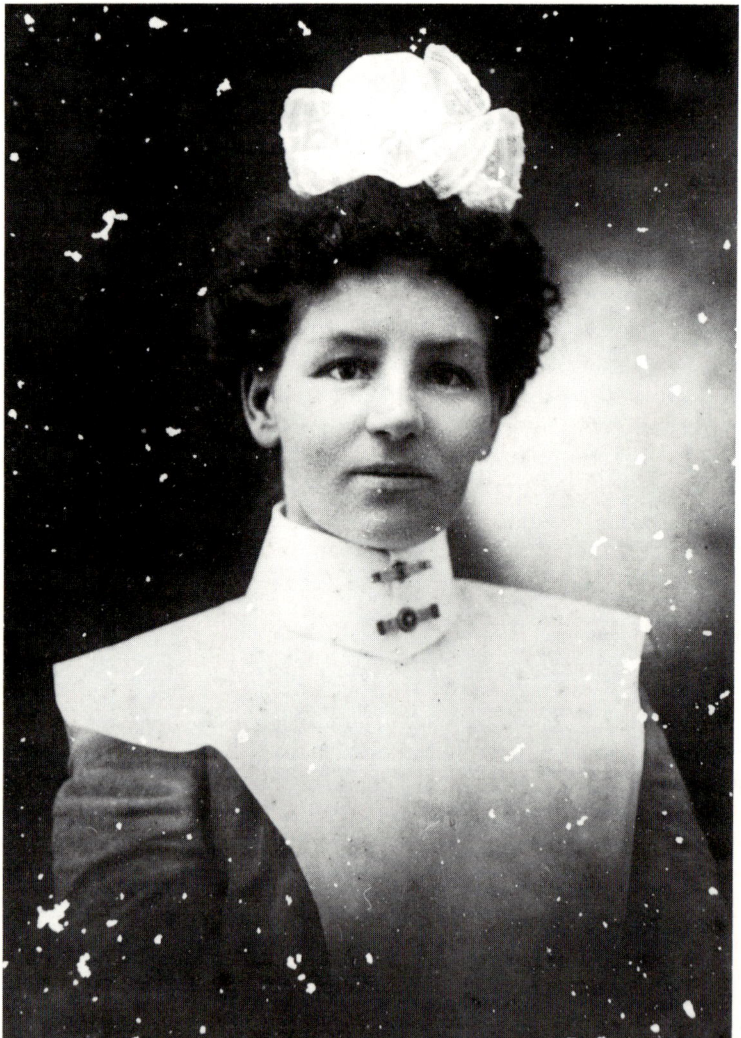

Figure 9.1. "ESSENTIALLY A LADY"
Nurse at Bowen Hospital, circa 1910
Photograph, courtesy of the John Oxley Library, Brisbane

FEVERS AND FRONTIERS 9

NURSING – ACROSS THE FRONTIER

Lori Harloe

From the bush to tertiary education, at last!

Controversy has always surrounded nursing educational changes. Debate has revolved not merely about the obvious need for improved education of nurses[1] but has centred on issues such as the treatment of patients, power games and status, aspirations to professionalism, and concomitantly, career structure. The medical profession has not yet accepted the need for higher and better education. Several members have erroneously believed that nurses might make incursions into the medical domain, untrained and lacking in the skills supposedly imparted by tertiary instruction. But the prejudice and fears have no foundation. Of particular focus, in this discussion, is the improvement of practical standards, and the ability of nurses currently practising and studying their chosen profession to really nurse: concerns, valid and logical have often masked insecurities and reactions both within nursing circles and the various disciplines of health care professionals.

In adjusting the height of the lamp nurses have seldom held it high enough to illuminate themselves. Traditionally the patient, the procedure, and the system have been weighed as more important than the nurse who effects the daily caring. It thus follows that the incipient aspirations of nurses for the twenty-first century have not been examined in the clearest light. Within the increasingly better educated community, nurses can no longer afford to stand modestly in the shadows of ignorance and apathy. Instead, nurses must absorb the light of higher education; and by continuing to care and develop the best qualities of nursing, participate in a more enlightened professional world.

Traditionally nursing education had been a State responsibility. In the wake of an 'in principle' agreement made by the Commonwealth in 1984 to provide funding, the glimmers of a national nursing identity emerged. However, all the States have retained a degree of autonomy; all commenced transferring nursing education from the the hospital to tertiary institutions. The pace of change varied across the nation. For example, in 1984, New South Wales unilaterally decided to commence the transfer of nurse education from hospitals to tertiary institutions. All nurses in that state are now educated in tertiary institutions. In the Australian Capital Territory and the Northern Territory, the transfer is also complete. This programme of transition is proceeding smoothly in Western Australia where the final intake into the old apprenticeship hospital system took place in 1987. In Tasmania the final intake was in 1989, and Victoria and South Australia ceased taking hospital-based trainees in 1990. Queensland

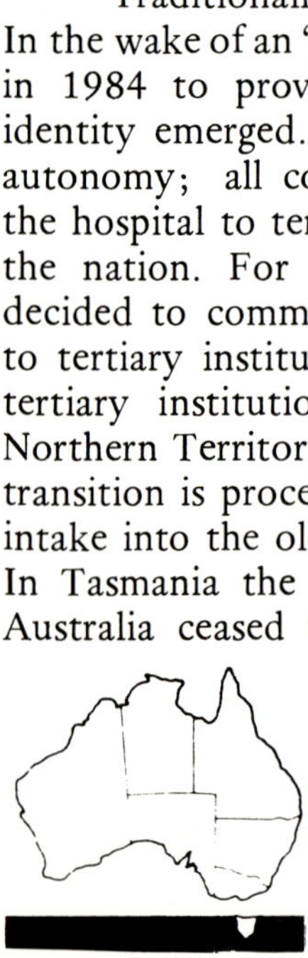

was the last state to follow what is a national pattern. In July 1988, the Queensland State Government eventually signed an agreement with the Commonwealth whereby the teaching of nurses would be transferred from hospital-based Schools of Nursing to tertiary educational institutions.[2] After the end of 1990 Queensland enrolled no more students in hospital-based nursing education programmes. In 1989 ten hospital nursing schools closed in Queensland. The phasing-out of pre-registration education was anticipated to occur over the four-year period 1990 to 1993.[3]

Within five years after the Federal Government approved the transfer of registered nursing education to CAEs and Universities (in 1984), there were already indications that the struggle for education reform would not be easy.[4] The tendency for exclusion and discrimination in educational matters has always been, and remains, a feature of nursing education. The *ad hoc,* piecemeal, and frequently irrational provision of educational opportunities have varied from state to state.[5] This has been best exemplified by the various attitudes to the potential global shortage of trained nurses.[6] South Australia recognised the problem as early as 1970 and commenced workforce planning.[7] The Queensland Health Department as late as February 1990 denied all idea of the projected shortage of trained nurses in that state.[8]

Furthermore, there had been no co-ordination between the Commonwealth Tertiary Education Commission, the Advanced Education Council or the individual colleges to consult with nursing unions and other professional bodies. Such has always been essential to achieve standardization and to reduce variations in education which threaten employment mobility and professional competence. By 1987, these themes were being addressed by a committee formed by the various state boards of registration. By 1990, there was still no national registration board which might ensure uniformity of standards and education opportunity.

As a result of the obvious lack of coherence in 1987 a national federation of nineteen State and Federal unions (with members in the health care industry) formed the National Council of Health Organizations. The focus of this group – which represented 85,000 nurses – encompasses five main themes. One major objective was that nursing educational initiatives should be of a high professional standard and be standardised nationally; and that such be comparable with practice in other related disciplines according to the criteria of the Australian Council of Tertiary Awards. Another objective was that career progression for nurses had to be restructured; and without prejudicing the quality of courses that affirmative action principles should be mobilised. The latter was necessary to ensure that hospital trained nurses were not discriminated against in their access to post-registration courses at tertiary level.

The Nature of Nursing

In order to examine these changes it is well to reflect upon the nature of nursing. When discourse turns to nursing, the result is often a complex mixture of emotional, non-rational, primaeval, and deep-seated responses. A common issue which has always characterised such dialogue has been the recognition of what constitutes the very core of nursing itself. Whatever this core is, it is that which sets nursing apart. However, a fundamental component of nursing is the

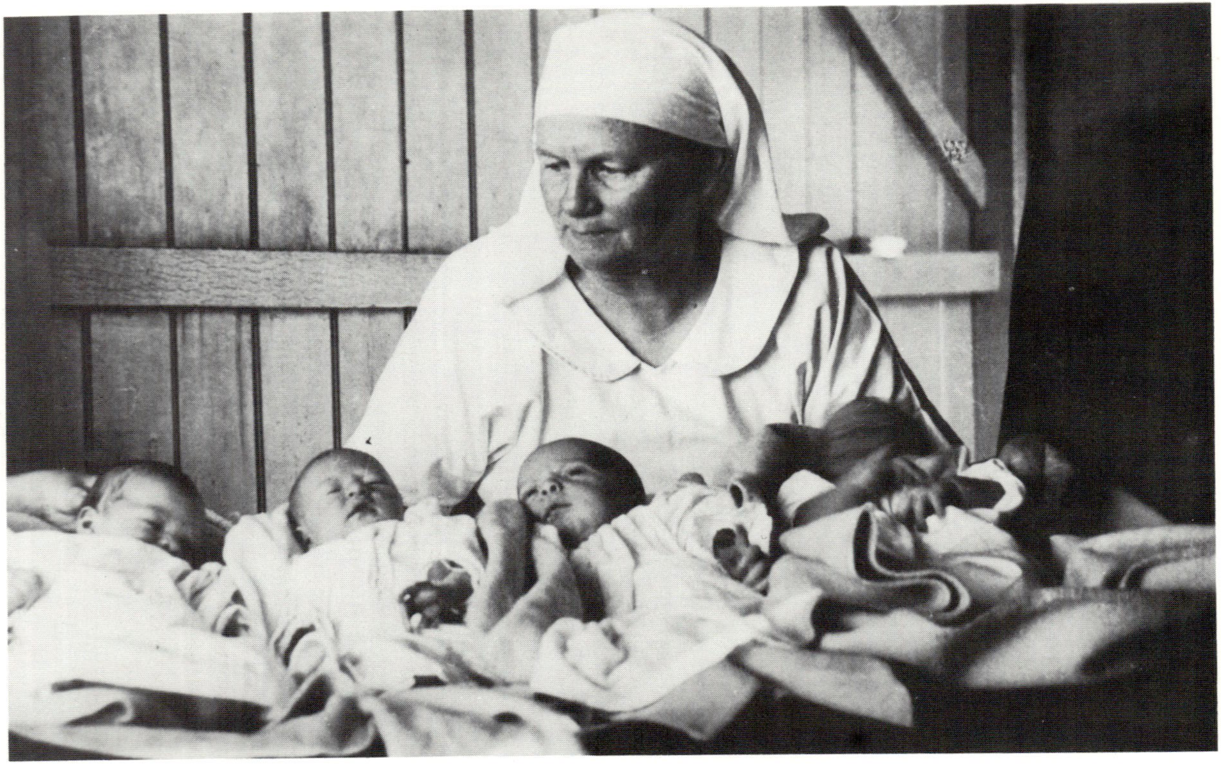

Figure 9.2. "*Motherly Care*". *Matron Whitehead, St Aubyn's Hospital, Kingaroy, circa 1925. Photograph reproduced by permission of the John Oxley Library, Brisbane.*

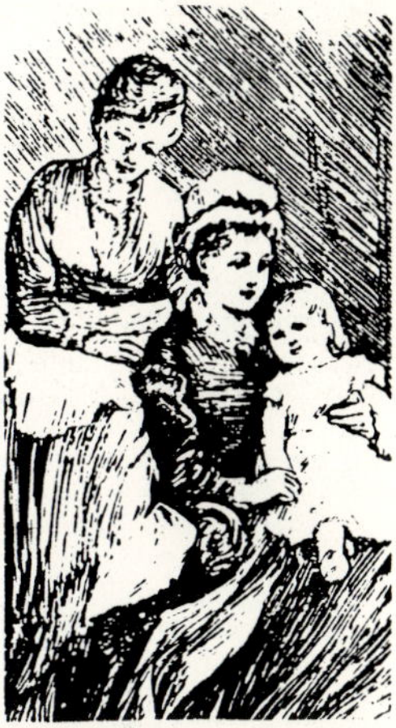

intimate human contact which comprises its essence. The intensely personal nurse-patient relationship can be equated with the type of care given by most mothers and is therefore understood and appreciated by all.

Another, less readily understood type of 'basicness', which touches a chord in this world of flux and violence, is the adaptability and responsiveness which nurses need in order to survive in a professional capacity. One may compare this 'basicness' with the response to horrid situations of human suffering in war, as patients confront their own particular duel with disease or infirmity. Nursing and nurses are very much part of the battle between the individual and his or her innermost fears about survival. Professional reassurance and care, on the most basic human level given to those in need, is the special commodity which nursing delivers.[9]

Perhaps it is a subconscious perception of the yearning for inspiration, reassurance, and care in times of physical and mental crisis which clouds objective discussion of the true nature of nursing. Nevertheless, it is not unreasonable to reiterate that nursing occupies a singularly important intermediary role between patient and treatment. As a personal advocate, the nurse acts as a bridge between the alien world of sickness or incapacity and the familiar every day world of health. The nurse can only change the quality of caring by improved knowledge of the true nursing situation. Throughout history education has radiated an enlightening effect: why should nursing not participate in better education, which is after all only part of the human struggle for truth and justice?

Anonymity, a dominant feature of the history of nursing, has simultaneously been beneficial and detrimental. The greatest benefit overwhelmingly, has been the focus of concentration in word, thought, and deed, upon those in need of restoration to health and upon the care of the sick and dying. On the other hand, anonymity has tended to stifle individuality and innovation. By far the greatest drawback has been the high number of displaced, disaffected, and disenchanted nurses, who leave the profession because of lack of intellectual and professional development. By restricting nursing education to a

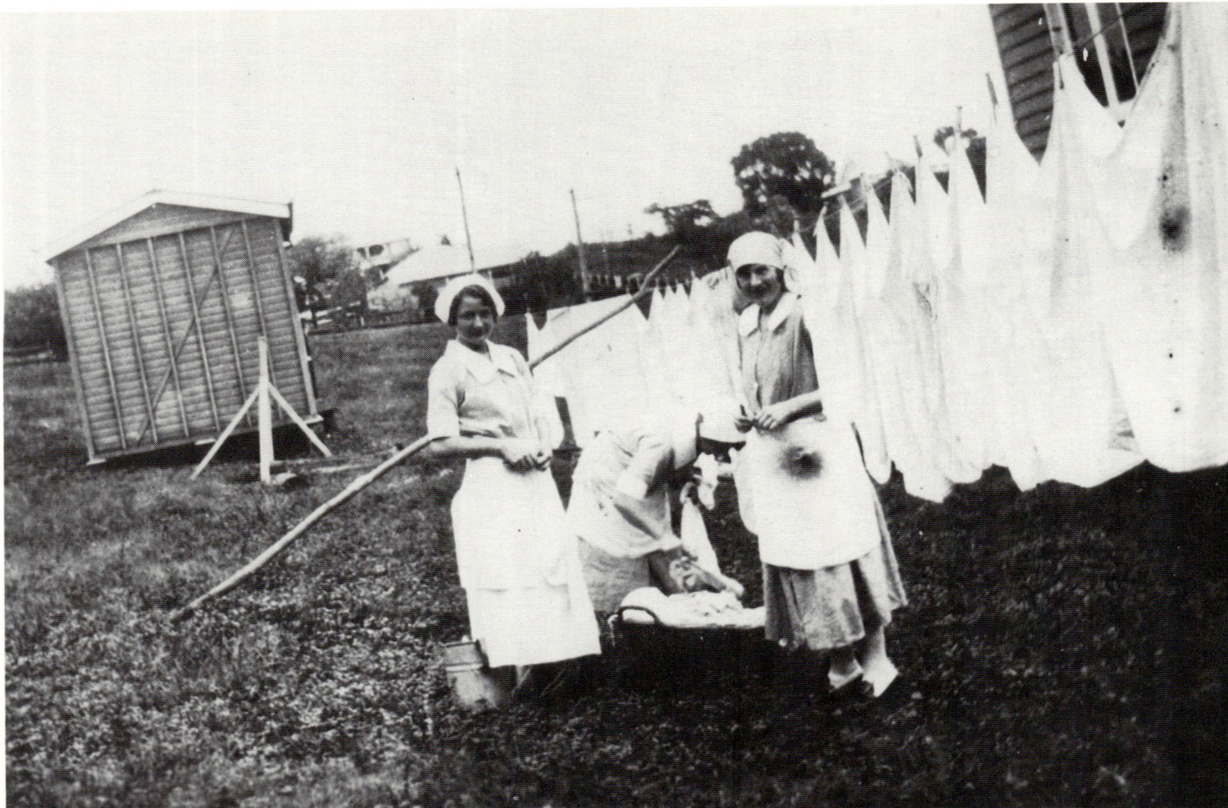

Figure 9.3. Nursing Staff hanging out washing at the Boonah Hospital, circa 1930. Photograph reproduced by kind permission of the John Oxley Library, Brisbane.

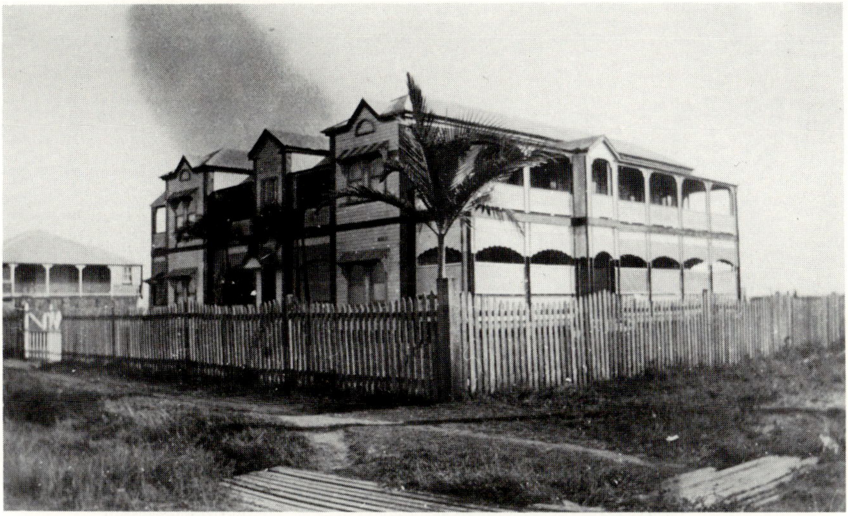

Figure 9.4. Lister Hospital, Mackay, North Queensland, 1910
The larger towns had bigger hospitals, but characteristically, no trees providing shade from the relentless tropical heat.
Photo, courtesy of the John Oxley Library, Brisbane.

purely vocational, old fashioned, unenlightened 'means to an end' approach, the future of nursing care will be out of step with the treatment delivered by other health professionals; and will also be further eroded by declining standards.

At the public level, until the advent of the feminist revolution of the 1970s, perception of women in our society has been largely managed and controlled by men who dictated what was safely acceptable to the *status quo*. Nurses have been defined by this masculinized world view. It is not an insignificant fact that nursing is predominantly a female occupation. In Australia only about 4% of all practising nurses are male.[10] From the time when Attic morality banished women from the public life of Athens, cultural codes, rather than specific political events, set the tone for our conflicts of gender in society. In early literature, the trilogy *The Orestia* stands as a symbol of a patriarchal takeover of public life[11] which continues to reverberate in our nursing history. It is argued that in this drama,

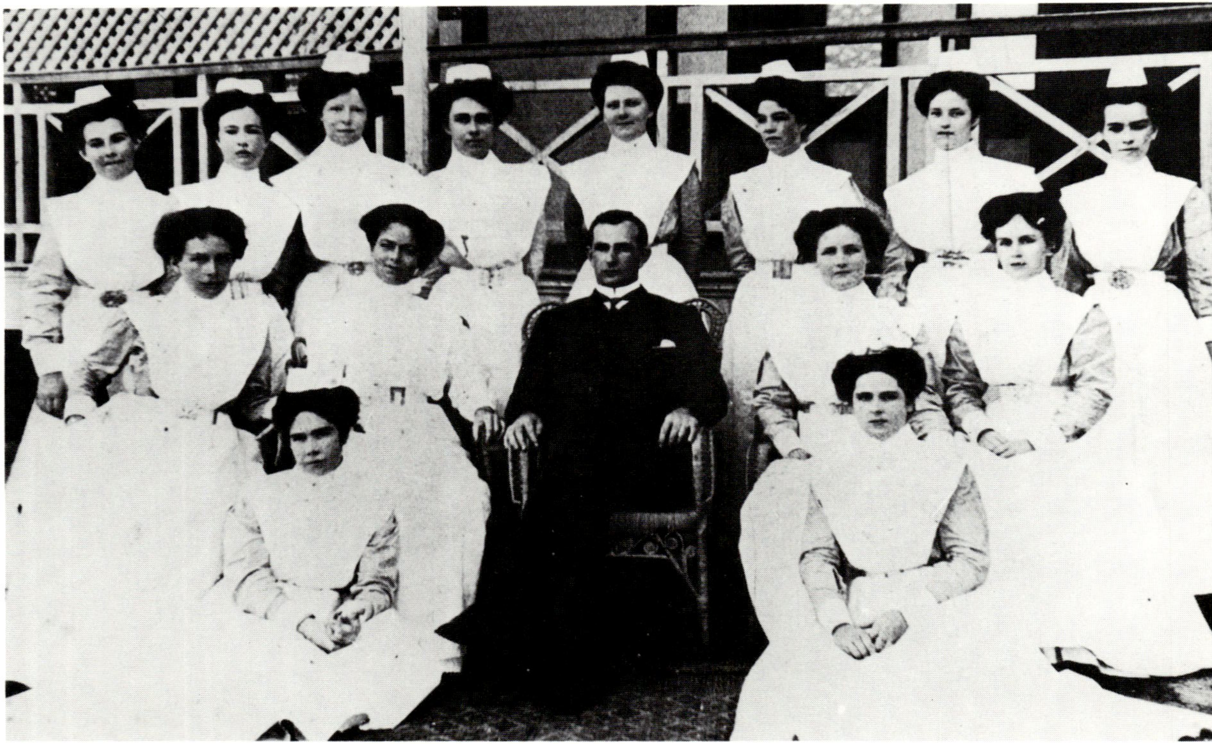

*Figure 9.5. 'Mandated Polygamy'. A group of nurses with the medical superintendent of the Townsville Hospital, Dr T. Gordon Ross, in 1910. **Photograph**, courtesy of the Townsville Hospital Archives.*

which formalised misogyny, the female gender has always been associated with sexuality and nature, and with those forces which must be contained and tamed in outside activities, and in the inner person, for the survival of the *polis*.[12] One writer claims that it is about winners and losers.[13,14]

This dramatisation of gender conflict stands as a reminder that things are changing. Under the influence of feminist analysis there has been a significant displacement of the central masculinized world view.[15] No longer is there quite the formal distinction between public life, which has been traditionally the provenance of men, and the private, often powerless, sphere to which women have been relegated.

Evolutionary Trends

From time immemorial, woman's role has centred on birth and nurturing: throughout history women have held special healing knowledge. At no time was this more dangerous than during the great European witch hunts. Between 1480 and 1750 half a million people were executed; most of these were midwives and the most common civil crime imputed to witches was infanticide. At that time even the influential medical faculties at the University of Paris were ineffectual in defending any female students against persecution for heresy.[16]

The Papal Bull *Malleus Maleficarum* (*The Hammer of Witches*), first printed in 1487, explicitly connected witchcraft with women because they were 'more credulous, had poor memories' and because witchcraft comes from 'carnal lust which is in women insatiable'.[17,18] For hundreds of years witches were identified, by Protestant and Catholic alike, in numerous re-issues of *The Hammer*, as women with the gift of healing (traditional empirics) and midwives. Clearly it seems that representation of women in history, in art, on the stage, and in myths, relies very much on male cultural perceptions of gender values; men's perceptions of women, rather than stories, feelings and ideas of actual women. Nurses as actual women have been caught in a fictionalized male construct.

Hospitals, it seems have been a private part of the public world and usually male dominated. In this privileged position, male doctors have had sufficient interest to define the role of the nurse as inferior, subordinate, and private (hence silent, powerless and anonymous). Very rarely has true recognition of the distinctiveness of nursing ever emanated from the medical professions.

A further complication of the public definition of female nurses was made by Florence Nightingale. Ironically, Nightingale, as a prime-mover in the power games of the times, for herself demanded an active role in a male world. Nevertheless, she expected her trainee nurses to be, what remains, a stereotype of a nurse as a woman (rather than a man) – a woman whose role as wife and mother has been extended to the hospital or clinic.

In Florence Nightingale's extraordinary drive for success and reform she exhibited some male traits. Rather disconcerting was her desire to control. Barry Smith in his story of Florence's 'thoughts in action' notes that 'only seriously ill deserved hospital care', and 'trifling hysterical or incurable cases were excluded because such patients tended to push their individual needs and were difficult to control'.[19] Her patriotic canonization was a diversionary tactic used by the authorities to cover for 'the muddle and national shame of a war that failed public expectations of early glory'. Smith goes on to say that –

> *... Miss Nightingale projected herself and was projected by others as a mature, maternal symbol, the embodiment of common-sensical housewifely virtues, in contrast to infantile male parliamentary and military blundering. She became a neutral, safely non-political diversionary focus for the discontents that might otherwise have been concentrated by J.A. Roebuck, Augustus Stafford, Charles Dickens and other radical critics in their attacks on aristocratic dominance and mismanagement.*[20]

Contrary to popular belief Florence Nightingale was not the originator of modern nursing. Her famous regimen ordering nurses lives and the control and surveillance of patients had been features of a gradual increase in efficiency in both religious and secular hospitals for at least twenty years previously.[21] Nevertheless, her exceptional gift of identifying nursing in the public mind with sanctified duty is undeniable. Victorian Britain appreciated her reputation and power. Colonial New South Wales sought her assistance in educating Australian nurses. Parkes envisaged that Nightingale trained nurses would spread out from the Sydney Infirmary to all parts of the continent.[22] However, progress was slow.

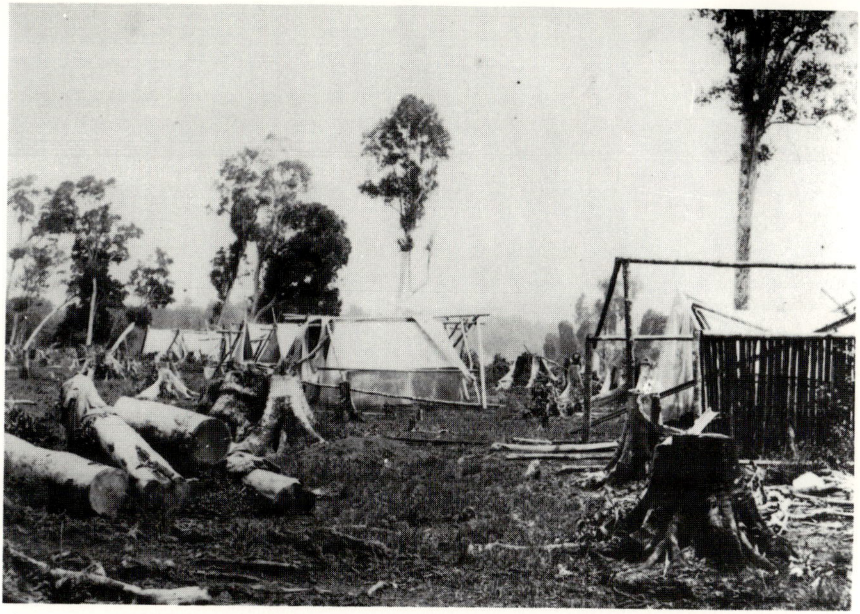

Figure 9.6. Government Hospital, Innisfail, circa 1885. Innisfail, North Queensland, was at that time named Geraldton. Photograph by courtesy of the John Oxley Library, Brisbane.

On 1 January 1884 the Queensland Government initiated the system of Government Kanaka hospitals. By September 1886 the Polynesian Labour Inspector, Sholto Stillingflat Bowles set up the first hospital for Kanaka sugar plantation workers, a 10' x 12' tent on the Johnston River bank adjacent to the tent hospital. Prior to 1886 and to the building of more substantial accommodation, hospital subscribers received medical attention at the tent hospital. Dr. Bancroft of Queensland medical history fame was the superintendent until he became exasperated by the objections of the townspeople to the extension of hospital services to Polynesians.

Early Nursing in Northern Australia

By 1887, in answer to an urgent call from Townsville for Nightingale trained nurses to replace a wardsman and his wife, the matron, who had been at the centre of a sensational court case involving mismanagement and assault of a female fever patient, the local hospital committee was informed that such nurses were only available from Sydney, not Brisbane. By the following year the Townsville Hospital had become a training school for nurses and lectures were given by the Matron and the Resident Surgeon. It was not until 1905 that the Queensland Branch of the Australian Trained Nurses Association recognised Townsville as a training school with Charters Towers remaining the examination centre for North Queensland. It also compiled a register of trained nurses working in the colony.[23]

As it happened Nightingale had a higher interest than the practice of nursing. Her gaze was directed towards the challenge of developing nursing as an honourable occupation. Those probationers accepted under the Nightingale Fund for Nurses were indeed, 'ladies', differentiated from those 'women' accepted as midwifery trainees who 'intend to pursue the calling as a business'.[24]

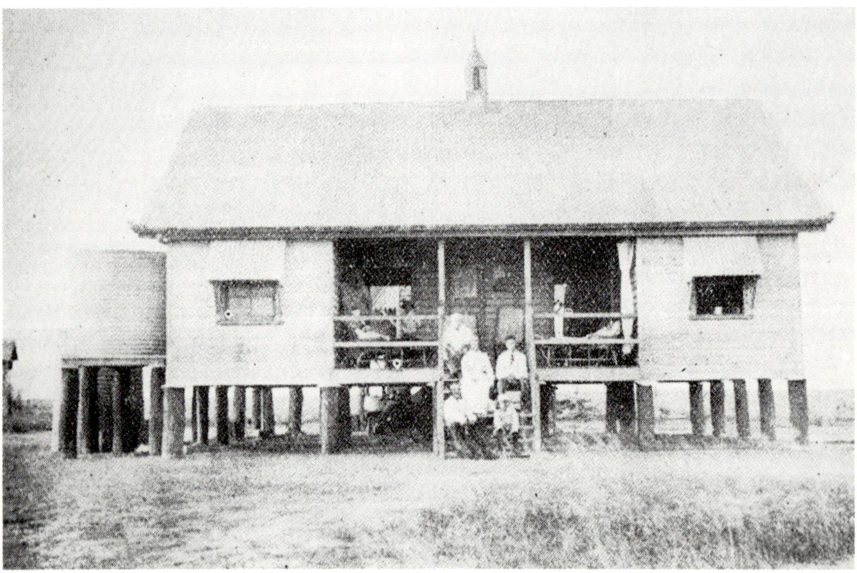

Figure 9.7. Burketown District Hospital, North Queensland.
'This hospital is situated about one mile from Burketown and is highly appreciated in the district, having a splendid record for its efficiency. The officers are – Medical, Dr E. Culpin; Secretary, R.H. Shadforth; Matron, Mrs Crank; Wardsman, U. Crank'.
(So described in the North Queensland Register, 14 May 1906.)
Photograph reproduced by permission of the John Oxley Library, Brisbane.

At the turn of the nineteenth century, with the exception of a few trained nurses at the hospitals in Charters Towers and Townsville, most nurses in tropical Queensland were untrained. Most who worked in hospitals did so to survive the harsh economic times which prevailed. In fact, not uncommonly, illiteracy is a feature of the composite profile of the early nurse in north Queensland. These informally trained women attended the sick at home, acting rather as nursemaids, providing comfort and doing a little cooking. Their idea of giving solace to their charges often included obtaining alcohol for them. Nurse Annie L... of Charters Towers, who possibly received her training from her husband Dr Joseph Henry L... could not read or write, fits into this category. Her contribution to home nursing care is recorded by the courts when she and the doctor gave evidence into the untimely death of Jane R... alias Mrs Monoghan, alias Mrs Lowe, a twenty-seven year old barmaid who died at the Central Hotel from 'compression of the brain' caused by 'the excessive use of alcohol'.[25]

Another, Mrs H... , with only general knowledge, and made redundant as a telegraph officer at the Antimony Works at Stannary Hills, was compelled to supplement the family income by rabbit catching and home nursing.[26]

Hospital and Reception House nurses and matrons were usually under the direct control of the wardsman who managed the institutions. The matron's duties, performed more often than not in uncomfortable facilities, were directly proportional to the involvement of medical knowledge and leadership given by the doctor. At Thornborough Hospital, in 1889, Dr Blanchard recorded some appalling conditions. His diary reads –

> ... [the hospital was] *an iron building, consisting of General Ward, Fairly cool in Summer and Cool in winter and generally draughty and windy. Female ward two beds in a corner, partitioned off General ward by canvas and framework. It is poky* [sic], *close in Summer and dismal. Off one end is Surgery, Small and hot – Stock of drugs fair for the field. Instruments very shabby. Off side is a bathroom, no bath is fitted up, It is very draughty for a bath room, Detached from building is a small building with two beds in. Sides of bark and roof iron, it is the Kanaka war or Dead or P.M. house. At present is not fit for a black to lie in, but only wants new sides and end. Also to side is wardsman & Matrons house and kitchen. A small poky* [sic] *iron house with kitchen and bedroom.*

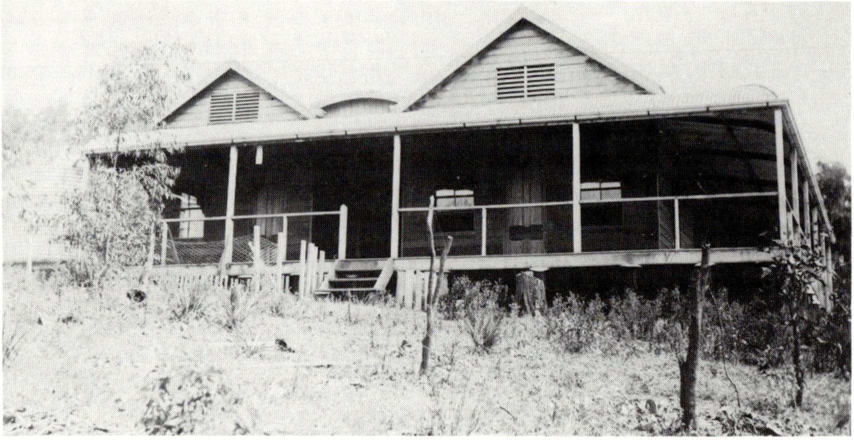

Figure 9.8. Hospital, Stannary Hills. A common hospital architectural style built in many isolated tropical locations in northern Australia. Photo by F.R. Dawson, 1 July 1907, courtesy of Queensland State Archives.

> *Kitchen fireplace open cooking done by campoven, at back are goat yards, hen houses etc, both fairly clean condition and do not cause any nuisance.*[27]

Matron K... of Thornborough Hospital, Blanchard describes as a 'slightly delicate person, but seems contented enough, does not care for nursing, but makes splendid bread and does her best to feed the patients well'. Her husband, the wardsman, also perhaps not suited to his duties was 'kind to patients but has not mastered the strict idea of cleanliness'.[28]

A dramatic increase in formal nursing knowledge in Queensland country districts is determinable by the 1920s. On the health and medical front the second decade of the twentieth century was one in which structural changes and closer examination of constitutional provisions of care were becoming issues influencing the national lifestyle. With the formation of the Nurses Registration Board the character of nursing in isolated hospitals throughout the tropics became more professionally recognised. However, those women often succeeded against impossible odds. At the Croydon District Hospital Matron Thomas[29] was representative of that new breed. She deputised for a medical practitioner; and assumed a responsibility which in the ordinary course of events, city or town nurses would have found unacceptable.

Contemporary Nursing

As nursing becomes more scientific the 'art versus scientific' debate will almost certainly be settled by an integrated approach to nursing. Such will co-ordinate research, theory and practice.[30] It is argued that well-developed nursing theories will give nurses in clinical practice the information necessary to choose specific nursing actions for predictable outcomes.[31] It can be further argued that no resolution of the complex humanitarian and scientific interaction of nursing can be achieved without more research into the historical and philosophical foundations of nursing.

In a book dedicated 'to the many expert nurses who know more than they can tell and who taught us in their caring' and entitled *The Primacy of Caring: Stress & Coping in Health & Illness,* Patricia Benner and Judith Wrubel have articulated ideas about the unique nature of bedside nursing. Their ideas are remarkable in that they are a highly developed distillation of centuries of nursing experience. This book fulfills its claim in addressing –

> *... the cultural and ideological background that lies at the root of the nursing shortage – the devaluation of nursing care and other caring practices. In a highly technical society that values autonomy, individualism and competitiveness, caring practices have always been fragile, but this societal blindness causes those who value technological advances to overlook the ways these advances are rendered dangerous and unfeasible without a context of skilful, compassionate care.*[32]

Discussion of the art and of the science of nursing advances maturation of nursing as a profession with its own discrete characteristics and its own special place in society by building on the empiricism of the past with well thought out and rational solutions to the ever-increasing technological developments. Nothing in the literature suggests that nursing is contemplating abandoning any favourable attributes learned throughout the centuries.

One hundred years ago, doctors were trained by 'walking the wards'. A marked rise in professional standards and identity came once the study of medicine was introduced into universities:[33] for some of the same reasons nurses today choose to study in tertiary institutions. Up to a point nursing has served medicine quite well by remaining in the subordinate and service role. By forging ahead and managing to keep nurses informed only to the extent that they were useful by controlling the content, the scope and the application of the nursing curriculum, medicine has created a major inter-professional problem. It is as though the medical quest for power, status and control has been achieved at the expense of a large female labour force which makes a lot of doctoring viable. This form of medical protection has had a negative effect; it has retarded over-due developments in nursing by encouraging dependence at the expense of an intelligent active role in the health care team. Although the medical profession has been dominant in nursing education, nurses have also failed to see that the outworn philosophies of the historical Nightingale tradition have shielded nurses. Such protection has prevented them from accepting the notions of responsibility intrinsic in professional determinism.

Current trends are that nurses have more scope for introspective analysis of concepts which were once considered sacrosanct. For example, it is possible to examine the sources of power and authority in health delivery teams. Most nurses now accept that the masculine world view is only half the story, and more importantly that knowing of an option does not necessarily mean that it must be exercised. Some nurses nowadays recognise that the use of power is necessary to change the *status quo*.[34] Undoubtedly, it is important to acknowledge that nursing decisions and nursing controls are essential to the nursing profession. These changes are part of professional development rather than a threat to medical knowledge *per se*, although such changes inevitably will bring forth reaction and resistance. Canadian studies have shown that under the old system (whereby doctors were participating in a form of doctor-nurse game) often the doctors were told what they wanted to hear. Rather than being an ally in the health team, the nurse was subconsciously jeopardising the care of patients by playing games to the extent that communication was often subliminal, and mistrust and conflicts for power and territory were dominant themes.[35] It is anticipated that definition of the unique role of the nurse will better serve the health needs of patients by focussing on the use of power and power relationships, which have tended in the past to undervalue the nurse. This theme remains a professional frontier.

The sociological views espoused by Emily Mumford and others about nursing being somehow or other a pale reflection of medicine is quite ludicrous. Nursing, modern nursing, is not doctoring, nor does it see itself as a rival for that role. Nursing is unique and fulfils a special place in the care of the sick and in preventative and other avenues of health care. To say as Mumford does that there –

> *... is no career ladder that allows nurses an uninterrupted line upward, for example to nurse practitioner and then to physician*[36]

denies not only the professional integrity of nursing but the real value of nursing, which is to nurse. The old hierarchial thinking – that one group is better or worse – is economically, culturally and tactically inappropriate. Such attitude validates a value judgement which is out-dated.

There are new ways of perceiving the worth of nursing as a profession. It is now ready to change and acknowledge within its own ranks the clinical nurse who, in the past, had no option for advancement other than through administration. This chance of developing higher clinical standards to act as the patient's nurse, efficiently assuming a time-honoured role of personal assistant and advocate, can only be improved by better access to appropriate comprehensive education. Career paths which simultaneously enhance the individual nurse (educationally, financially and professionally) must surely influence the entire system favourably.

In a position statement prepared by the National Council of Health Organisations in response to the DEET Working Party Report, *Review of the Initial Qualification for Nurse Education* (October 1989), a major concern about nursing competence on completion of a university nursing degree was highlighted. Most States have addressed this question. For example, The Queensland Nurses Union recognises the difficulties inherent in the acquisition of the development of clinical skills. Most nursing unions accept that the central problem appears to be what should be expected of the new graduate in the workforce.[37] Registration does not instantaneously convey the capacity to be able to function immediately as an independent autonomous practitioner. A model of progressive skill acquisition described by Benner follows logically through at least five stages of development from 'Novice' to 'Expert'.[38] This reasoning differentiates between what can be taught by precept and what must be learnt experientially from comparison of similar and dissimilar cases. Thus it is generally agreed that experience is vital for any nursing graduate to work safely in an unstructured, or unsupervised environment.

With a preceptorship programme of more experienced nurses to guide new graduates, a supportive structured continuation of learning in clinical situations will be possible. It has been recommended that due to the clinical requirements of the nursing degree, the National Board of Employment, Education and Training should consult with nursing academics on the funding arrangements essential to ensure an adequate span of clinical practice and supervision.

Conclusion

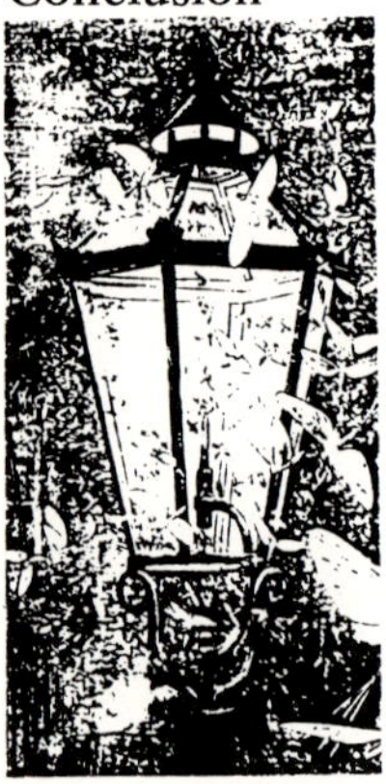

It is salutary to recognise that any changes to the method and content of Australian nursing education will not necessarily occur without some degree of anxiety within the nursing community itself. Historical analysis shows that such has always been the case when innovation and the lifting of standards is attempted. To a large extent these changes will be integrated into what has been traditional nursing practice. But, as can be expected with such a large group of individuals socialised into accepting the status quo, learning to think abstractly, laterally and independently will not be without problems. For nursing to advance satisfactorily, the first lesson considered will have to be recognition of the awareness of the value of nursing; the second, acknwledgement of the wider world and participation in the intellectual life of the community, a feature which has been sadly lacking in nursing circles; and thirdly, professional interaction with medical and paramedical groups and individuals, in a manner befitting the new found status, not in an attitude of inferiority or conflict.

It is anticipated that this new found confidence, within the profession, will generate more informed, more intelligent nursing, enabling a truly twenty-first century response to community nursing needs. The main worries about acknowledged competence, the development of nursing awareness which could threaten the power source of other professionals, and the significance of nursing professionalism should be negligible if one remembers the past and the reason for the existence of nurses – the patient.

FEVERS AND FRONTIERS 10

MATERNITY HOSPITALS AND BABY CLINICS

A Twentieth Century Australian Frontier

Wendy Selby

They left the vine-wreathed cottage and the mansion on the hill,
The houses in the busy streets where life is never still,
The pleasures of the city, and the friends they cherished best,
For love they faced the wilderness – the women of the West.

In the slab-built, zinc-covered homestead of some lately taken run,
In the tent beside the 'bankment of a railway just begun,
In the huts of new selections, in the camps of man's unrest,
On the frontiers of the Nation – live the women of the West.

And there are hours men cannot soothe, and words men cannot say,
The nearest woman's face may be a hundred miles away.
While men have hearts to do and dare, and yet o'er all the rest,
The hearts that make the Nation are the women of the West.

George Essex Evans

Emotions ran high during the second reading of the Maternity Bill as the Secretary for Mines, Mr A.J. Jones, read sections of George Essex Evans' poem, *The Women of the West*, to parliament in September, 1922.[1] This Bill, which became law on the 14th October, 1922, authorised the Queensland Government to build maternity hospitals, baby clinics, antenatal clinics and hospitals for the treatment of diseases peculiar to women.

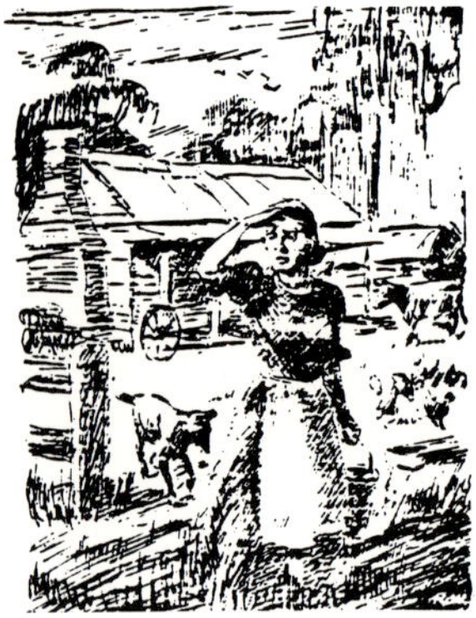

Building began immediately and the Northern and Western regions of the State were specifically targetted for maternal and infant welfare facilities. It was the women living in Queensland's frontier regions whom the Labor government claimed they wanted to help. It was thought that by providing medical services to these 'noble and splendid women' during a 'very trying period' of their lives,[2] the [white] women on the frontier would do everything possible to increase the population in the State's remote and unprotected regions.

The extent to which these services helped Queensland's pioneering women is the subject of this paper. Did the building of public maternity hospitals throughout the State help the women to give birth more safely and in greater comfort? Did the baby clinics assist mothers in raising healthy children? Were all women to benefit by the ambitious plans of the Labor government's 1922 *Maternity Act*? Using oral evidence of the women's experiences of these government maternal and infant welfare facilities,[3] as well as archival documents and medical inquiries, it will be argued that there were a number of negative aspects to these new healthcare facilities. Only white women will be considered because the Act was specifically designed for them. Despite the pretence of universalism by the Labor government, the Aboriginal women were usually actively discouraged from using these new hospitals and baby clinics.

Most existing Queensland histories of either obstetrics or infant welfare present the changes which took place during the first half of the twentieth century in a positive light. These histories of 'progress and achievement' usually support their arguments by using evidence collected from medical records and the annual reports of health departments.[4] It could be argued that the records of these official groups of middleclass professionals are likely to have highlighted only the changes which showed their work favourably, taking credit for decreases in infant mortality or maternal mortality rates, and blaming others (usually the mothers) if these mortality rates increased. Furthermore, the experiences of women are completely absent from these records. The annual reports of the Infant Welfare Section of the Queensland Home Office reflect these tendencies.[5] By using a wider range of sources and by attempting to consider how the women, for whom these services were designed, used (or avoided using) the government maternity hospitals and baby clinics, I hope to show another aspect of the maternal and infant welfare schemes in the first half of the twentieth century in frontier Queensland.

The use of the concept of 'frontier' is meant only to refer to the relatively harsh living conditions and sparsely populated regions of Northern and Western Queensland. Many historians, such as Russel Ward,[6] have used this concept to suggest that the frontier experience was a dominant influence on the peoples' values and social institutions. It is not my intention to enter into this historiographical debate. The term will be used loosely, referring simply to the general knowledge that Queenslanders who lived in the earlier part of this century were more likely [than other Australians] to be less urbanised and more dependent on unstable or seasonal rural industries for their survival. Together with the tropical climate and their remoteness and isolation from many facilities, it is fair to say that most of these women faced many hardships.

The 1922 Maternity Act

The 1922 *Maternity Act* was an Act to make better provision for the establishment and maintenance of maternity hospitals, baby clinics and for other ancillary purposes. In the second reading, Mr Jones states that the four aims of the Bill are to decrease the death rate of mothers and babies, to increase the birthrate, to increase outback settlement and lastly, to train mothers in how to care for children.[7] Careful planning for the building of maternity facilities had begun in 1920 by the [soon to be appointed] Assistant Under Secretary of the Home Office, Charles Chuter.

Chuter remained the key bureaucrat behind the implementation of the Act over the next fourteen years and was the chief advisor to William McCormack, James Stopford, James Peterson and Edward Hanlon, the four successive Home Secretaries responsible for the administration of the Act. The Act became obsolete with the introduction of *The Hospitals Act of 1936* which made maternity accommodation a part of the State Public Hospital Service.[8]

The Act was to provide, at the government's expense, fully equipped maternity hospitals or cottages which catered for both public [both paying and non-paying] and private patients.

Once completed, the building belonged to the local hospital board who was required to meet the staffing and on-going administrative costs. It was intended that the local people should maintain and manage the institution with the aid of government endowments. However, the local community had to obey a set of administrative rules issued from Brisbane. All women unable to pay were to be provided with free maternity services, but it was left up to the individual boards to determine their ability to pay. Another rule, and the one to cause the smaller, remote regions such as Camooweal and Herberton the most problems, was that the maternity ward must be headed by a double certificate nurse and that the staff were only to work in the maternity section of the hospital. In 1922 double certificated nurses were rare and not easily enticed to live in remote regions. Another rule was that the local doctor or resident medical officer would be remunerated by way of salary for his services to patients in public wards. By necessity, all of these rules were continually broken by various hospital boards.

In regard to the baby clinics, the government provided not only the fully equipped building but also all the expenses to do with the staff and the administration. Unlike the maternity hospitals, the baby clinics did not cost the local community a penny in local taxes or fund raising activities. Active participation by local women's groups was discouraged, with the exception of the Country Women's Association providing rental space in their halls and announcing the arrival of the baby clinic train in their town. The clinics aimed to contact every Queensland mother with the hope of winning her support to follow 'the clinic ways'. To make the job easier, legislation was introduced in 1932 which made it compulsory for all births to be notified to the district registrar within forty-eight hours. The registrar had to then inform the nearest clinic about the birth within twenty-four hours.[9]

Interestingly, the government failed to provide 'hospitals for the treatment of diseases peculiar to women' and I can find no evidence of why this section of the Act was ignored. One reason may have been the unexpected cost of building the maternity hospitals. It was thought that £200,000 was sufficient to meet all the expenses but, by 1925 and with only half of the first part of the programme completed, it was estimated that another £180,000 was required.[10] The funds came from the Motherhood and Child Welfare and Hospital

Fund, which were the profits of the Golden Casket, a State-run lottery. Even though the Home Secretary had full control of the Caskets' profits from 1920 and the power to allocate them as he saw fit,[11] the Labor government had many other demands on its limited resources. Another reason might have been that the intended women's hospitals had no use in directly raising the birthrate of the State, which was one of the major aims of the Act. Two antenatal clinics were started in Brisbane at the Valley and Woolloongabba baby clinics in 1929 but the government was reluctant to do much more other than recommend that the women attend outpatient facilities or their private doctors.[12]

Monuments to Motherhood

The building programme of the maternity hospitals was divided into three parts. Part one focussed on providing for remote regions, particularly those where no maternity hospital beds existed. Places such as Boulia, Emerald, and Winton received five bed hospitals attached to their existing hospital facilities, whilst places such as Mount Mulligan and Millaa Millaa received two bed cottage hospitals with nurses' quarters. Part two aimed at the perceived needs of larger towns such as Innisfail, Cloncurry and Ayr where five or nine bed hospitals were built. Part three provided much larger hospitals for the major cities, including Cairns, Townsville, Mackay and Rockhampton.[13] Within eighteen months, twenty-eight hospitals had been built and after three years there were fifty-seven maternity hospitals, with another ten in the process of being constructed.[14] The government had originally planned to build fifty hospitals and eleven maternity cottages. By 1938, however, they boasted the completion of ninety-four maternity hospitals in all parts of the State. (*See map*)

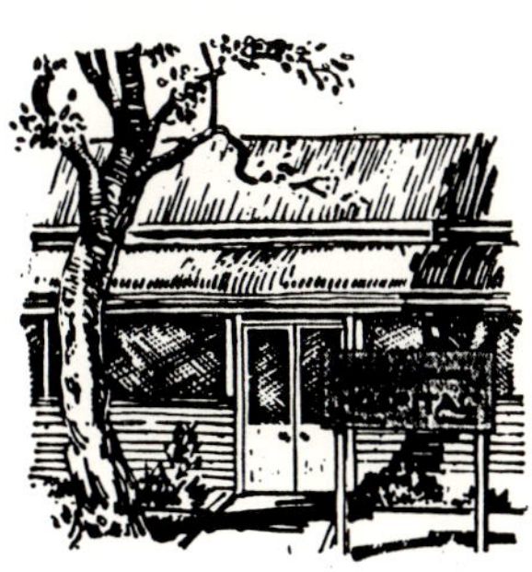

Although the costs of building baby clinics were much cheaper, the government was less enthusiastic in providing these services during the 1920s, especially to women in remote regions. Four clinics had been in existence in Brisbane since 1918, under the supervision of Florence Chatfield, the Superintendent of the Diamantina Hospital for Chronic Diseases. The government did provide Queensland nurses

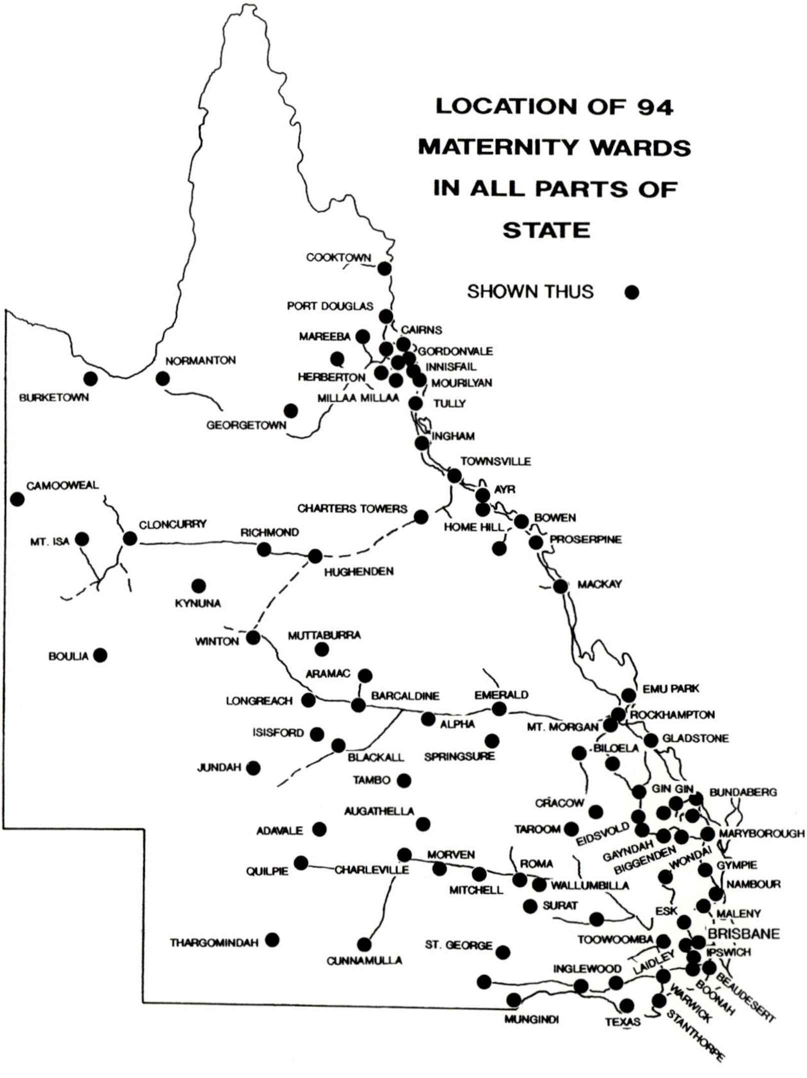

Map of Queensland, showing location of Maternity Wards in all parts of the State.
(Reprinted from Department of Health and Home Affairs, 'At Your Service', Brisbane 1938, p.8)

with a training school for the certificate in Child Welfare from 1924 but by 1927 had only built ten clinics in the major cities such as Rockhampton and Cairns. Expansion of the clinic services really began in the early 1930s, with the establishment of thirty-one clinics and one hundred and four sub-clinics by 1940.[15] There was also a travelling baby clinic railway car, with a staff of two baby clinic sisters, in operation from 1930.

All the Queensland Labor governments between 1915 and 1957 attempted to gain political mileage out of the maternity wards and baby clinics. Most opening ceremonies were gala occasions, often with the whole township attending. Everything possible was done to ensure that the Home Secretary was the guest of honour at the opening, even if this meant delaying the official opening for several weeks after the building had been in use. Grand speeches were made and the building, be it a maternity ward or a baby clinic, was usually described as 'a monument to motherhood', and the Labor government was praised for its foresight and humanitarian outlook towards the women of Queensland.[16] A silver cup, a symbol of achievement, was presented by a Labor politician to the mother of the first baby born in a maternity hospital.

At the opening of the Rockhampton baby clinic in 1923 [the first to be built outside Brisbane], James Stopford made numerous references to the work his government was about to undertake so that Queensland women would raise 'a pure white race of good living citizens'.[17] Eugenist overtones were always apparent in the Labor politicians' speeches and the most frequent slogan was that –

A Native born Child is the State's Best Immigrant.[18]

Probably Hanlon most typified the feelings of his party when he declared in parliament that –

> *... the sick mothers, babies and poor of this State are looked after here by a Labor government better than they are in other parts of this Commonwealth or of the world.*[19]

The extent to which the women agreed with the Labor government's belief is the subject of the rest of this chapter.

The Experiences of Queensland's Women

Queensland women who married and raised children in the 1920s have fascinating stories to tell about their lives. Droughts, floods, depressions and wars were all a part of their lives but the daily problems of hand milking thirty cows before breakfast or washing napkins in a cut-down kerosene tin on an open fire or caring for a child with whooping cough were more immediate concerns for them. Husbands were often absent for long periods, cutting cane or working on the railway and it may have been weeks before they would receive any money to pay off the 'tick' at the local store. However, Mrs Ward, of Bowen, summed up the general feeling of these women: 'We never worried about it. It was a life!'[20]

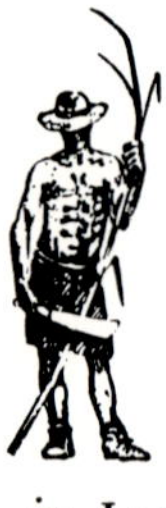

My sample of interviews was taken from all the major towns and cities of the State as well as from some of the more remote areas such as Boulia and Winton. The average age of the interviewee was eighty-four years old and the average number of children per woman was 4. Their first child was usually born in the early 1920s. Most women came from a working-class background where money was scarce, especially after World War I and in the late 1920s. Forty per cent of the women had rarely seen a doctor in their lives before motherhood, and twenty-five per cent had never been to a doctor until one of their pregnancies. All the interviewees had clear memories of their lives and could recall very exact information about their birthing and child raising experiences.

Prior to the government's maternity hospitals, or in areas where one was not built, the women often had a number of choices when they became pregnant. The most typical choice was to 'book in' at the nearest nursing home. These nursing homes served multiple needs: typically the midwife who ran them might also have kept one State child, as well as her own family and perhaps an aged person or a person recovering from a major illness. Eighty per cent of the State's nursing homes had only six rooms or less and could accommodate one or two maternity cases.[21] All the midwives were registered after 1911 but many were not trained if they had been in practice for three years prior to the 1911 *Health Act Amendment Act.*[22] It was not uncommon for the midwife to work together with the local doctor, as Nurse Harrison did in Charters Towers. All the women I spoke to have fond memories of these 'homes away from home'. Mrs Davids came down to Nurse Gregory's nursing home in Cairns in 1916 and nearly seventy-five years later recalls the midwife 'as a lovely woman: gentle and considerate'.[23] The most common praises the women express about these nursing homes are that they were conveniently placed and that the midwives were caring and 'motherly'.

A second choice for the women was to engage a midwife [and sometimes also a doctor] to come to their home. Many midwives with nursing homes also provided these domiciliary services. Women from Charters Towers and Townsville remember Nurse Wells who delivered hundreds of babies in her lifetime. Even though she had never been trained and had delivered her first child using a book, she always wore a light grey uniform with stiffly-starched collar and cuffs and travelled to her patients by horse and sulky.[24] The midwife always stayed with the woman for the duration of the labour and then made daily visits for the next fortnight. It was not uncommon for her to take home the washing or to cook the family a meal. Mrs Campbell recalls Nurse Wells brushing her hair and helping her to get ready for school after she had finished delivering her mother's ninth child.[25] Payments for these services were small and certainly much less than a doctor's confinement charge of between £5 and £10. Once again these midwives and their services are fondly remembered by all the mothers I interviewed.

Women confining in larger towns or cities usually had these services plus a range of small private hospitals from which to choose, such as the Lucina, Hillcrest and Tannachy Private Hospitals in Rockhampton. In six major urban centres there were also older, more established lying-in hospitals [for example, the Lady Goodwin at Rockhampton and the Lady Chelmsford at Bundaberg] where nurses were able to complete their midwifery certificate. Services in the private hospitals were usually more formal than in the nursing homes, and the hospital rules less likely to be broken. Most were run by trained nurses and owned by a local doctor, such as the Lister Private Hospital in Mackay. All women using these private hospitals engaged their own doctor to attend the birth: in fact, it was usually the doctors who recommended the hospital to the woman when she came to the doctor to confirm her pregnancy. If she had the money, she often took the advice as there was a certain amount of prestige thought to be gained by using these hospitals.

The Government's Maternity Hospitals

There is little doubt that these new hospitals and maternity wards did much to change the birthing experiences of Queensland women. In 1928, 16% of all births were in government-provided beds but by 1930 this had risen to 28%.[26] By the end of World War II over 67% of Queensland births were in public maternity beds.[27] One reason for the steady increase in useage was that their existence often forced the closure of the nursing homes and smaller private hospitals in the area, despite the government's assurances that this would not happen.[28] It was common amongst the interviewees to find that their third or fourth baby was born in a government hospital only because their favourite midwife had moved away or retired. With the new beds came new experiences. Mrs Posselt's fourth baby was born in the new maternity facilities at Charters Towers in 1931 and she recalls Matron Henry not allowing her other children to sit on her bed: 'the Matron was very strict and once the quilt was put on it was to remain just so!'[29]

As well as the stricter rules in the wards, the women were the first generation to receive the 'standard' hospital birth, managed and controlled by doctors. Doctors conducted most of the deliveries in these hospitals and came to rely on the maternity cases as an important part of their practices. It is remarkable how similarly the confinements were managed in all parts of the State for public, intermediate and private patients. On arrival at the hospital, the labouring woman was usually given a dose of castor oil, an enema and a shower. She was then put in a room 'to get on with it'. Attention from the nursing staff depended upon how busy they were and the hour of the day. If it was a night-time birth then she was likely to remain alone for much of the time as there was usually only one nurse on duty for the whole maternity section. The doctor was called when a digital examination showed the woman had reached the second stage of labour and she was moved on to a narrow delivery bed. On doctor's arrival, chloroform or ether was usually given and the woman more often than not awoke to find it 'all over'. Forceps deliveries and episiotomies were common: the women have sharp memories of the pain and discomfort of the stitches and the funny marks on their baby's head and their baby's 'bunged up' eyes.

The high incidence of medical intervention in normal deliveries was the subject of many inquiries during the 1920s and 1930s and these inquiries were often conducted by the medical profession. The fundamental issue was that neither neonatal mortality rates nor maternal mortality rates had decreased with the involvement of doctors in obstetrics: if anything, these mortality rates had increased. Doctors trained in the 1920s or earlier at Sydney University only received two weeks' obstetric training where they attended a few lectures and watched and assisted with some births.[30] In 1925 Dr Sydney Morris published his results of an intensive inquiry in New South Wales where he found that –

> *... the parturient woman is most safe when FURTHEST removed from centres of population ...* [where there is] *skilled care and treatment.*[31]

Although he criticises some midwifery practices, his overall impression is that 'the medical profession must assume a considerable amount of responsibility for the unsatisfactory state of affairs'.[32] Top of his list of concerns was the important part forceps was playing in the causation of puerperal mortality and morbidity and he called on medical men to show 'less inclination to indulge in the passing craze of the moment'.[33] Dr Marshall Allan published similar thoughts in 1928 when his investigations showed that –

> *... the majority* [of maternal deaths] *was traceable to some obstetric procedure or failure of aseptic technique during labour on the part of the doctor.*[34]

Queensland did not conduct any major inquiries until after the formation of the Department of Health and Home Affairs in 1935. Dr Raphael Cilento, the first Director-General, was particularly concerned with the number of death certificates showing 'prematurity' or 'birth injury' as the cause of death: these categories accounting for 50% of all infant deaths. In a personal letter to the minister he expressed his concerns:

> *... the diagnosis of 'birth injury' is a blunt and obvious one. It means, in a great majority of cases, injury through casual handling on the part of the attending doctor.*[35]

He also thought that only one in eight deaths diagnosed as 'prematurity' were genuine, the rest being mismanaged births or cover-ups for abortions. Dr Fryberg, whilst undertaking his duties as Inspector of Private Hospitals in 1937, investigated 195 infant deaths in the Brisbane region. Again, obstetric skills came under criticism and he found that the two main reasons for the misuse of forceps were because the doctor was underpaid and therefore delivered in a hurry and secondly, because the patient asked for the doctor to speed up the birth.[36]

It is not possible in this paper to further discuss the various aspects of these inquiries as they cover a very complex set of issues that remain controversial fifty years later. There were many caring doctors who always tried to act in the woman's best interests and there were some nursing homes that deserved to be closed down. Nevertheless, Queensland's *Maternity Act* was unique because women in the more remote regions of the State were given access to hospitalised births and all that this meant in the 1920s. My aim in briefly highlighting these medical inquiries is to argue that, because of the government policy of the day, many Queensland women using these facilities had traumatic birth experiences in comparison to their babies' births in other places. Coupled with the less personal and less 'homely' environment than that of the smaller nursing homes, many women remain confused as to why all the modern facilities did not always make their births easier and their lying-in more comfortable. The women hold little resentment towards their doctors: on the contrary, they continue to hold the doctor in high regard long after his death. However as Mrs Winter, of Home Hill, said of her third baby's birth when she learnt that the doctor 'sort of slipped' using forceps for the first time:

> ***I said to him, 'you could have practised on someone else!'***[37]

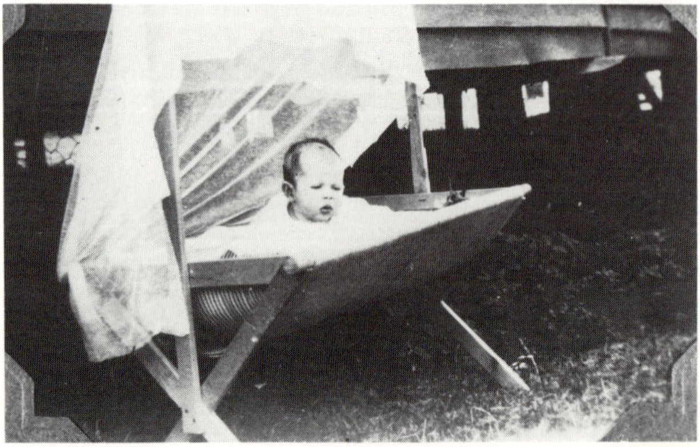

Photograph, courtesy of the John Oxley Library.

Baby's Health: Nation's Wealth

Like so many similar middle-class professional groups in the Western world, Queensland's Infant Welfare Division was intent on educating mothers in the new 'scientific' ways of raising a healthy baby. Officially the new section of the Home Office began in 1926 under the Directorship of Dr Jefferis Turner [who held this position until 1937] but direct government involvement in infant welfare work began in 1918 with the opening of four baby clinics in Brisbane and the training of its staff at the Tresillian School in Sydney. Unlike other similar organisations, however, the Labor government wanted to completely finance and control the baby clinic work and attempts by women's groups to work with the Home Office were generally thwarted, much to the regret of Dr Turner.[38] Much has been written about the impact these new 'experts' had on women and the construction and surveillance of the modern family.[39] In this section my aim is to briefly show some of the women's experiences of the Queensland baby clinics and to show how their evidence contradicts some of the claims made by Turner and others about the department's work.

A close reading of the Annual Reports of the Infant Welfare section [called the Maternal and Child Welfare Section from 1939] reveals the major preoccupations of Turner and the clinic sisters. Turner stated in his 6th annual report that –

> *... our objective is the building-up of a new generation more sound in body and mind and more resistant to disease than the present.*[40]

and this objective was to be primarily achieved through educating women with a better knowledge of mothercraft. Turner was deeply worried about 'the refusal of so many married women to become mothers'[41] and, for those who were mothers, their lack of regular attendances at the baby clinics and antenatal clinics. Underlying these concerns was the belief that the infant mortality rate could be decreased [if not practically eliminated] if all mothers could be brought under their influence and learn 'the clinic ways'.[42] Turner was obsessed with the perceived correlation between the clinic's work and Queensland's infant mortality rate: his eleven annual reports contain forty-seven tables and thirteen graphs to do with infant mortality, as well as long discussions about the statistics. Any reduction in infant mortality was always partially attributed to his staff's work but any increases [as there were in both 1932 and 1933] were blamed on the mothers' ignorance, the lack of antenatal care and on the lack of baby clinics in the remote parts of the State.[43]

The women I interviewed showed a mixture of feelings towards the baby clinics. Considering only those women in my sample who had access to a baby clinic, 42% of the women felt the clinics were a help while they were raising their children and they attended the clinic regularly and attempted to follow most of the advice. Thirty-one per cent, however, were completely aganinst the clinics and would have nothing whatsoever to do with them. Of special interest are the remaining 27% of my sample: women who attended the clinics but who were fairly cautious in their praise of the service. These women did not attempt to follow the clinic advice unless it agreed with their own opinions. Instead, they used the clinic service to have their baby weighed or to meet their friends and have a social outing.

This means that about 40% of the women who attended the baby clinics took little or no interest in making up the clinic formula of 4 ounces of milk and 6 ounces of water and 2 level tablespoons of sugar of milk, or of introducing the baby to only 2 drops of egg yolk at a time, or in following the advice against dummies, or of keeping to a strict schedule of 4 hourly feeds, or of obeying any of the other clinic advice given in the 1920s and 1930s. These women believed that their own views on caring for infants were just as important. Mrs Posselt, who attended the Proserpine clinic, sums up this way of thinking when she claims that –

> *... the clinic sister can tell you things but you've got to use your own judgement, you know, with your kiddies.*[44]

One of the main complaints which the women expressed about the clinics was the insistence on breast feeding. Mrs Winter recalls the Mackay clinic sister spending over an hour with her trying to re-establish her breast milk. She recalls this exercise being a total waste of time but she otherwise enjoyed going to the clinic:

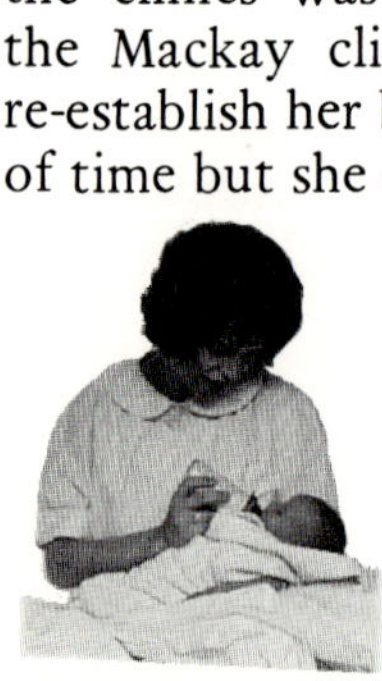

> *... I always tried to take their advice but not as far as feeding the baby because you know what you can do and what you can't do.*[45]

An ex-clinic sister stated that the nurses were taught to advise the mothers to continue breast feeding even if they were only producing a half an ounce of milk per feed because 'weaning a baby was the greatest moral sin that anyone could possibly do'.[46] It was a fine line that women walked in this new 'science' of mothercraft because the other sin was to overfeed the baby, even with breast milk. Mrs James remembers the clinic at Malanda warning her that her baby was too fat from breast milk. Mrs James was very hurt by this comment and she never went back.[47] Many practising doctors, including Dr Felix Arden, the Medical Superintendent of the Hospital for Sick Children, Brisbane, 1938 to 1946, were concerned about the underfeeding of 'clinic babies' and Dr Arden believes that the clinics gave this advice because they were scared that overfeeding caused gastroenteritis.[48]

The evidence of these women suggests that any attempt to correlate attendance figures at the clinics with a reduction in infant mortality is fraught with problems because it is based on the assumption that the women attending the clinics were following the instructions they were given on infant care. While this may have been the case for some mothers, my sample showed this was far from typical. The women may well have enjoyed the company of the clinic sister and the outing to town to meet their friends. Their attendance, however, does not mean that they disregarded their mother's or neighbour's advice. If arrowroot biscuits mashed up with milk kept the baby quiet then they were likely to feed the baby this food in spite of what the clinic sister said. Turner's claims that his staff's work did much to reduce Queensland's infant mortality rate cannot be assumed to be correct if the women's evidence suggests the clinics' limited influence.

Conclusion

The 1922 *Maternity Act* was unique because it provided many facilities to the frontier women of Queensland earlier than in other States of Australia and also because the services were fully funded and controlled by the government. The extent to which the Act made childbirth a safer and more comfortable experience and the extent to which mothers learnt how to care for children using the advice of the new infant welfare 'experts' has been examined in this essay.

Despite the good intentions of the politicians and the administrators, this analysis has shown that the implementation of the legislation was to have some negative consequences.

It was found that many women did not have more comfortable births. Instead they were to have many unpleasant experiences as the 'guinea pigs' in the developing speciality of obstetrics. It was also found that many women did not 'learn' how to care for their children because they felt that they already knew how to look after their families. They may have attended the clinics but many women either ignored all the advice or made careful selections with the advice they chose to follow. The infant mortality rate for children between one month and one year does not appear to have been greatly affected by the Queensland women's belief in their own skills: it had been steadily decreasing since the 1870s, long before the new 'science' of mothercraft was constructed.[49]

Based on the evidence of women who were having babies and rearing children in frontier Queensland in the 1920s and 1930s a very different history can be written. This history does not see the changes in maternal and infant welfare as a movement from ignorance [of the midwives and mothers] to enlightenment. This whig view of medical history where all changes are seen to be progressive is not supported by the women's evidence.

On the other hand, the evidence is not suggesting that the traditional methods of midwifery and child rearing were uniformly better. What I have attempted to show, through a critical analysis of the effects of a specific piece of legislation in the 1920s, is another perspective to the debate on health-care. This analysis suggests that it is important to consider more than the official reports and medical documents before making an assessment of the worth of any new medical practice. The women's stories provide valuable insights into how these changes affected the women in ways neither predicted by the government nor seriously considered by the healthcare professionals.

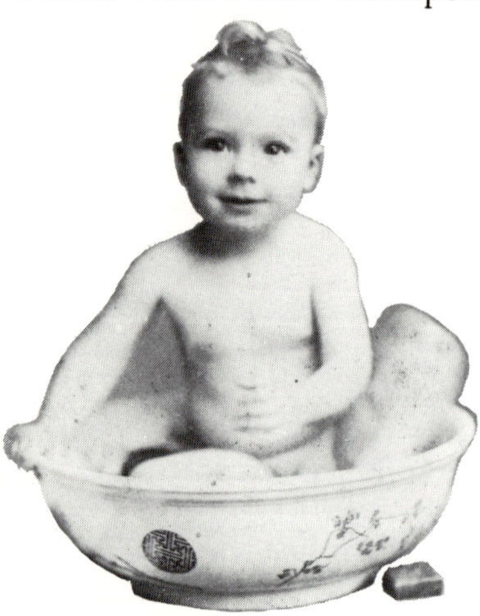

Photograph, courtesy of the John Oxley Library

FEVERS AND FRONTIERS 11

AMBULANCE TRANSPORTATION

Pushing back a Technical Frontier of Patient Carriage

Vincent Little

The development of efficient casualty transport has surmounted a series of logistic and technical frontiers. The history of the evolution of better casualty evacuation is an intriguing study of ingenuity in the service of sick and injured victims. The extra problems of casualty transport in outback Australia have given a distinctive flavour to their solutions.

The history of transport services for the sick and injured began in the First Century BC, when the Romans established a regular military service. Physicians attended the sick and wounded and accommodation was provided for them in Hospitals or *Valetudinaria.* The first record of a body that one might identify as a prototype of a Field Ambulance is that of the Roman Army in imperial times. After that brief appearance of an organised casualty evacuation unit, the concept of systematic casualty retrieval disappeared for one thousand years in the western world. At the end of the Sixteenth Century, in addition to introducing 'Fixed' hospitals, Henry of Navarre (1553–1610) established portable hospitals, called 'Ambulances'.[1] Ambulances, sometimes known as 'Marching' or 'Flying Hospitals', were much in use in the late Seventeenth Century, in the reign of William and Mary; and, as a harbinger of those vehicles needed to traverse terrain of the Australian Outback included springed ambulance wagons. After Marlborough's campaigns they were discontinued until early in the Nineteenth Century, when Sir James McGrigor (1711-1858) persuaded Wellington, during the Peninsula War, to allow him to set up Regimental in addition to Base, Hospitals.

The systematic hand-retrieval and formalised casualty-carriage of war wounded date essentially from the mobile ambulances (*Ambulance Volante*) developed by the French Military Surgeon, Baron Dominique-Jean Larrey (1766–1842). Their worth was first proven in the Napoleonic wars culminating in the awesome morbidity and mortality at Waterloo, in 1815. With the experience of the South African campaign (1899–1902), the British Army included in its order of battle, a Casualty Clearing Hospital. The new unit was to have this novel concept (the carriage of casualties to a definitive point of treatment) integral to it. Thus modern ambulances had their origins in military units.

The rapid collection of casualties has been a major goal since modern surgeons recognised the need to stem the flow of blood as rapidly as possible, and to resuscitate patients. In parallel with resuscitation itself, the transportation of casualties has become progressively sophisticated. Collection has evolved from the most primitive forms of conveyance, which for millennia consisted of carrying or dragging (or any other means that could be devised) to transport the victim home, or to a place of shelter where a physician or surgeon could be summoned; or to the nearest charitable institution or inn where (always for a fee), the victim could be left to recover.

The Nineteenth Century saw the first groundswell of interest to ensure more humane carriage of the sick and injured. The Industrial Revolution sparked many movements of social reform, and many secular bodies undertook worthy social 'causes'. One of those was an evolving civil awareness of the need for compassion for the actuely ill and injured, and their transport. In Victorian times special attention was focussed on this subject, and earlier military experience influenced the wider civil community. As the medical profession became more sophisticated in resuscitative skills, so too did the need to get the doctor quickly to the patient, or the patient more expediently to the doctor. Hospital development then brought about a need for transport to the doctor and then to the hospital, or in some cases directly to the hospital. But by what means? Conveyance by hand-stretcher has existed since recorded time. The Victorian era however saw the beginnings of experimentation with a stretcher which could be part of a vehicle-based casualty transport system.

Hand Stretchers in the Ambulance Context

Litters or hand-carried stretchers are all based on the original military stretchers, of which the famous Mark II pole-and-canvas stretcher is still in current use. Other specialty stretchers include the Stokes Litter, the Neil-Robertson Stretcher, the Jordan Frame, and various types of 'scoop' stretchers.

In Charters Towers, in north Queensland, the specialised Scott-Treacy mining ambulance stretcher was conceived in 1903, whereby an injured person could be safely and comfortably raised from any depth to grass level regardless of the nature of his injuries.

Most modern stretchers are of simple but ingenious design, as it has been found that complexity in construction (no matter how theoretically logical) adds little to their efficiency in practice. One of the most sophisticated stretchers was invented in 1926 by Sister Elizabeth Kenny, of poliomyelitis fame.[2] Sister Kenny had had extensive wartime experience of casualty evacuation and transport. She had been a nurse (and after 1917, a nursing sister) in the No. 1 Sea Transport Section in the period 1915–1918. In the civilian world of outback Australia in 1926, she perceived a need for a sophisticated 'community' casualty stretcher. With her wartime nursing experience, and the encouragement that followed her role in successful management of bush trauma, she conceived the idea of an all-purpose casualty stretcher for rural use. She designed a new stretcher (*Figure 11.1*)

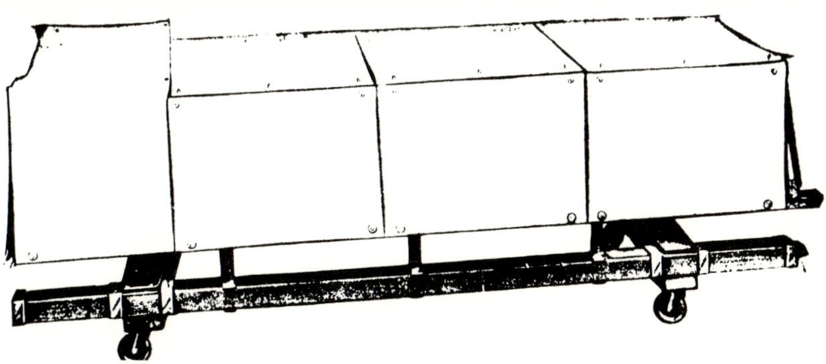

Figure 11.1. The Sylvia Stretcher, invented by Sister Elizabeth Kenny as an 'improved transport stretcher', in 1926.

on her farm at Nobby, in Queensland. The prototype incorporated springs to reduce shock during handling and transport, a box encasement to protect the victim, wheels for mobility, a rigid three-ply base in place of the usual canvas hammock, and places for hot water bottles. The Queensland Country Women's Association assisted greatly in promoting the use of the stretcher, in the special role of a 'community stretcher'. The patent for her 'improved transport stretcher' was accepted by the Commonwealth Government on March 15th, 1927. Patents also were secured in India, the United Kingdom, South Africa, France, Canada and New Zealand.

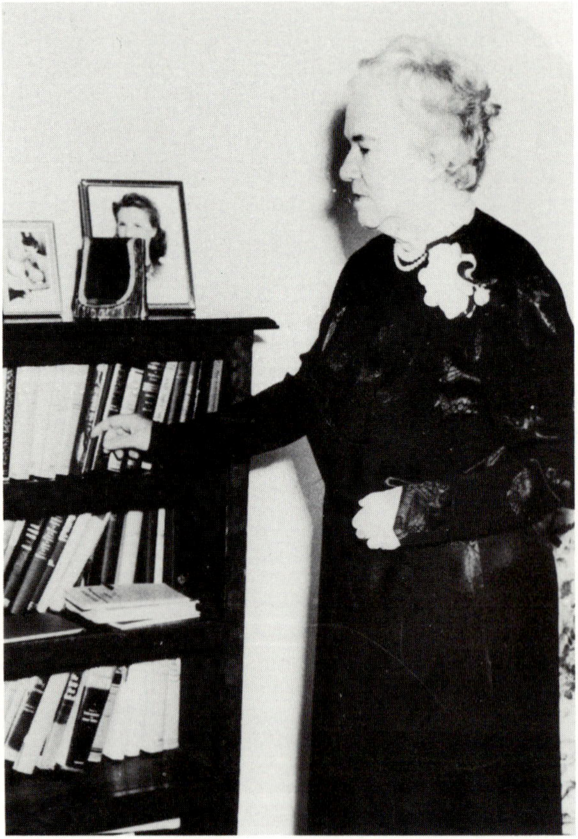

Figure 11.2.

Sister Elizabeth Kenny (1880–1952)

inventor of the Sylvia Stretcher, at her home in Toowoomba, circa 1950.

Photo, courtesy of Mrs Mary McCracken (Sister Kenny's adopted daughter), with acknowledgements.

The new stretcher was accepted by the NSW Branch of the St John Ambulance Association on March 17, 1927; and by the Queensland Ambulance Transport Brigade for use on a trial basis in the same year.

For her invention, Sister Kenny was made a Member of the Institute of Patentees (of London) (*Figure 11.2*), and subsequently was awarded the Certificate of Merit by that body, for her humanitarian invention.

It soon became apparent that the new stretcher had two particular design problems. First, it was too cumbersome and too complicated for routine use. Most casualties do not have complex wounds and do not require special equipment. The box panels for encasing the patient also were difficult to use and, in practice, it was found that it was rare for a casualty on a stretcher to need intrinsic protection from the elements. Shade always is provided by bystanders, and protection from rain and wind is uncommon. Closed ambulance cars were already in use when the stretcher first was sold. The day of emergency transport in exposed vehicles already had passed by the time that the new stretcher was being promoted. Secondly, the complicated stretcher with its crevices and crannies was difficult to clean. The latter was especially a problem if contaminated with blood or vomitus, or with the black or red soil that is so characteristic a feature of much of the Australian Outback.

Sister Kenny's invention, like a number of other complex litters, was a good idea, an innovative response to a specific problem of casualty transportation, and it was unassailably logical. However, it lost money for its manufacturers, and was not accepted by the ambulance and first-aid workers who were to use it. With a certain hint of Heath Robinson complexity, its features were too specific for most occasions when an all-purpose stretcher was required; and the development of better motor ambulances and changed first-aid practices made its special features redundant.

Hand-carried stretchers required strong and willing hands to carry them. In the 1890s, in Brisbane, the bearers who were on night duty were accommodated in the *Courier* Newspaper building. This enabled the bearers on night duty to shelter from the weather; in fact, they slept on rolls of newspaper on the floor amidst the din and industry of newspaper production. Later, blankets were supplied by the Immigration Department and the first uniforms were presented by

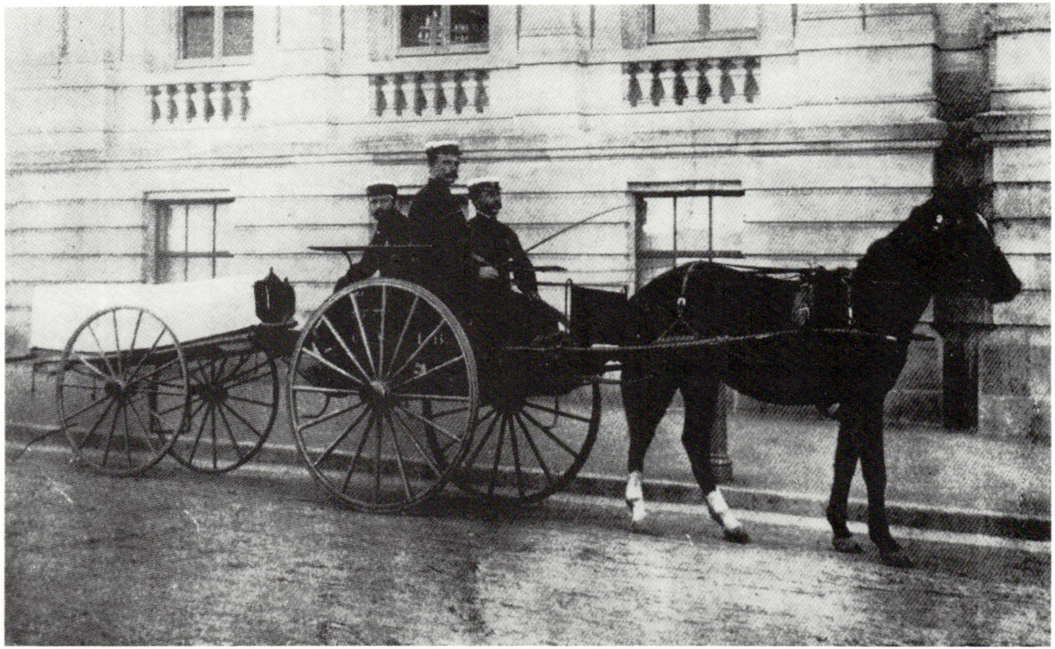

Figure 11.3. Horse-drawn wheeled litter of the Queensland Ambulance Transport Brigade, showing the horse-drawn sulky with three Bearers.
Photo, outside the Treasury Building, Brisbane, at the end of the 19th Century.

Finney, Isles and Company, a Queensland retail store. The first patient transported by the civilian Ambulance Corps in Queensland was carried from Taringa to a private hospital. He was carried on a military stretcher strapped to the shoulders of the bearers. Lady friends of the patient walked alongside holding sunshades over his head to protect him from the hot sun. The bearers trudged along taking turns at carrying the burden together with their meagre supply of first aid equipment. Often when returning from hospital the bearers were allowed to sit on the steps of buses and tow the litter behind them along the roads. Perhaps this universal type of practice gave rise to the next move in the progress of casualty transport – the attachment of wheels to the litter, which facilitated both hand traction and the use of a horse-drawn sulky. (*Figure 11.3*)

In the 1990s new litters have continued to be invented. The latest in contemporary hand-litters is a compact, disposable, inflatable stretcher which can be carried in a small bag. (*Figure 11.4*)

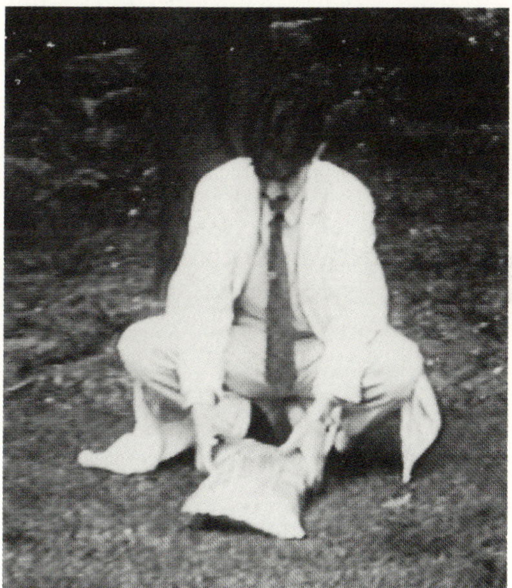

***Figure 11.4.** The St John Compact Inflatable Stretcher, 1990. Compact, inflatable and disposable.*

Hand-Litters on Wheels

A major innovation was to equip the hand-held litter with wheels. Wheeled frames were developed from simple beginnings, and subsequently came to be fitted with springs and later with pneumatic tyres. (*Figure 11.5*)

Since the early days of the hand carriage of patients on stretchers (*see cover*), various State Ambulance Departments adopted a variety of vehicles suitable for the task of transporting patients. These vehicles included Wheeled Stretchers, Sulky and Pony Litter Carriages, Horse-drawn Ambulance Wagons, motor vehicles, rail vehicles and aircraft.

In Queensland, the Civil Ambulance Transport Brigade (CATB) received its first hand stretcher as a loan from the Defence Department. According to the late Superintendent, W.G. Daniel, (one of the early bearers in Brisbane before his appointment to Rockhampton as Superintendent) the first two collapsible stretchers used when the Brigade was housed in the *Courier* Building were paid for by the bearers themselves. Often the bearers removed the stretcher from the litter after conveying a patient to hospital and slept on it. In Brisbane, early in 1893, a hand litter with detachable buggy wheels and movable legs was devised by Captain E.M. Jack and Mr Edward Slaughter. The Federal Carriage Company of Elizabeth Street, Brisbane, built the litter from plans and drawings submitted by Captain Jack, whilst the iron work was made by Mr Slaughter who was a blacksmith. The stretcher had a special spring design developed by Captain Jack and Inspector Warrian to provide a smoother ride for the patient. This vehicle, when completed, weighed three-quarters of a hundredweight, and is believed to be one of the first of its kind in Australia. It was housed in the vestibule of the old *Courier* Building in Queen Street.

The transporting of patients by way of these hand litters was arduous and challenging – no doubt almost as arduous for the patients as well as the bearers when one considers what had to be done to get both patient and litter to the hospital. In bad weather conditions ingenuity often took a hand in achieving the objective, and the anecdotes are many and monumental. Calls involved considerable train travelling. In such cases the stretcher was disconnected from the wheels and placed on the verandah of the railway carriage. The wheels were strapped over the rails, the 'off' wheel usually resting

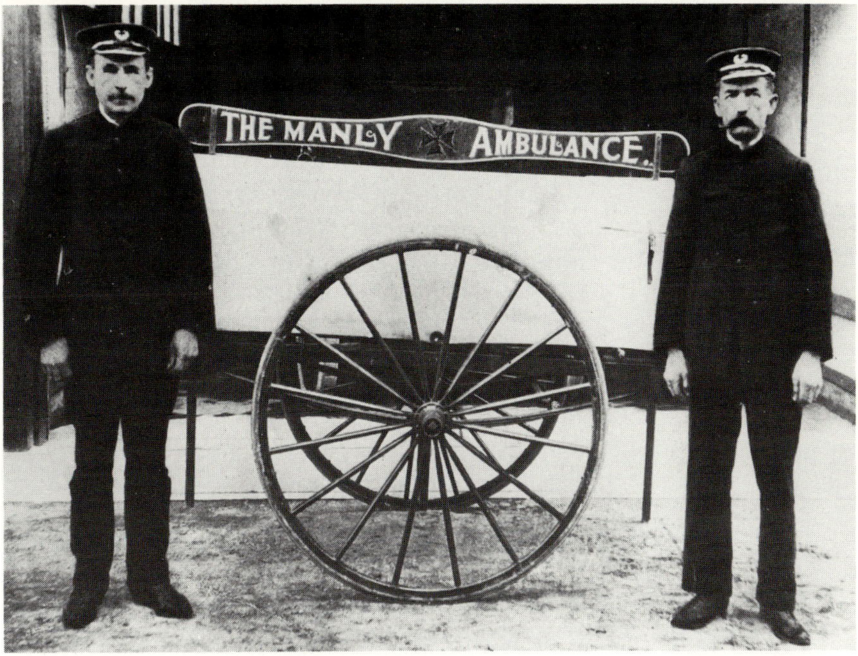

Figure 11.5. 'THE MANLY AMBULANCE'
A wheeled litter used in Sydney in the pre-Federation era. The ambulance bearers, A.W. Wilkinson (left) and J. Ellison, wore a charzcteristic 'lion-tamer' uniform.

for safety on the Westinghouse brake-pipe. After travelling to the casualty, the bearers had to wait for the train to return from the terminus to complete the journey. Arrangements were made with the station master to hold the train for the bearers' return. The job generally took the bearers three or four hours, depending on the distance to the victim, and the train schedules involved. On a hot day the pushing of a litter (with an average 60 kg patient) for four or five miles was strenuous work. In Queensland in 1896, an invalid chair was purchased from penny subscriptions received from children attending the sixty-six Sunday Schools in and around Brisbane. This mobile chair was used to transport patients suffering from asthma and allied troubles and 'was much appreciated'. Ten years later a second invalid chair was donated by convalescents.

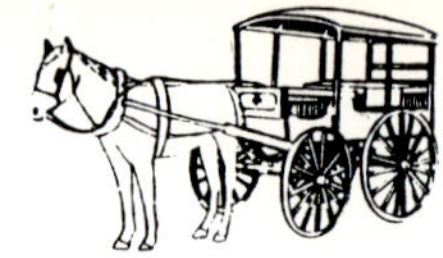

Frontiers for Ambulancemen

In Australia, the first organised civilian ambulance service was formed in 1881. Called an 'Ambulance Corps', the new service was hospital-based.[3] The first such Corps was situated at the Coast Hospital on Little Bay, near La Perouse, fourteen kilometres south of Sydney. We now know that Hospital as Prince Henry Hospital.

The duties of that first Ambulance Corps included the disinfection of infected premises, the removal of patients from infected houses, the making of coffins, and the burying of the dead. The members of the Corps were at first housed in tents on ground belonging to the Police Force at Botany. Following the opening of the Coast Hospital the Ambulance Corps was shifted to special quarters in the grounds adjacent to the Hospital buildings. In the newly formed New South Wales Board of Health, special constables were appointed to guard quarantined houses and arrange for provision of food, new clothing, furniture and bedding to householders during the period of quarantine and disinfection of their premises.

In these services the Ambulance Corps proved to be of great assistance. The ambulance service maintained at the Coast Hospital (Sydney) comprised six ambulances, twelve horses, and four drivers. The annual cost of this inaugural service was £1,136. It was the only complete ambulance service in the Colony and was –

> *... ready at a moment's notice for use in case of an epidemic of infectious disease and it performed in addition to the ordinary services for the Coast Hospital much useful work for the metropolitan hospitals and the Asylums for the Infirm.*

If a medical practitioner from Gordon (a northern suburb of Sydney) for instance, telephoned requesting the urgent admission to hospital of a patient suffering from typhoid fever, the Superintendent of the Coast Hospital rang the ambulance quarters and gave the ambulance man on duty the relevant details. He harnessed the two horses to the horse ambulance and drove down to the Coast area. The nurse on 'Ambulance duty', already alerted, was ready with the emergency medical basket containing necessary drugs and equipment and together they drove in the ambulance the twenty miles to Gordon.

Upon arrival at the patient's home, the nurse helped the ambulance man lift the patient on to the stretcher and load it into the ambulance. She nursed the patient during the exhausting return trip over sandy rutted tracks, down stony inclines and often through creeks which in wet weather became flooded and treacherous. The Harbour was crossed on the horse ferry at McMahon's Point. The construction of bridges allowed the vehicular carriage of casualties to be extended from the central suburbs of Harbour-side Sydney – Pyrmont Bridge (built in 1857), Gladesville Bridge, Iron Cove Bridge and Lane Cove Bridge (1881) allowed horse drawn ambulances to extend their radius of operations further afield.

The Coast Hospital in those days was in every sense an isolation hospital – an oasis of humanity in a wilderness, but one not without its beauty, especially on the coast itself. After such a journey, a casualty would encounter* the stone lodge and entrance gates at the top of the stiff rise and the straight sandy hospital road bordered with the young pine trees. With home in sight the ambulance horses quickened pace and had to be checked by the mechanical braking on the steep descent. In 1903, it was recorded that –

> *... at easier gradients than the old ones,* [there was less] *wear and tear on the horses.*

Wear and tear on the ambulance men was also a consideration. It was a not infrequent occurrence in the early Nineteenth Century for a sick patient to arrive at a hospital on a hand litter, having been pushed four or five miles along lonely sandy tracks. Behind the pre-Federation statistics of the NSW Board of Health Reports lie many epic ambulance journeys and many stories of family tragedy when such journeys were in vain.

Nurses also played an integral part in the early Nineteenth Century ambulance services in Australia. This role continued well into the Twentieth Century. For example, Miss Dickson who started training at the Coast Hospital (Sydney) in 1909 and was Assistant Matron and then Matron in 1936 and 1937, recorded that –

> *... ambulance duty for young trainee nurses was quite an ordeal, this often being the first time they had come into contact with real squalor and destitution.*

*The casualty could not see the approach to the Hospital, as the horse-drawn ambulance was totally enclosed.

She clearly remembered her first call on ambulance duty to a desperately ill child choking with diphtheria, who was rushed to the Children's Hospital where an immediate tracheotomy was performed. On another occasion, with the horses galloping at top speed and the foot bell clanging, the ambulance careered across Pitt Street intersection (in central Sydney) against the traffic policeman's halt sign, taking a seriously ill woman from Church Hill along King Street to Sydney Hospital.

In the pre-Federation era before motorised ambulances had been developed, many roads in Sydney and its suburbs were little more than stony rutted tracks. The road to La Perouse was particularly notorious. For many years it caused much suffering to ambulance patients. Despite repeated requests by the hospital authorities for its repair, little was done until the day the New South Wales State Director of Health had to be taken in an ambulance to the Coast Hospital suffering from an attack of renal colic. Within a very short time, the road had been improved almost out of recognition.

In Queensland the Civil Ambulance Brigade (CATB) was formed in Brisbane in 1892. However, before the formation of the CATB the Queensland Turf Club had engaged the services of a military detachment from the Queensland Defence Force Ambulance Corps. The soldiers attended in military uniform at the principal race meetings. This practice is thought to have originated some three and a half years prior to the formation of the CATB. The members of this Military Ambulance Corps initiated the Queensland Ambulance Service, as a result of a horse-riding accident which occurred at the Exhibition Grounds in 1892. Transport to hospital (in a 'Molly Brown' horse-drawn cab) proved inadequate, and this led to agitation for a better casualty carriage system.

When the new civilian ambulance was formed in Brisbane, donations for the purchase of equipment soon followed. Sir Thomas Brassey of Sunbeam fame donated an Ashford Litter, then the latest design in patient conveyance for bearers on foot. By way of gratitude for the services rendered by the military bearers, Dr John Thompson in May 1889 gave a series of lectures in First Aid and Nursing. These were conducted at the Brisbane School of Arts and certificates were issued to successful examinees. The ambulancemen, mainly unemployed workers, volunteered for duty on Saturdays and holidays under the command of a non-commissioned officer. Free passes were granted for railway travel and entry to the racecourse, where they were given access to all parts of the grounds. When necessary,casualties were driven to hospital in a two-horse military wagon, the drivers being members of the permanent artillery from the Petrie Terrace Barracks. For this service the driver was paid 6s.0d (60 cents) and the NCO 7s.0d (70 cents) – with a first class dinner thrown in for good measure.

Horse-Drawn Ambulances

The 1890s saw the evolution of a further milestone in casualty transport, the development of the sulky-litter. This system was characterised by a single horse vehicle, with the litter detachable and towed separately (*Figure 11.3*). This system was very unsatisfactory and did not improve the lot of the patient. It did, however, constitute one very important advance in that it transported the bearers to the patient, thus preserving their energies for the return journey.

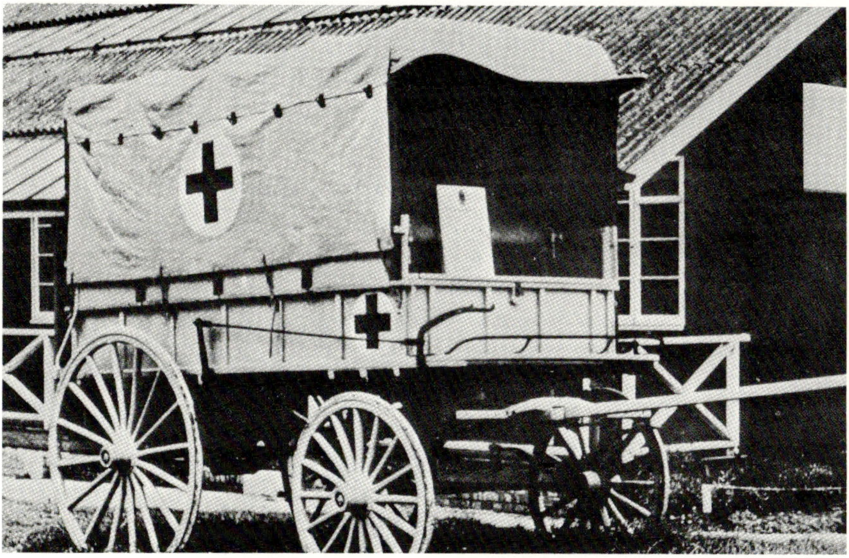

Figure 11.6. A Military horse-drawn ambulance of the wagon type. First used in the South African War (1899–1902). Photo courtesy of the Forces Press (Naafi), with acknowledgements.

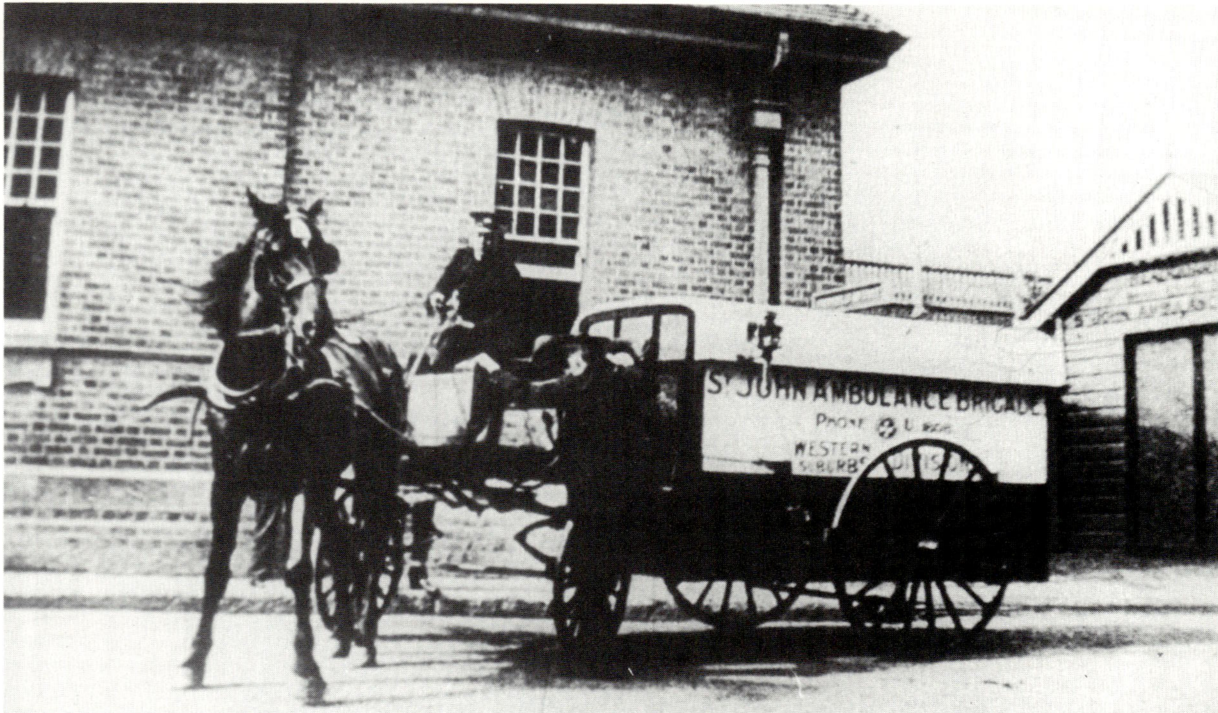

Figure 11.7. *A St John horse-drawn wagon ambulance at the turn of the twentieth century.*
Photo, Summer Hill Railway Station, Sydney, Australia.
The author served as an Ambulance Officer at the Summer Hill Ambulance Station in the mid 1960s.

The sulky provided the bearers with a means of transport to the case, but the patient was then pushed to hospital on the litter, after which the bearers returned immediately to the ambulance centre for further similar duty. At times the men were completely prostrated owing to the sheer exhaustion consequent on the extraordinary physical exertion entailed in the carriage of the patient.

Early in 1897 – five years after the foundation of the Queensland Ambulance service – the first of the white ponies and sulkies, soon to be well known at Brisbane and other State centres, were purchased. In 1904 there was a further change in ambulance transport ideas. It was generally agreed that, notwithstanding the value of the sulky-litter, it had to give way under altered conditions to the field wagon, which had been developed in the preceding decade, in the Royal Army Medical Corps. (*Figure 11.6*)

The wagons proved to be a great boon and in the country districts of Australia they increased the distance of effective operations, the bearers being able to travel over many miles of rough roads without inconvenience to the patient. The field wagon relieved much of the onerous work for the staff under inclement weather conditions and the patient had more protection, his environment being partly controlled for the first time. (*Figure 11.7*)

By 1907, ambulance wagons were being used for the retrieval of patients over long distances in the bush, the first of such services in Queensland being at Charters Towers and Cairns.

Motor Ambulances

Motor ambulances were first introduced in the period just prior to 1908. Their practical use depended on the invention of springs, and the protection these gave to the casualty. Springs ensured a smoother ride than the bone-shaking, jolting passage which was the lot of the victim being carried prior to the Twentieth Century. Countless wounded patients have cause to bless the success of the spring, especially the shock absorbers and pneumatic suspension of the first motorised ambulance vehicles. The doctrine of speed versus patient stability currently remains an issue of considerable debate.

In May 1908, the first motor ambulance was put into use in Queensland. The car had a 10–16 four cylinder Clement Talbot chassis. The body was built in Brisbane, and was specially designed to carry a wheeled litter (*Figure 11.8*).

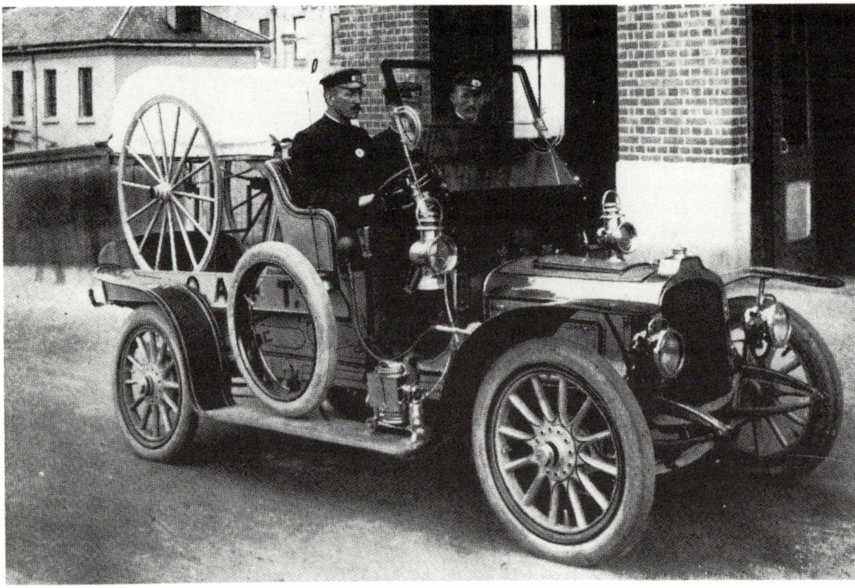

Figure 11.8. An early Q.A.T.B. motor ambulance of the first decade of the twentieth century. The three bearers rode in the front, with a hand-drawn wheeled litter carried on the rear chassis tray. Photo, in Brisbane, of a Q.A.T.B. Clement Talbot ambulance, circa 1908.

The car was not intended to transport a patient, but to carry bearers and litter to the scene of the accident. Subsequently other motor ambulances were introduced, not only at the Brisbane centre, but at other centres throughout the State, provision being made to transport the patient and thus dispensing with the pushing of litters.

Centres throughout Australia tended to modify motor vehicles according to local tastes and needs. (*Figure 11.9*)

In Rockhampton, Queensland, the first motor ambulances were supplied by the local agent for the Ford Motor Company, the late Theo Kingel, who was for many years a member of the Rockhampton centre ambulance committee, and was the latest standard four-cylinder 30 horse power car fitted with oversize Barnett Glass tyres and tubes. The body was built by the late Mr M.J. Ryan, a well known coachbuilder in Alma Street, Rockhampton.[4]

The Rockhampton wagon was capable of carrying the driver and an assistant bearer and two patients, one patient at full length and the other in a reclining position. Inside the wagon rests were fitted to hold two collapsible stretchers, with springs and rubber wheels. The entrance was at the rear by means of a step which folded up when the wagon was in motion. The hood was of American Duck, with side blinds of the same material, which could be raised or lowered as required. The wagon interior was equipped with electric light, a copper water tank and two cupboards for first aid material, and was painted yellow, with the Brigade sign on both sides and a red cross in a circle on the blinds.

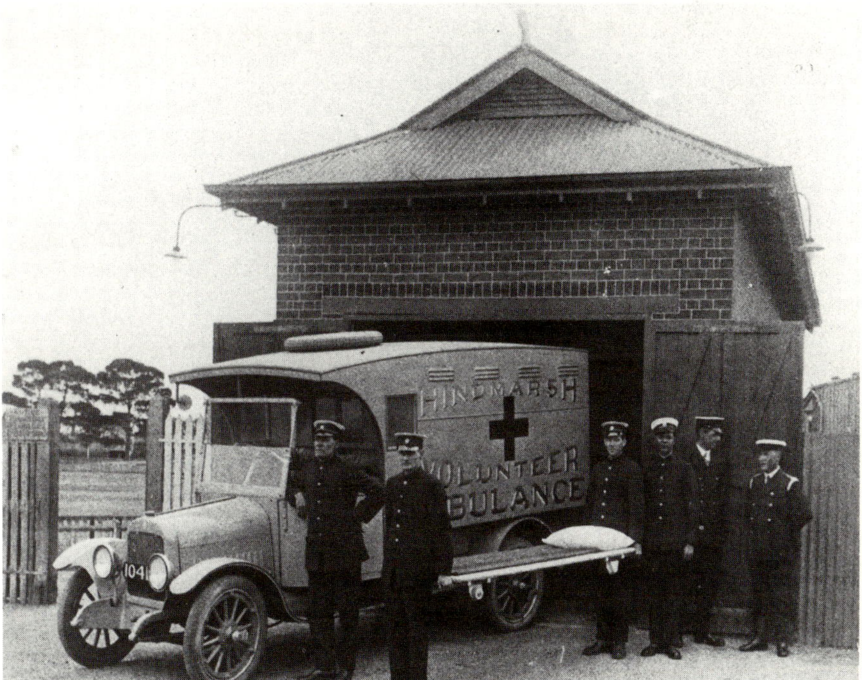

Figure 11.9. The motor ambulance in service in Hindmarsh, South Australia, circa 1925.

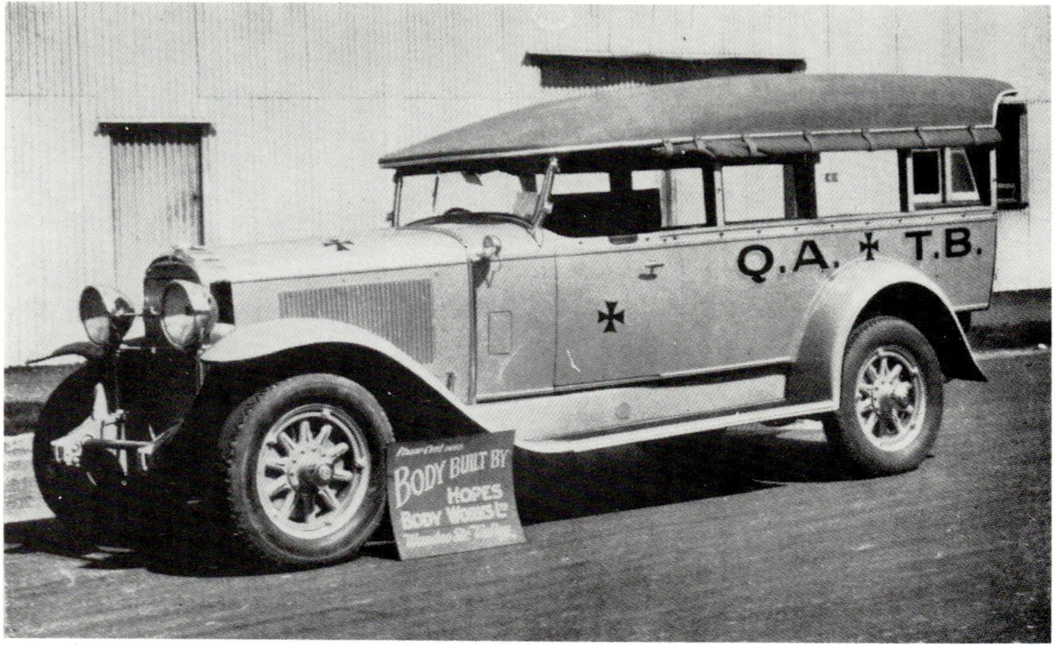

Figure 11.10. The evolution of modern motor ambulance transport.
A Buick 'Silver Anniversary' modified by the Hope Engineering Company of Fortitide Valley, Brisbane. This model featured the Hope Patent Roller Curtain, appropriate for vehicles operating in the heat of the Australian Outback. Photo, at the Mt Isa Q.A.T.B. centre.

The Rockhampton vehicle was somewhat on the lines of those in use in Brisbane and Mackay, but the centre's aim was to provide a conveyance to be 'the last word in comfort'. By 1914, it was certainly the very latest in accident transport vehicles. This trend of continual improvement in design was seen in many centres throughout Australia. (*Figures 11.10 and 11.11*)

A further development in motor ambulances was the invention of devices that would enable the motor vehicle to run on railway lines, so necessary in outback Australia where there were no roads, or when such things as floods had precluded the use of roads for casualty transport. Later a vehicle was developed which could travel on railway lines of different gauges. Called a motor 'quad', it had the approval of the Commissioner for Railways for travel on Queensland Railways, and had a gauge changing device so that it could be quickly transferred by one man from the railway gauge to the tramline gauge in the northern sugar districts. Some of these vehicles travelled considerable distances; for instance, one built at the Ipswich Railway Workshops for the Dalby centre in 1917 travelled 60,000 miles before it was replaced ten years later. One was even built privately for the Charters Towers centre by Douglas Webb, a native of the town and nephew of the then Ambulance Superintendent.

The Chinchilla ambulance jeep proved invaluable in many cases. During floods people marooned in leaking boats were rescued by this means. It was frequently used to rescue people and to carry medical supplies and food in emergencies, and proved its worth many times in travelling along washed out roads and through flooded country.

The Kidson ambulance sub-centre in the North also made history in 1916 by using an ambulance boat to carry provisions, including flour and potatoes, across the Cooperfield River in high flood to residents sorely in need of foodstuffs.

Today the use of rotary wing and fixed wing aircraft as ambulances has now developed into a very sophisticated means of safe and effective patient management, reducing the need for long hours of road or rail transportation.

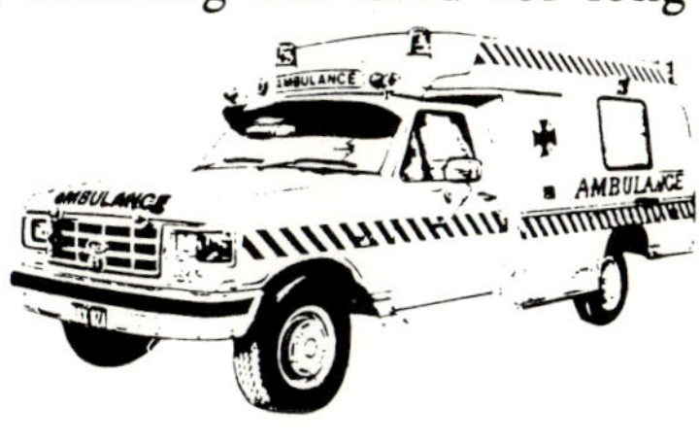

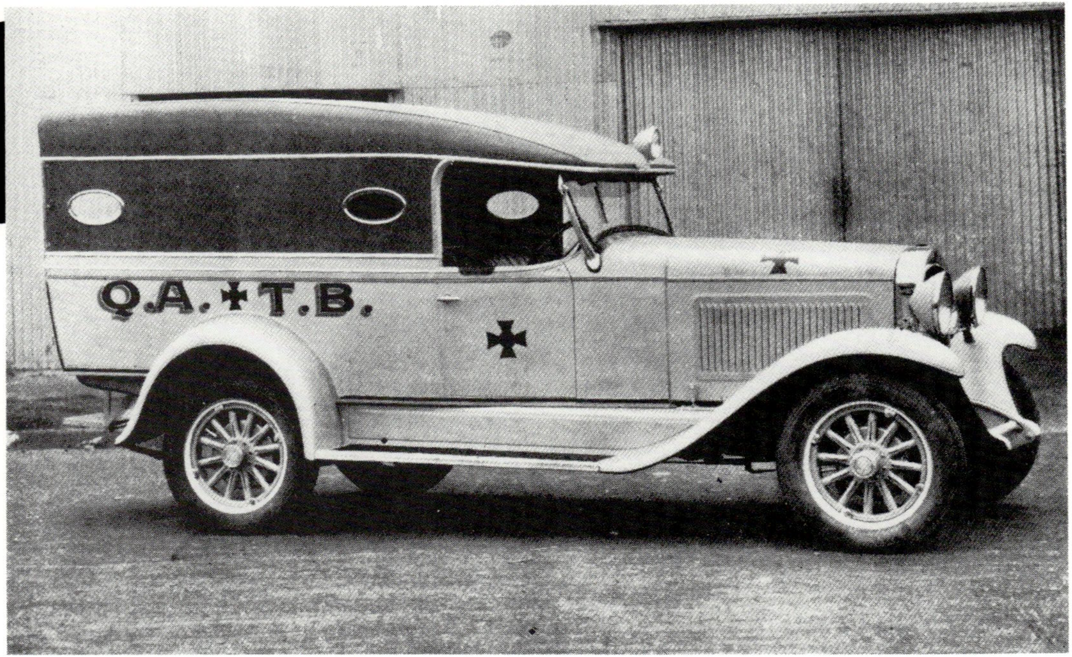

Figure 11.11. The evolution of modern motor ambulance transport.
A 'Whippet Six' chassis modified as an 'Open Tourer Front Fixed Side Type' ambulance, of the 1930s.
Photo at the Q.A.T.B. centre, Caboolture, Queensland.

FEVERS AND FRONTIERS 12

"A CHANGE IS AS GOOD AS ..."

Changing Frontiers

Berenice Wright

Health support institutions evolve at the changing frontiers of community attitudes. Much can be learnt from an appraisal of individual case studies of the rise and fall of individual sanatoria, hospitals and welfare homes. One account – the battles over a children's orphanage in Mackay, Queensland – teaches much about the politico-sociological frontiers of the past.

St Joseph's Orphanage, Merara, via Mackay, was established by the remarkable Breten priest, Father Pierre-Marie Bucas. Father Bucas had been appointed the first resident Catholic Parish Priest of Mackay in August, 1869. A few months later, he began negotiations to bring to Mackay some members of the congregation of the Sisters of St Joseph of the Sacred Heart, an Order of religious sisters which had been founded in South Australia only a few years previously. The special work of the Sisters was the education and care of the poor, and they were responsible for the establishment in June, 1871, of the first formal school in Mackay.[1]

After nine years of settlement, Mackay was declared a Municipality on September 22, 1869.[2] Founded as a port for a pastoral district, it was hardly a wealth township; instead it was on the threshold of becoming a thriving sugar producing area, although the development of the sugar industry was still in the embryonic stage.

It would seem from the correspondence of Father Bucas in 1885 that poverty existed in the township and the surrounding district. The natural drift of the poor was near to the priest and to the sisters who were accommodating orphaned and abandoned children from the time of their arrival in Mackay. (Their convent was located on the bank of the Pioneer River on the western side of Gregory Street, in the 'town house' of the generous T.H. Fitzgeralds of Alexandra plantation. All that remains to mark the site – allowing for river erosion – is a stand of ancient fig trees between St Patrick's College and St Patrick's Church.)

Father Bucas demonstrated a deep compassion for the Islander (Kanaka) and aboriginal people. He had been associated with pastoralist-philanthropist G.H. Bridgman in the establishment of Queensland's first aboriginal reserve at Mackay. This reserve, a strip of land three miles wide by eight miles deep, extending inland from the estuary of Sandy Creek, was gazetted in 1871. Bucas and Bridgman planned another reserve at Cape Hillsborough.[3]

Between July 1876 and December 1877, Bucas selected a total of 2880 acres of land in the area of Shoal Point, again with the idea of establishing an aboriginal reserve. It is noteworthy that several adjacent portions were taken up by Bridgman. The land selected at Merara (later named Seaview, and, in more recent times, Bucasia, after the pioneer priest) was classified as second quality grazing land.[4] Much of it was mangrove swamp, though a long strip was sand-dune country edged by a fine long beach, and is today (1990) prime residential and tourist real estate.

The call on the Sisters to care for increasing numbers of children led Bucas to reconsider developing the Merara land not as an aboriginal reserve, but as a permanent site for the Orphanage. The date of the latter's establishment is not clearly recorded, but it was certainly inhabited by early 1879, as a contemporary account of an accidental death of a workman, Martin Lorenz, while fencing, indicates.[5]

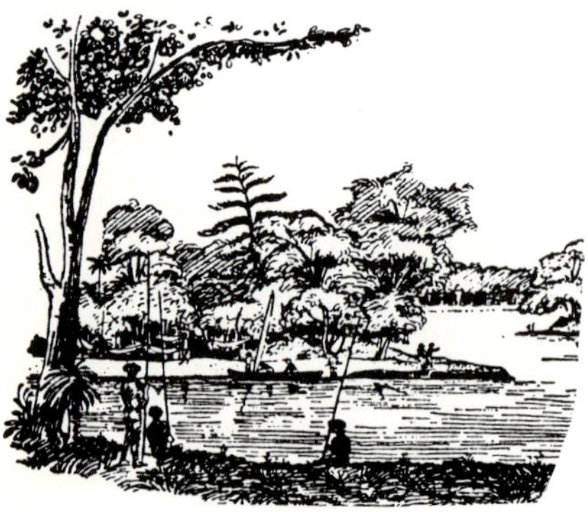

By the time of the first available Report of the Inspector of Orphanages (1882), St Joseph's Orphanage at Merara, Mackay, was under the control of the Sisters of Mercy, the Sisters of St Joseph having withdrawn from most of their Queensland establishments in late 1879 because of a dispute with Bishop Quinn, then Catholic Bishop for the whole of Queensland, involving the jurisdiction of the Order.

The 1882 Report nominates three State Orphanages – the Diamantina, Brisbane, with its Infants' Home, and the Townsville and Rockhampton Orphanages – and two under Catholic auspices, at St Vincent's, Nudgee (founded in 1866) and St Joseph's, Mackay. All were registered under *The Orphanages Act of 1879*.

Apart from the report of a bazaar held in 1879, the Mackay Orphanage did not become a newsworthy item again until April 18, 1885, when a small paragraph in the *Mackay Mercury* alluded to a 'disturbing rumour' that the Orphange was to be removed to Rockhampton. A reiteration of the rumour occurred in the edition of April 29, 1885, with threat of action if such a move were contemplated. Little did Mackay residents know that by then, the decision to close St Joseph's Orphanage had been well and truly made!

In its 130 year history, Mackay has known several notable confrontations with government officialdom. One such clash with authority occurred quite early when, in 1885, the Government Medical Officer, with the concurrence of the Catholic Bishop of Rockhampton, decided that an orphanage which had been conducted by Catholic authorities for several years, should be closed for health reasons and re-established in a more salubrious environment near Rockhampton.

Consternation among the citizens of Mackay and district at the loss of 'their' orphanage was rife, and undoubtedly inflamed by the realisation that the decision was a *fait accompli* before they were even vaguely aware that the issue was under discussion.

One of the chief characters in the drama associated with the closure of St Joseph's Orphanage, indeed the instigator of the whole affair, was Dr Arthur Henry Cutfield, who had been appointed Government Medical Officer in 1884.[6] At the time of his appointment, the Resident Medical Officer at the Mackay District Hospital, Dr Robert McBurney (who had been in charge since the hospital's inception in 1871) took a well-earned year's holiday in England. Perhaps Cutfield saw himself as the proverbial 'new broom', since his first twelve months seemed to teem with improvements in various areas of health care and management. Meetings of the Hospital Committee and the Hospital Subscribers' Committee reported tightening of previous laxity, and Dr Cutfield, with the help of Dr Clarkson, assumed responsibility for the establishment of a separate Islander Hospital within the Mackay District Hospital Reserve.

Another area to cause concern to Dr Cutfield was the precarious state of health of many of the inmates of St Joseph's Orphanage. In a letter to Mr Anderson the Under Secretary of the Department of Public Instruction, dated October 27, 1884 (a full six months before the story 'broke' in the press), Cutfield commented that four children, aged between nine and eleven years, 'though of sufficient age and size, are physically unfit for service'. Cutfield was obviously unaware that the provisions of the *Orphanages Act of 1879* prevented the hiring of children under the age of twelve years, the previous limit having been eight years of age. His letter continued –

> *... I have also to report that a large number of the children have an extremely unhealthy appearance, and several suffer or have suffered from an affection of the heart produced by debility; I believe them to be suffering from malarial disease produced by the situation of the Orphanage, which lies between a swamp and the sea – the swamp, in which there is almost always stagnant water, being immediately behind the buildings.*

He further suggested that all children be brought to him for a medical examination prior to admission.

Mr Anderson immediately informed the Catholic Bishop of Rockhampton, the Most Rev. Giovanni Cani (in whose Diocese the Orphanage was situated) who added courteously –

> *... I may be allowed to remark that for years past the said buildings have been in the present locality, which has not been considered objectionable except by Dr Cutfield ... Probably the long drought may be the cause of the unhealthy appearance of the children.*

Dr Cutfield carried out monthly inspections of the Orphanage together with Mackay's Police Magistrate, Thomas Mowbray.

Following the inspection of January 23, 1885, Mowbray painted a very gloomy picture indeed, giving instances of the condition of specific children, and quoted Dr Cutfield's summation of the state of one young girl –

> *She is a very good type of Orphanage child, suffering from peculiar pallor, breathlessness and heart disease.*

Mowbray could cast no aspersions on the Sisters' treatment of the children, but commented –

> *... there is reason to believe that to the situation and the locality of the premises is the mischief alone attributable.*

Dr Cutfield himself reported on the same visit –

> *... the general health of the children remains extremely unsatisfactory, a large number of them suffering from a peculiar intense state of anemia, which I can only ascribe to malarial poisoning.*

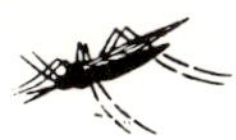

On the siting of the buildings, he commented –

> [They] *are situated on a low sandy ridge, separated from the sea in front by a strip of forest, and closely surrounded on all the other three sides by a large swamp, the surface of which is only a few feet lower than the ground on which the Orphanage buildings stand.*

> *It is easy to see, then, that if this swamp be malarious the inhabitants of the Orphanage must be exposed to the malarial poisoning in an intense form.*

> *I could not find, on enquiry, that any of the Sisters had suffered in a similar manner to the children, but it is a well-known fact that the malarial poisoning is most dangerous at night, and that it does not extend far from the surface of the ground in a vertical direction; now, the sleeping apartment of the Sisters is the only portion of the buildings not situated on the ground, being placed at a considerable height over the children's dining place and this, I think, would go far to explain their immunity from the disease as compared with the children, whose power of resistance to malaria would be much less, and who sleep at a height of two feet from the ground.*

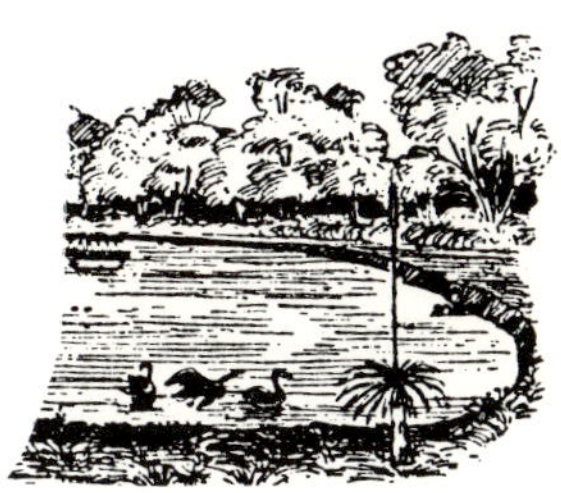

The reaction of Government officials to the reports was to recommend that the Orphanage be closed and the children transferred to St Vincent's Orphanage, Nudgee. Bishop Cani, however, suggested another solution – that a suitable site be found near Rockhampton, possibly for no other reasons than that the Mackay Orphanage was now under his jurisdiction (the Catholic Diocese of Rockhampton having been founded in 1852) and that the Sisters of Mercy who were in charge of the Mackay Orphanage were now a separately constituted congregation from those at Nudgee in the Brisbane Diocese.

Within a few days, the Bishop had selected the new location –

> *... high land along the Central Railway, twelve miles from Rockhampton and a short distance from Stanwell ... It has been free from fever, even during the late epidemic at Rockhampton. I could not desire a more suitable place.*

Approval for the new location was readily given by Government authorities.

The reaction in Mackay was swift, with a public meeting of protest directing the Mayor, Mr John Harney, to request verification of the rumours.[7] The Mayor's blunt telegram received an equally blunt and quite erroneous reply –

> *The removal of St Joseph's Orphanage to Rockhampton is the spontaneous act of Bishop Cani.*

This was rebutted a few days later, stating the concurrence of the Government officials and Bishop Cani.

A further result of the initial public meeting was a letter from Mr M. Hume Black, MLA, Member for Mackay, asking if the Orphanage was to be shifted, and suggesting that it remain at least in the district, since it enjoyed private benefaction. A second meeting rallied the 'Catholic Body' in protests on Sunday, May 10th ("The better the day, the better the deed" was the rallying cry),[9] which led to inspection by the Mayor, Dr Cutfield, and the Police Magistrate (Mr Mowbray), and a further request that the Orphanage be left at Mackay, the inhabitants being willing to fund its removal 'to a better site'.

Bishop Cani was equal to any challenge, and remained undeterred in his decision to proceed with the Stanwell institution already under construction. Further pleas from Mayor Harney,

Mr Black and even Dr Cutfield that a better site had been found at Mackay, seemed only to strengthen the Bishop's determination.

The Report of the Inspector of Orphanages, Mr Charles Horrocks, for July, 1885, is detailed and most favourable to the Sisters of Mercy in their conduct of the institution, in every respect. The death rate had, however, increased, and the Health Report stated in part –

> *They* [the children] *were nearly all in good condition and spirits but their faces were pale and sallow, and those marked on the list were decidedly delicate.*

Of the increase in mortality, he commented –

> *The Sisters state that these children were in a very emaciated state when they were admitted, and ought, properly speaking, to have been sent to hospital.*

As late as August, 1885, a delegation on Mackay Council matters, including the Orphanage issue, was sent to Brisbane. Premier Griffith declared that he was willing to grant a new Orphanage licence to Mackay, provided that a 'religious sisterhood' could be found to conduct it. The delegation, with fresh hope, approached Bishop Robert Dunne, the Catholic Bishop of Brisbane, for help. Dunne telegraphed Bishop Cani, but the reply must not have been favourable, as Dunne's shrewd and kindly advice to the two men was 'not to go to Rockhampton'. In reporting back to Mackay Municipal Council, the delegates were forced to admit defeat.

The last word on the file of correspondence rested with Father Bucas, labouring that year in North West Queensland. Bucas agreed with a comment from Sister M. Augustine Hardiman (who had been in charge of Mackay Orphanage from February 1880 until December 1884) that little had been done for the Orphanage by the people of Mackay. He stated that he had paid the rents on the land out of his own means, and that he had provided 'every article in connection with the Orphanage', except for eight head of cattle.

Because of the outcry that the nucleus of a charitable institution was being formed in 1870 which might develop and saddle the parish 'with uncalled-for responsibilities', Father Bucas said that an undercurrent of opposition had existed against the Orphanage. The press commented that Father Bucas' remarks would not find favour with the people of Mackay.

AGE (Years)	SEX	CAUSE OF DEATH	DURATION OF FINAL ILLNESS	ATTENDING DOCTOR	DATE LAST SEEN BY DOCTOR	DATE OF DEATH
4	M	Consumption of Glands	5 months	Dr Swayne	21. 7.1881	2. 8.1881
2	M	Croup	–	–	–	26. 4.1881
5	F	Continued Fever	18 days	Dr E.H. Byrne	15. 7.1881	18. 7.1881 (Buried Mackay Cemetery)
5	M	Dysentery	10 days	Dr R. McBurney	27. 2.1882	3. 3.1882
12	F	Disease of the Heart	6 months	Dr R. McBurney	27. 2.1882	25. 3.1882
4	F	Disease of the Heart of long standing	2 hours	Dr R. McBurney	2. 6.1883	2. 7.1883
4	M	Disease of the Heart	18 months	Dr R. McBurney	2. 6.1883	8. 7.1883
1	M	Mumps and teething	–	Dr A.H. Cutfield	–	5. 3.1884
11	M	Spinal Disease	1 yr 9 mths	Dr A.H. Cutfield	7. 6.1884	8. 6.1884
9		Lingering Consumption	12 months	Dr A.H. Cutfield	7. 6.1884	13. 6.1884
6	F	Heart Disease	–	Dr A.H. Cutfield	11. 7.1884	19. 7.1884
9	M	Heart Disease	14 days	Dr A.H. Cutfield	30.11.1884	7.12.1884
3½	M	Dysentery	1 month	Dr A.H. Cutfield	30.12.1884	2. 1.1885

AGE (Years)	SEX	CAUSE OF DEATH	DURATION OF FINAL ILLNESS	ATTENDING DOCTOR	DATE LAST SEEN BY DOCTOR	DATE OF DEATH
3	M	Dysentery	1 week	Dr A.H. Cutfield	22. 1.1885	27. 1.1885
9	M	Consumption	–	Dr A.H. Cutfield	–	6. 2.1885
2	F	Dropsy	–	Dr A.H. Cutfield	28. 2.1885	29. 3.1885
6	M	Dropsy	12 months	Dr A.H. Cutfield	25. 5.1885	2. 6.1885
6	M	Dysentery	3 weeks	Dr A.H. Cutfield	–	10. 8.1885
5	M	Paralysis	3 days	Dr A.H. Cutfield	30. 9.1885	2.10.1885
8	M	Malarial Anaemia	9 months	Dr A.H. Cutfield	8.11.1885	16.11.1885

FOOTNOTES:

All the children listed died and were buried at the "Cemetery at Mackay Orphanage", with the exception of one whose death occurred at the District Hospital, and who was buried in Mackay Cemetery. No indication remains of the actual site of the Orphanage buildings or of the Cemetery itself.

There are no records of deaths of "Orphanage Children" noted prior to 1881. It is probable that deaths occurred, but they would be difficult to extract from an official record if, for instance, the death/s occurred in the District Hospital, and no residential details or other clues were given.

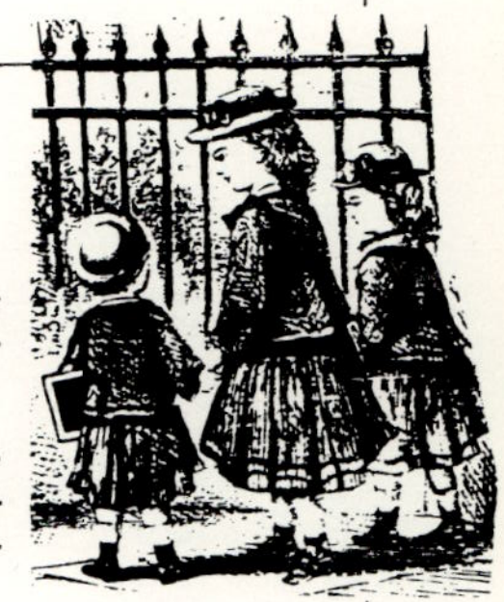

DEATH REGISTER FROM ST JOSEPH'S ORPHANAGE, MERARA, VIA MACKAY, QUEENSLAND
(See Note 12.11 in Notes and References)

A sad little paragraph in the *Mackay Mercury* of December 23, 1885, completed the Mackay portion of the story –

> *By the 'Yaralla' on Sunday last, the children, who had been removed from St Joseph's Orphanage, left for Rockhampton, and the last scene of this unpleasant business is over.*[11] *A few of the children who have gone south are doomed to die within the next few years, but it is hoped that change of air will restore many of them to health.*

Then, on a practical note –

> *On the Estimates, there is 12,000 pounds for the removal of the Orphanage buildings, and, if this money is to be utilised, it is time steps were taken to push the matter forward.*

In the Register of the Merara Park Orphanage (St Joseph's Orphanage, Neerkol, Rockhampton), the following was recorded –

> *Why admitted:*
> *Merara Orphanage was becoming more unhealthy every year, through its position. The children grew delicate so our Bishop, Rt Rev. Dr Cani, built this Orphanage to receive them. Fifty-seven of them came here on 22nd December, 1885. Of that number, only five (5) are under State Control at present time.*

Unfortunately, the names of only nine children are registered against the admission date of December 22nd, 1885. No state of health is recorded, though it is interesting to note that all lived to be discharged at dates which would have made them eligible for service in the wide world, thus vindicating the action of Dr Cutfield, supported by Bishop Cani. The Orphanage was to become the special care of the Bishop, and it is recorded that every day he was in Rockhampton, he would take a 'constitutional' out to Neerkol to visit the orphans.

St Joseph's Orphanage, Neerkol, went from strength to strength, enduring for a further ninety years until changes in the care of orphaned, abandoned and neglected children led to its closure in 1975. It now serves a wide area of Central Queensland as a Conference Centre, still under the care of the Sisters of Mercy.

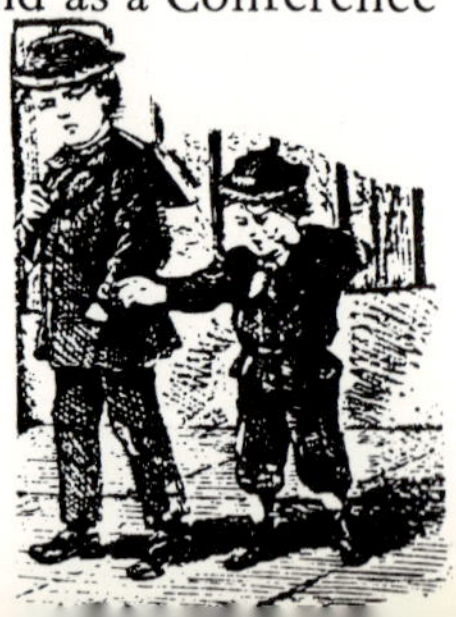

REFERENCES AND NOTES

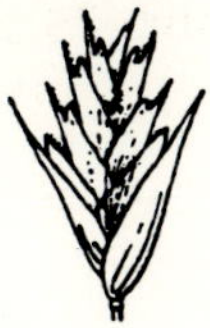

CHAPTER 1

1. 1 **Harmstorf, I.** Basedow, Herbert (1881-1933): **In:** *Australian Dictionary of Biography,* Volume 7; 1891-1939. A-Ch. General Eds. Nairn B and Serle G. Melbourne, Melbourne University Press 1976: 202-203.

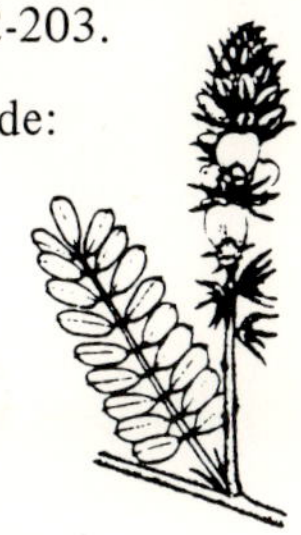

1. 2 Plants named after Dr Herbert Basedow (1881-1933) include:
Basedowia tenerrima (a monotypic genus)
Acacia basedowii
Eragrostis basedowii – Basedow's Love grass
Indigofera basedowii
Pandanus basedowii
Triodia basedowii

1. 3 Plants named after Dr Hermann Beckler (1828-1914) include:
Acacia beckleri
Archithodomyrtus beckleri
Dendrobium beckleri
Eurybia beckleri
Hibiscus beckleri
Myrtus beckleri
Ozothamnus beckleri
Streptothamnus beckleri

1. 4 The living memorials to Dr Hans Herman Behr (1818-1904) in Australia include:
Eremophilia behriana – Behr's Emu Bush
Eriochlamys behrii – Woolly Mantle
Eucalyptus behriana – Behr's Gum
Glischrocaryon behrii – Golden Pennants
Malva behriana
Senecio behrianus – Behr's Groundsel

1. 5 Dr Daniel Curdie (1810-1884) was a keen naturalist. The plants and seaweeds which bear his name include:
Curdiea spp (e.g. *Curdiea laciniata, Curdiea obtusata*)
Hymenena curdieana – a rose-pink seaweed
Limosella curdieana – Large Mudwort
Nitophyllum curdieanum

CHAPTER 1 (continued)

1. 6 Dr John Ravenscroft Elsey (1834-1857) has a number of animals and plants named after him, including the tortoise *Elseya*, and Elsey's Supplejack, *Ripogonum elseyanum*, a rainforest climber of North Queensland.

1. 7 Dr Ludwig Leichhardt has at least thirty plants and trees named after him. These include:

Leichhardtia australis – 'Bush banana', 'Native Pear', 'Doubah', 'Alunqua', 'Cogola bush'
Leichhardtia brockmaniana
Leichhardtia cinerascens
Leichhardtia velutina
Leichhardtia viridiflora

Soft Leichhardt (*Nauclea orientalis*)
Hard Leichhardt (*Neonauclea gordiniana*)

Acacia leichhardtii – Leichhardt's Wattle
Duboisia leichhardtii – Pituri
Rauwenhoffia leichhardtii (form. *Melodorum leichhardtii*)
Gmelina leichhardtii – White Beech
Datura leichhardtii
Commersonia leichhardtii
Euphorbia leichhardtii
Harpullia leichhardtii
Bauhinia leichhardtii
Chorizema leichhardtii
Macropteranthes leichhardtii
Psoralea leichhardtii
Sarcopechalus leichhardtii
Anthocercis leichhardtii
Parsonsia leichhardtii – Leichhardt's Silkpod
Marsdenia leichhardiana
Prostantheria leichhardtii - Leichhardt's Mint-bush
Ammania occultiflora Var. Leichhardtii
Bridelia leichhardtii
Ficus leichhardtii – Leichhardt's Fig
Liverstona humilis (form. *Liverstona leichhardtii*)

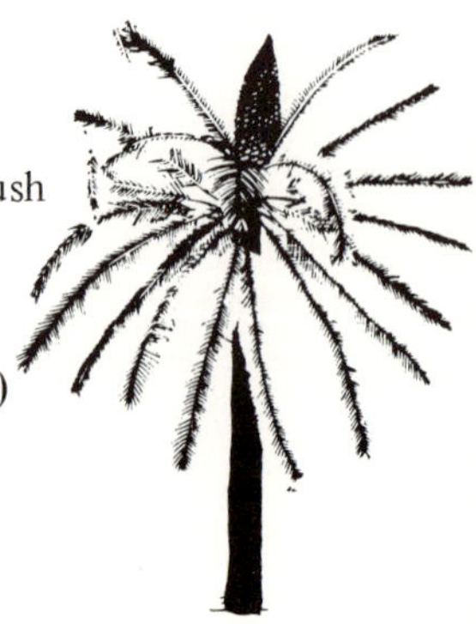

CHAPTER 1 (continued)

1.8 The last resting place of Dr Johann Lhotsky (1800-*c.* 1861) is unknown, but is possibly in London. The fish genus, *Lhotskya*, commemorates him; the beautiful plant genus, *Lhotskya* (the Fringe-myrtles), and one species of Button Daisy *Leptorrhynchos lhotskyanus*, also note his work.

1.9 It is important to note that James Patrick Murray, and his botanical memorials, are to be in no way confused with those of Johann Andreas Murray (1740-1791) after whom the genus *Murraya* is named; or with Sir George Murray (1772-1841), who was Secretary of State for the Colonies and after whom *Santalum murrayana* has been named; or with John Murray (1851-1916) who was a Premier of Victoria in 1909-1912, after whom *Kochia murrayana* has been named.

CHAPTER 2

2.1 **Hagger J.** 1979. *Australian Colonial Medicine*. (Rigby Ltd.: Adelaide).

2.2 **Covacevich J.** 1988. Australia's dangerous snakes. **In** *Venoms and Victims.* Eds. Pearn J and Covacevich J. (Queensland Museum and Amphion Press: Brisbane).

2.3 **White J.** 1987. Elapid snakes: aspects of envenomation. **In** *Toxic Plants and Animals. A Guide for Australia*. Eds. Covacevich J, Davie P, and Pearn J. (Queensland Museum: Brisbane).

2.4 **Covacevich J.** 1987. Two Taipans! **In** *Toxic Plants and Animals. A Guide for Australia.* Eds. Covacevich J, Davie P, and Pearn J. (Queensland Museum: Brisbane).

2.5 **Pearn J.** 1988. Human snakebite – effects and first aid. **In** *Venoms and Victims*. Eds. Pearn J, and Covacevich J. (Queensland Museum and Amphion Press).

2.6 **Cunningham P.** 1827. *Two years in New South Wales*. Vol. 1. (Henry Colburn: London).

2.7 **Cann J.** 1986. *Snakes Alive! Snake Experts and Antidote Sellers of Australia.* (Kangaroo Press: Sydney).

2.8 **Bennett G.** 1860. *Gatherings of a Naturalist in Australasia: Being Observations Principally on the Animal and Vegetable Productions of New South Wales, New Zealand and some of the Austral Islands*. (John Van Voorst: London).

CHAPTER 2 (continued)

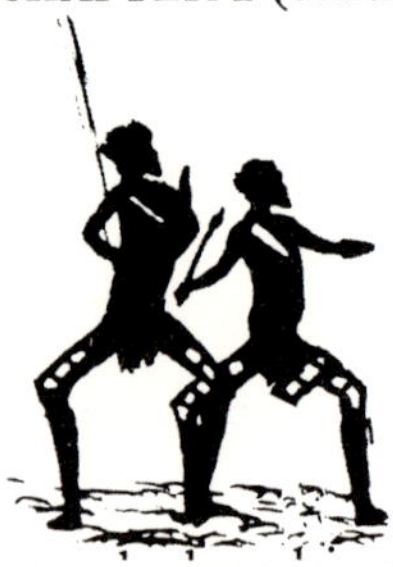

2. 9 **Agnew JW.** 1864. Notes of the poison of venomous snakes. *Pap. Proc. Roy. Soc. Tas.* 9-13.

2.10 **Dawson J.** 1881. *Australian Aborigines. The Languages and Customs of several Tribes of Aborigines in the Western District of Victoria, Australia.* (George Robertson: Melbourne).

2.11 **Foelsche** P. 1882. Notes on the Aborigines of North Australia. *Trans. Roy. Soc. S. Aust.* 5:1-18.

2.12 **Curr EM.** (ed.) 1886. *The Australian Race: Its Origin, Languages, Customs, Place of Landing in Australia, and the Routes by which it spread itself over that Continent.* Vol. 2 (Government Printer: Melbourne).

2.13 **Lumholz C.** 1889 (Facsimile reprint 1980). *Among Cannibals: Account of four Years Travels in Australia, and of Camp Life with the Aborigines of Queensland.* (Australian National University Press: Canberra).

2.14 **Maiden JH.** 1895. A reputed antidote to snakebite. *Agric. Gaz. N.S.W.* 5: 473.

2.15 **Stirling EC.** 1896. Horn Expedition Results. Vol. IV. p. 131.

2.16 **Roth WE.** 1897. Ethnological Studies among the north-west central Queensland Aborigines. *The Queensland Aborigines*, Vol. 1. (Government Printer: Brisbane) Chapter XI, p. 157.

2.17 **Macpherson J.** 1902. Ngarrabul and other Aboriginal tribes. Part I – Medical and surgical practices. *Proc. Linn. Soc. N.S.W.* 27: 637-647.

2.18 **Macpherson J.** 1926. The treatment of snakebite. *Australasian Nurses Journal* 24: 54-58, 108-110.

2.19 **Bennett MM.** 1927. Notes on the Dalleburra tribe of northern Queensland. *J. Anthrop. Inst.* 57: 399-415.

2.20 **Webb TT.** 1933. Aboriginal medical practice in East Arnhem Land. *Oceania* 4: 91-98.

2.21 **Winterbotham LP.** 1951. Primitive medical art and primitive medicine men of Australia. *Med J Aust* 1: 461-68.

CHAPTER 2 (continued)

2.22 **The Australian Encyclopaedia** (1963). Aborigines Vol. 1. (The Grolier Society: Sydney).

2.23 **Webb LJ.** 1969. The use of plant medicines and poisons by Australian Aborigines. *Mankind,* 7: 137-46.

2.24 **Anonymous.** 1982. Bites and stings. *The Aboriginal Health Worker* 6(1), March, 4-13.

2.25 **Covacevich J, Irvine T, and Davis G.** 1988. A rainforest pharmacopoeia. Five thousand years of effective medicine. **In** *Pioneer Medicine in Australia*. (Ed.) Pearn J. (Amphion Press: Brisbane).

2.26 **Krefft G.** 1869. *The Snakes of Australia; an illustrated and descriptive Catalogue of all the known Species.* (Thomas Richards: Sydney).

2.27 **Pearn JH, Covacevich J, and White J.** (in press). Snake venom poisoning. Australia and New Guinea. **In** *Snake Venom Poisoning.* (Ed.) Russell F.

2.28 **Campbell CH.** 1976. *Snake bite, snake venoms and venomous snakes of Australia and New Guinea. An annotated Bibliography.* School of Public Health and Tropical Medicine, The University of Sydney. Service Publication No. 13. (Commonwealth Department of Health: Canberra).

2.29 **Agnew JW.** 1864. Notes on the poison of venomous snakes. *Pap. Proc. R. Soc. Tas.,* 9-13.

2.30 **Hood AJ.** 1887. Notes on Australian snakebite. *Australasian Med. Gaz.* 6: 265-6.

2.31 **Martin CJ.** 1893. Observations of the poisonous constituents of the venom of the Australian Black Snake (*Pseudechis porphyriacus*). *Proc. Linn. Soc. N.S.W.* 7: 319-22.

2.32 **Martin CJ.** 1897. On the advisability of administering curative serum by intravenous injection. *Intercolonial Med. J. Australasia* 2: 537-8.

2.33 **Bancroft TL.** 1894. Some further observations on the physiological action of snake venom, together with a reference to the strychnine cure of snakebite. *Australasian Med. Gaz.* 13: 228-30.

2.34 **Welsh DA. and Chapman HG.** 1910. Concerning snake venom. *Australasian Med. Gaz.* 29: 344-9.

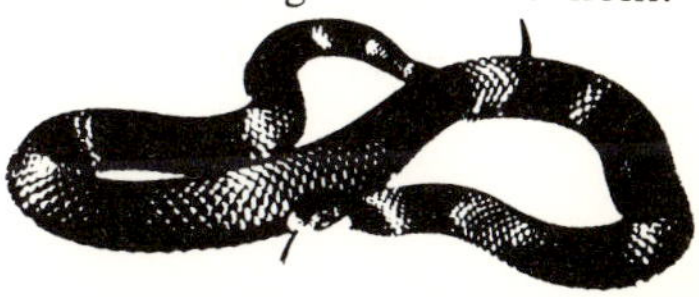

CHAPTER 2 (continued)

2.35 **Fairley NH.** 1929. Criteria for determining the efficacy of ligature in snakebite. (The subcutaneous-intravenous index). *Med J Aust* 1: 377-94.

2.36 **Sutherland SK, Coulter AR, and Harris RD.** 1979. Rationalization of first-aid measures for elapid snakebite. *Lancet* 1: 183-6.

2.37 **Sutherland SK, Coulter AR, Harris RD, Lovering KE, and Roberts ID.** 1981. A study of the major Australian snake venoms in the monkey (*Macaca fascicularis*). 1. The movement of injected venom, methods which retard its movement, and the response to antivenoms. *Pathology* 13: 13-27.

2.38 **Sutherland SK, Harris RD, Coulter AR and Lovering KE.** 1980. A simple method to delay the movement from the site of injection of low molecular weight substances. *Med J Aust* 1: 81.

2.39 **White J, Pounder D, Pearn JH and Morrison JJ.** 1985. A perspective on the problems of snakebite in Australia. **In** *Biology of Australasian Frogs and Reptiles.* (Eds.) Grigg G, Shine R and Ehmann H. (Royal Zoological Society of N.S.W.: Sydney).

2.40 **Cleland JB.** 1953. The healing art in primitive society. *Mankind* 4(10): 395-411.

CHAPTER 3

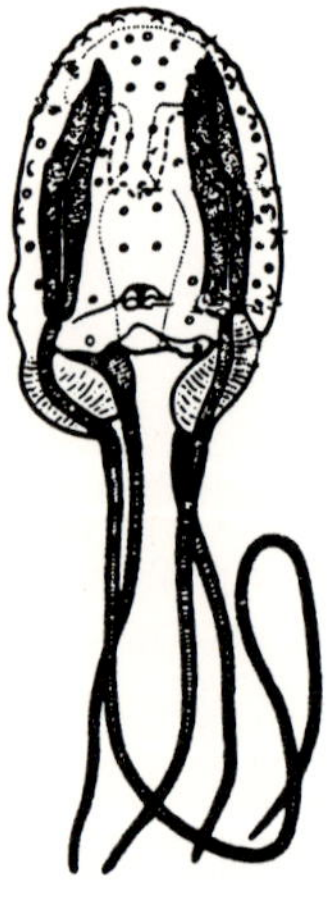

3. 1 **Cleland JB Sir, Southcott RV.** Injuries to man from marine invertebrates in the Australian region. Canberra: NHMRC, 1965; Special report series No. 12.

3. 2 **Williamson JAH.** *The Marine Stinger Book.* 3rd edn. Brisbane: Queensland State Centre, Surf Lifesaving Association of Australia, 1985.

3. 3 **Flecker H.** 'Irukandji' sting to north Queensland bathers without production of weals but with severe general symptoms. *Med J Aust* 1952;1:89-91.

3. 4 **Barnes JH.** Cause and effect in 'Irukandji' stingings. *Med J Aust.* 1964; 2:993-999.

CHAPTER 3 (continued)

3. 5 **Fenner PJ, Williamson JAH, Callanan V, Audley I.** Further understanding of, and a new treatment for, 'Irukandji' *(Carukia barnesi)* stings. *Med J Aust* 1986;145:569-574.

3. 6 **Fenner PJ, Williamson JA, Burnett JW, Colquhoun DM, Godfrey S, Gunawardane K, Murtagh W.** The 'Irukandji syndrome' and acute pulmonary oedema. *Med J Aust* 1988;149:150-156.

3. 7 **Barnes JH.** *Chironex fleckeri* and *Chiropsalmus quadrigatus* – morphological distinctions. North Queensland Nat. 1965; 32:13-22.

3. 8 **Southcott RV.** Tropical jellyfish and other marine stingings, *Mil Med* 1959; Vol 124 No 8:569-579.

3. 9 **Southcott RV.** Studies on Australian cubomedusae, including a new genus and species apparently harmful to man. *Aust J Mar Freshw Res* 1956;7:254-280.

3.10 **Southcott RV.** Revision of some Carybdeidae (Scyphozoa:Cubomedusae), including description of the jellyfish responsible for the 'Irukandji syndrome'. *Aust Zoo* 1967;15:651-657.

3.11 **Flecker H.** 'Irukandji' sting to north Queensland bathers without production of weals but with severe general symptoms. *Med J Aust* 1952;1:89-91.

3.12 **Barnes JH.** Cause and effect in 'Irukandji' stingings. *Med J Aust* 1964; 2:993-999.

3.13 **Haeckel.** *System der Medusen* 1880:447.

3.14 **Kinsey B.** More Barnes on box jellyfish. Sir George Fisher for Tropical Marine Studies, James Cook University 1988.

3.15 **Hartwick RJ, Callanan V, Williamson JAH.** Disarming the box jellyfish: nematocyst inhibition in *Chironex fleckeri. Med J Aust* 1980;1:15-20.

3.16 **Barnes JH.** Observations on jellyfish stingings in north Queensland. *Med J Aust* 1960;2:993-999.

3.17 **Barnes JH.** Extraction of Cnidarian venom from living tentacle. *Animal Toxins.* Russell FE, Saunders PR (eds.) Pergamon: Oxford 1967:115.

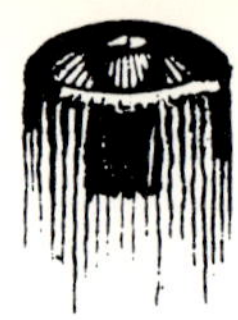

CHAPTER 3 (continued)

3.18 **Williamson JAH, Le Ray LE, Wolfhart M, Fenner PJ.** Acute management of serious envenomation by box jellyfish *(Chironex fleckeri). Med J Aust* 1984;141:851-853.

3.19 **Fenner PJ, Williamson JA, Blenkin JA.** Successful use of *Chironex* anti-venom by members of the Q.A.T.B. (Queensland Ambulance Transport Brigade. *Med J Aust* 1989;151:708-710.

3.20 **Burnett JW, Othman IB, Endean R, Fenner PJ, Callanan VI, Williamson JW.** Verapamil potentiation of *Chironex* (Box-Jellyfish) stings. *Toxicon* 1990;28(2):242-244.

CHAPTER 4

4. 1 A collection of archival and personal papers relating to Dr Cook made available by Ms Suzanne Saunders, 1990.

4. 2 **Austin T.** Exceptionally Assimilable: The Commonwealth and Half-caste Youth in the Northern Territory, 1911–1939. PhD Thesis, University of Queensland, 1989.

4. 3 **Cook C.** The Epidemiology of Leprosy in Australia. Commonwealth of Australia Department of Health, Service Publication No. 38, 1927.

4. 4 **Saunders S.** Another dimension: Xavier Herbert in the Northern Territory. *Journal of Australian Studies,* in press.

4. 5 **Saunders S.** A Suitable Island Site: Leprosy in the Northern Territory and the Channel Island Leprosarium. Historical Society of the Northern Territory Publications.

4. 6 **Lockwood D.** *The Front Door. Darwin 1869-1969.* Rigby Limited, Adelaide. 1968.

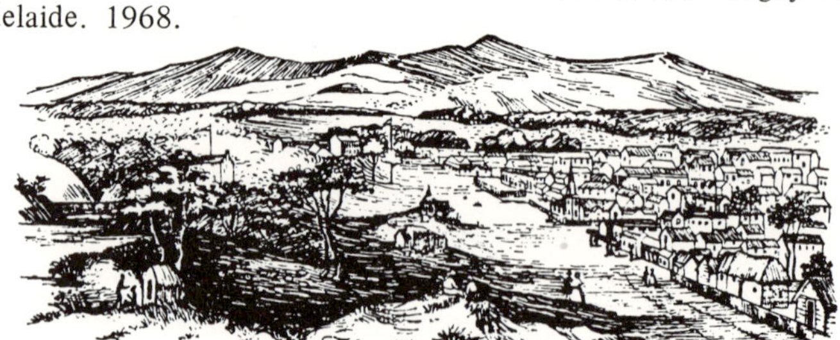

CHAPTER 5

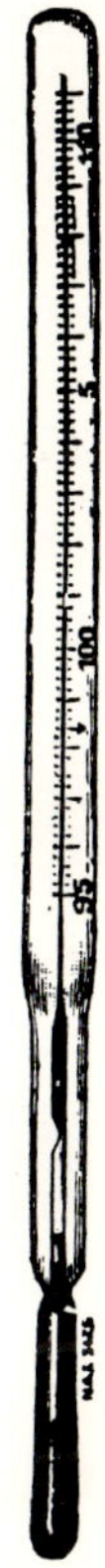

5. 1 Quoted in Strauss M. *Familiar Medical Quotations,* Boston, Little Brown, 1968, p 181.

5. 2 *The Bible:* Deuteronomy 28, verses 21 and 22.

5. 3 **Hutchinson R.** *Clinical Methods,* London, Cassell, 1924, pp 41-46.

5. 4 **Davis A.** *Medicine and its Technology,* Westport (USA), Greenwood, 1981, pp 61-85.

5. 5 **Lyons A. & Petrucelli R.** *Medicine, An Illustrated History,* Melbourne, Macmillan, 1979, p 510.

5. 6 **Scurr C. & Feldman S.** *Scientific Foundations of Anaesthesia,* London, Heinemann, 1976, pp 9-10, 81-84.

5. 7 **Toulmin S.** *The Philosophy of Science,* London, Hutchinson, 1960, pp 129-133.

5. 8 **Parkinson C.** *Breakthroughs,* London, Mansell, 1985, p 55 *et passim.*

5. 9 *New Encyclopaedia Brittanica,* Chicago, University Press, 1986 (15th Edition), Vol 23, pp 734-737.

5.10 **Pearsall R.** *Collecting and Restoring Scientific Instruments,* London, David & Charles, 1974, pp 146-153.

5.11 **Benedict R.** *Fundamentals of Temperature, Pressure, and Flow Measurement,* New York, Wiley, 1974, pp 5-8.

5.12 *World Book Encyclopedia,* Chicago, World Book, 1985, Vol 3, p 253; Vol 12, p 505; Vol 19, p 192.

5.13 **Newman H.** *An Illustrated Dictionary of Glass,* London, Thames & Hudson, 1977, pp 12-13, 133.

5.14 **Morton L.** *A Medical Bibliography,* Edinburgh, Morrison & Cribb, 1970, p 319.

5.15 **Druitt R.** *A Surgeon's Vade Mecum*, London, Renshaw, 1878, p 42.

5.16 **Allwood J.** *The Great Exhibitions,* London, Studio Vista, 1977, p 180.

5.17 **Dornette W.** *Monitoring in Anesthesia,* Philadelphia, Davis, 1973, p 7.

CHAPTER 5 (continued)

5.18 **Marion J. & Hornyak W.** *Principles of Physics,* Philadelphia, Saunders, 1984, p 344.

5.19 **Beck M.** *The Science and Art of Surgery*, London, Longmans, 1884, Vol 1, p 178.

5.20 *National Geographic Magazine*, Washington, 1982, Vol 162, pp 445, 470.

5.21 *Anaesthesia and Intensive Care,* Melbourne, 1988, Vol 16, pp F6, 44-47.

5.22 **Harpur P.** (Editor) *The Timetable of Technology,* London, Marshall, 1982, pp 169, 204.

5.23 **Phillips J.** (Editor) *MIMS Hospital Equipment & Supplies 1989/90,* Crows Nest, IMS Publishing, 1989, p 485.

CHAPTER 6

6. 1 **Stacey M.** *The sociology of healing: a textbook.* London: Unwin Hyman, 1988:154.

6. 2 **Gillespie R.** Conference Report. Searching for new perspectives in the history of medicine in Australia. *Journal of the Society for the Social History of Medicine* 1989; 2:251.

6. 3 **Fulder S.** *The handbook of complementary medicine,* 2nd edition. Oxford: Oxford University Press, 1988:15.

6. 4 **Illich I.** *Medical nemesis: the expropriation of health.* New York: Bantam, 1977.

6. 5 **Stacey**, *op cit*, 172.

6. 6 **The Webb Report.** Report of the Committee of Inquiry into Chiropractic, Osteopathy, Homeopathy and Naturopathy. Canberra: Australian Government Printing Service, 1977.

6. 7 **Australian Health Survey No. 4320.0.** Canberra: Australian Bureau of Statistics, 1977-78. Cited in Weisner D. *Alternative medicine: Australia's systems of alternative and natural medicine. A guide for patients and health professionals.* Kenthurst: Kangaroo Press, 1989:18.

CHAPTER 6 (continued)

6. 8 **Weisner D.** *Alternative medicine: Australia's systems of alternative and natural medicine. A guide for patients and health professionals.* Kenthurst: Kangaroo Press, 1989:18.

6. 9 **1988 Year Book Australia (No. 72).** Canberra: Australian Bureau of Statistics, 253-7.

6.10 Quoted by Weisner, *op cit*, 22-39, and taken from the 1984-1986 Report of the Social Development Commission of the Victorian Parliament, Vol. 2.

6.11 Opinions about natural therapists. Report of opinion research. Lagendijk: Foundation Central Bureau NWP, The Netherlands, 1980.

6.12 **Wharton R, Lewith G.** Complementary medicine and the general practitioner. *Brit Med J* 1986; 292:1498-500.

6.13 **Reilly DT.** Young doctors' views on alternative medicine. *Brit Med J* 1983; 287:337-9.

6.14 **Anderson E, Anderson P.** General practitioners and alternative medicine. *Journal of the Royal College of General Practitioners* 1983; 37:52-5.

6.15 **Fulder SJ, Monro R.** Complementary medicine in the United Kingdom: patients, practitioners and consultations. *Lancet* 1985; 2:542-45.

6.16 **Ackerknecht EH.** *A short history of medicine, revised edition.* Baltimore: The Johns Hopkins University Press, 1982:17.

6.17 **Kaptchik T, Croucher M.** *The healing arts. A journey through the faces of medicine.* London: Guild Publishing, 1986:43.

6.18 **Billroth T.** *General surgical pathology and therapeutics, in fifty lectures. A textbook for students and physicians.* Translated from the fourth German edition (1869) by Hackley CE, New York: D. Appleton and Company, 1871:226.

6.19 **Sheehan MC.** Alternative healing and medicine: the roles of naturopathy, homeopathy, osteopathy, chiropractic and medical practice in the health system. PhD thesis, University of Queensland, 1983:35.

6.20 **The Webb Report**, *op cit,* 30.

6.21 **Sheehan**, *op cit,* 38-39.

CHAPTER 6 (continued)

6.22 **The Webb Report,** *op cit,* 41.

6.23 **Nicholls PA.** *Homeopathy and the medical profession.* London: Croom Helm, 1988:3-4.

6.24 **The Webb Report,** *op cit,* 98.

6.25 **Willis E.** *Medical dominance. The division of labour in Australian health care.* Sydney: George Allen and Unwin, 1983:163.

6.26 **The Webb Report,** *op cit,* 103.

6.27 **Penn RG.** Adverse reactions to herbal medicines. *Australian Prescriber,* 1985, 2(1):16-18.

6.28 **Fulder, Monro,** *op cit,* 19.

6.29 **Editorial.** At the centre and on the fringes. *Lancet* 1981, 2:1209.

CHAPTER 7

7. 1 **Sandford Morgan E.** (1969). *A Short History of Medical Women in Australia.*

7. 2 *Sydney Morning Herald* 26.5.1891.

7. 3 *Courier Mail* 30.5.1891.

7. 4 **Summers HJ.** (1979) *They Cross the River,* University of Queensland Press.

7. 5 This Church was in John Street near the river bank. Mr Moffatt remained Rector of Kangaroo Point until 1870 and he was also the first Queensland Parliamentary Librarian. The present St Mary's Church was completed in 1873, but *Old St Mary's* was never used as its rectory.

7. 6 Records of Ipswich Girls' Grammar School.

7. 7 Personal communication, Keith Greenham.

7. 8 **Ure N.** (1988) *Brisbane Bound.*

7. 9 **Queensland Government.** (1915) *Pocket Queensland.*

CHAPTER 7 (continued)

7.10 Stanthorpe Historical Society.

7.11 Oxley Memorial Library OM68-25/108.

7.12 Oxley Memorial Library OM68-25/108.

7.13 **Queensland Parliamentary Papers.** Vol. II, 1911-12. Report of Medical Inspector of Schools.

7.14 **Queensland Parliamentary Papers.** Vol. I, 1912.

7.15 Oxley Memorial Library OM68-25/135.

7.16 Queensland State Archives. Report of Medical Inspector – Diphtheria outbreak in Mackay 4.12.1912. 38095/12 Health.

7.17 Oxley Memorial Library OM68-25.

7.18 **Brotherton H.** (1973). *A College is Built.* Baskerville Printing and Publishing Co.

7.19 Dr R.G. Bourne is her nephew.

7.20 **Hutton Neve M.** (1980). *This Mad Folly.* Library of Australian History, Sydney.

7.21 *Medical Journal of Australia,* July 6th 1946.

7.22 Boulia is 870 km west of Townsville. It meant a rail journey to Winton, then a coach trip of 315 km.

7.23 Adela Williams married Henry Porter and from 1909 practised at Moggill Road and later Swann Road, Taringa.

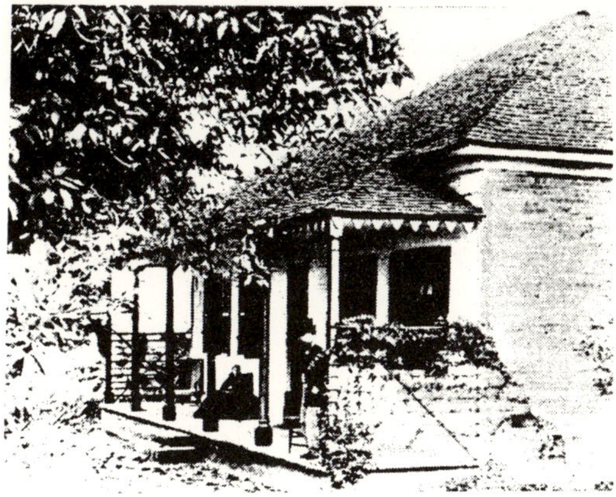

CHAPTER 7 (continued)

7.24 Alice Kirke (*nee* Miles) LPCP & S (Edin.) and LFPS (Glasg.) was married to Revd G. Kirke, a Presbyterian minister. She practised at Queenton, Charters Towers for many years before moving to Ipswich in 1917.

7.25 The Harlins resigned from Clermont in January 1911; they spent a short time in Crows Nest before moving to Killarney.

7.26 One of her brothers was Sir John Lavarack, former Governor of Queensland.

7.27 Personal communication. Mrs H. McCrea, daughter of Dr Jones.

CHAPTER 8

8. 1 **Robertson WH.** *An illustrated history of contraception.* Jersey: Parthenon Publishing Group, 1990: 67-70.

8. 2 **Siedlecky S, Wyndham D.** Chronology of birth control. Populate and Perish. Australian women's fight for birth control. Manuscript to be published, Sydney: Allan & Unwin.

8. 3 **Wyndham D.** Overview: the history of contraception and abortion in Australia. *Healthright* 1985; 5(1): 9-11.

8. 4 **Siedlecky S, Wyndham D.** *op cit*. Search for the ideal contraceptive.

8. 5 **Cilento P.** *Lady Cilento MB BS. My life.* Sydney: Melhuen Haynes, 1987: 129.

8. 6 **Jackson ES.** Speculations on some cases seen in the Outpatient Department. *Australasian Medical Gazette,* August 20, 1897; 16: 403-406.

8. 7 **Young CM, Ware H.** Contraceptive use in Australia. *Aust NZ J Obstet Gynaecol.* 1979; 19(1): 1-6.

8. 8 **Jackson ES.** Speculations on the prevalence of syphilis in Brisbane, and consideration of certain other matters in connection with public morality. *Australasian Medical Gazette,* July 20 1910; 29: 367-370.

8. 9 **Wyndham D, Needham R.** Family Planning Associations in Australia, key events from 1926 to 1983. *Healthright* 1983; 3(1): 7-18.

8.10 **Family Planning Federation of Australia Annual Report 1988/89**: 36

CHAPTER 8 (continued)

8.11 **Family Planning Association of Queensland Annual Report 1988/89**: 5.

8.12 **Family Planning Association of New South Wales Staff Bulletin,** February 1977: 2-3.

8.13 **Caldwell J, Ware H.** The evolution of family planning in Australia. *Population studies 1973;* xxvii(1): 22.

8.14 **Young CM, Ware H.** Contraceptive use in Australia. *Aust NZ J Obstet Gynaecol.* 1979; 19: 1-6.

8.15 **Caldwell J, Ware H.** *op. cit.*: 17.

8.16 **Caldwell J, Ware H.** *op. cit.*: 19.

8.17 **Cashman P.** The Law Report. Australian Broadcasting Commission National Radio 3 April, 1990.

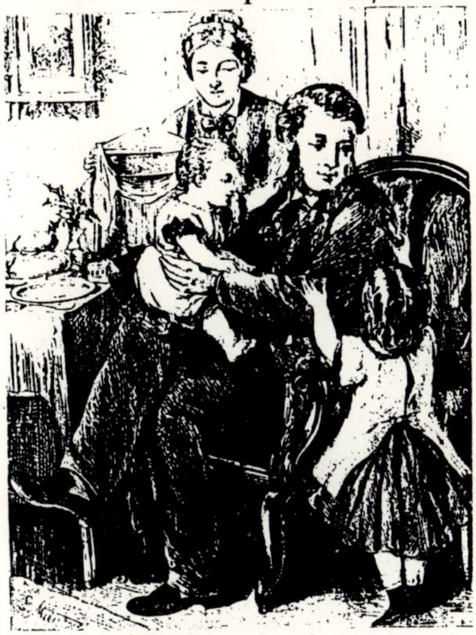

8.18 **Riisfeldt GD.** Personal communication, Schering Pty Ltd, NSW, 21 February 1990.

8.19 **Teitze C.** New estimates of mortality associated with fertility control, *Family Planning Perspectives 1977;* 9: 74-76.

8.20 **Fraser IS.** Depo-provera: a matter of public concern? *Mod Med Aust* 1988; 31(3): 14-27.

8.21 Royal Australian College of Obstetricians and Gynaecologists Policy Statement on Depo Provera. Adopted by Council, 28 November 1987.

8.22 **Selwood T, Leeton J.** Sterilization operations in Australia. *Med J Aust* 1980; 2(9): 499-501.

8.23 Health Insurance Commission, Actuarial and Statistics Branch, Canberra. Personal communication 18 April 1990.

8.24 **Caldwell J, Young C, Ware H, Lavis D, Davis AT.** Australia: Knowledge, attitudes and practice of family planning in Melbourne 1971. *Studies in Family Planning 1973;* 4(3): 49-72.

CHAPTER 8 (continued)

8.25 **Gerber P.** Vasectomies are legal – even in Queensland. *Med J Aust* 1987; 146: 84-87.

8.26 **Himes NE.** *Medical History of Contraception.* Baltimore. Schoken Books Inc. 1970: xii.

CHAPTER 9

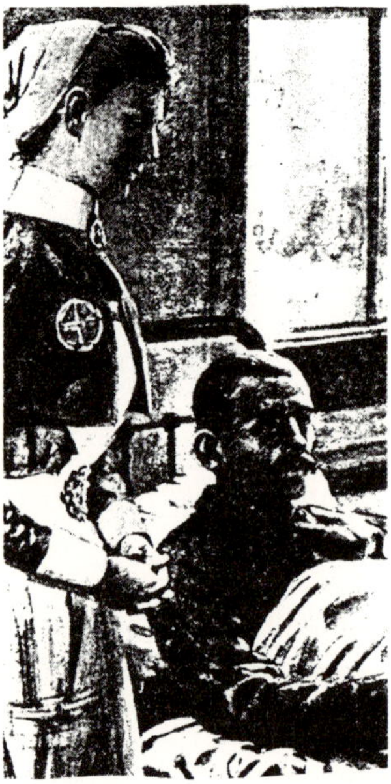

9. 1 Since World War II there have been in excess of twenty inquiries into how nurses should be educated. By the early 1970s the Sax Report on Nursing Education recommended, albeit cautiously, that pilot college based courses at diploma level be established across the country. The first of these was in Melbourne under the direction of Pat Slatter.

9. 2 Queensland Nurses Union correspondence file.

9. 3 In the fourteen pre-registration Schools of Nursing in the Queensland public hospital sector in 1989, there were approximately 152 nurse administrators and approximately 3000 student nurses.

9. 4 **Roy Drabble.** 'Equity Now'. A National Policy Statement on Nurse Education by the National Council of Health Organizations, February, 1987, pp 1-19.

9. 5 **Stuart Hamilton,** 'The Transfer of Nursing Education from Hospitals to the Tertiary Sector'. Progress Report to Parliament, June 1989, p 3.

9. 6 See *Nursing a New Tomorrow.* Proceedings of the International Council of Nursing Conference, Seoul, Korea, 1989, for information about the global shortage of nurses; when the projected shortage of nurses occurs in Australia it is possible that the tertiary education system could be nominated as the scapegoat by detractors of current nursing changes.

CHAPTER 9 (continued)

9. 7 **Vivian Griffin.** 'Workforce Planning for the Transfer of Nurse Education: when does it Happen?' *The Queensland Nurse,* July/August 1989, pp 8-9.

9. 8 This is evidenced by the lack of workforce planning and its disastrous effects on hospitals. The attrition rate in some hospital nursing schools has been as high as 42%, which has led to closure of beds, the practice of 'sweating' of nurses, waiting lists and unsafe nursing which in turn, leads to greater loss of nurses to an ever increasingly pressured system.

9. 9 For a Christian view of nursing regarding personal interaction see Rosalie Hudson, "Whole or parts – a theological perspective on 'person'." *Aust J of A N,* Sep-Nov, Vol 16, No. 1 pp 12-16.

9.10 **Gillian Briscor.** 'Thought, Action, Readiness & Responsibility', The Twenty Second Patricia Chomley Oration, College of Nursing Australia, Canberra, 28 May 1988.

9.11 **Sue-Ellen Case.** *Feminism and Theatre*, Methuen, New York, 1988, pp 12-19.

9.12 *ibid*, p 7.

9.13 **See Nancy Hartsock**, *Money, Sex and Power: Towards a Feminist Historical Materialism*, Longman, New York, 1983, p 192.

9.14 There is a great deal of re-organisation in the feminist morphology which seeks to re-define the existing, inherited order regarding interpretation of information in history. Luce Irigary describes the fashionable term 'contiguity' as "a nearness" which helps "constantly in the process of weaving itself ... embracing words and yet casting them off", concerned not with clarity, but with what is "touched upon". Helen Cixous, in *The Laugh of the Medusa* in Marks and de Courtivorn, *New French Feminists* (pp 245-264), calls it reading between the lines. These difficult concepts are in operation, it seems, without borders, often there seems to be a sense of no beginning, middle or end in the abandonment of hierarchical organising-principles of traditional form which has served to exclude women from discourse.
(**Sue-Ellen Case,** *ibid*, pp 128-129.)

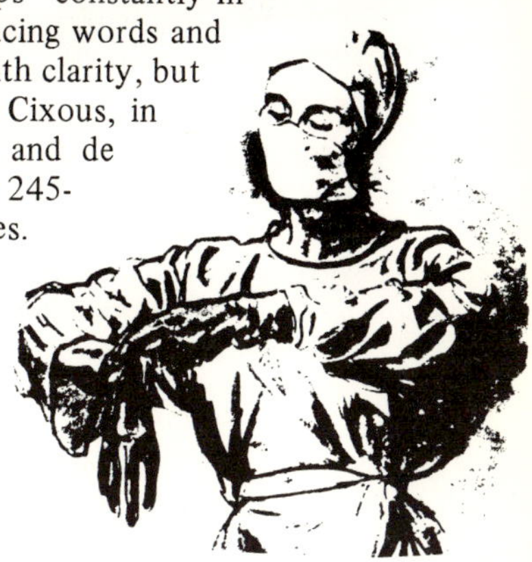

CHAPTER 9 (continued)

9.15 See **Kate Millett's** influential book *Sexual Politics*, New York, 1970 which gives a way to recognise and interpret the images of women in male literature as misogynic. The distinction is made between the historical woman and the male-produced fictional woman of male history and literature; see also, **Judith Fetterly's** *The Resisting Reader*, for a method of re-reading texts by men as they were conventionally read.

9.16 **E. Boulding**, *The Underside of History*, Westernview Press, Boulder, Colorado, 1976, p 57.

9.17 **Ben-Yehuda**, "The European Witch Craze of the 14 to 17 Centuries: a Sociologists Perspective". *American Journal of Sociology,* 86(1). July 1980, pp 1-32.

9.18 Until recently historians have shown little interest in who the women were who were accused of witchcraft. The stereotype of the English witch was of an old woman who cursed those who did not comply with her requests; the Continental witch was seen as an hallucinating psychopath obsessed with the notion of copulating with the devil. For an excellent book on the character, motivation and values of the last English woman to be executed for witchcraft see **Joyce Bigson,** *Hanged for Witchcraft: Elizabeth Lowys and her Successors*, Toudo Press, Canberra, 1988; see also **Barbara Ehrenreich**, *Witches, Midwives and Nurses*, Feminist Press, Old Westbury, 1973.

9.19 **F.B. Smith**. *Florence Nightingale: Reputation and Power*, Croom & Helm, London & Canberra, 1982.

9.20 *ibid*, p 52.

9.21 **Edward James Edwards** *Nursing Association For The Diocese of Lichfield,* London, 1867, p39 & **Mary Stanley,** *Hospitals and Sisterhoods*, London, 1954, pp 1-2, in **F.B. Smith** *ibid*, p 155.

9.22 The disillusionment and frustrations of early professional nursing in Australia are none more poignantly revealed than in the story of Lucy Osburn who was sent by Nightingale to found the Sydney Infirmary in 1868. See **Freda MacDonnell,** *Miss Nightingale's Young Ladies: the story of the Sydney Infirmary,* Angus & Robertson, Sydney 1970; also *Footnote – People in Australian History,* edited by Ann Atkinson, published by Fairfax Library in association with Daniel Publishing, Broadway, NSW, 1987.

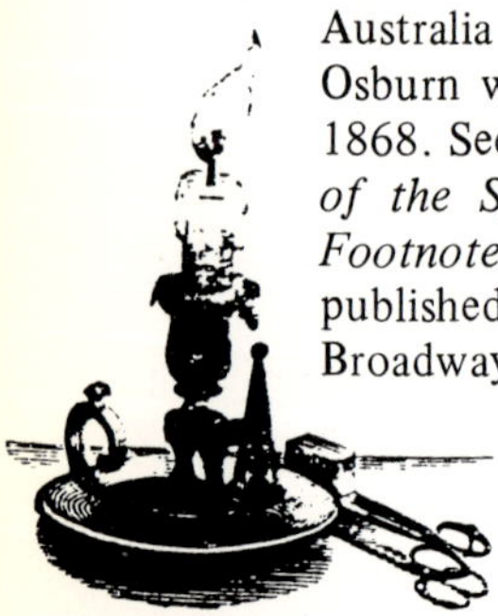

CHAPTER 9 (continued)

9.23 **Kay Jaumees**, *Century of Service 1881-1981*, Townsville General Hospital Centenary, Wilmetts, Townsville, 1981.

9.24 **F.B. Smith,** *ibid,* Ch. 5.

9.25 **Queensland State Archives,** Col A/233, 48/894, item 1602.

9.26 **George Blanchard**, Thornborough Diary 1889, John Oxley Library.

9.27 *ibid.*

9.28 *ibid.*

9.29 **Queensland State Archives,** "Croydon District Hospital". Col 14A/44. 1921, item 74/46.

9.30 **Judith Perry & Cheryl Moss**. "Generating Alternatives in Nursing: turning curriculum into a living process". *Aust J of A N*, Feb 1990, Vol 6, No 12, pp 35-40.

9.31 **Andrea C. Bostrom, Margaret Malnight, John MacDougall & Dina Hargis,** "Staff nurses' attitudes towards nursing research: a descriptive survey", *Journal of A N,* 1989, 14, pp 915-922.

9.32 **Patricia Benner & Judith Wurbel,** *The Primacy of Caring: Stress and Coping in Health and Illness,* Addison-Wesley Publishing Company, Menlo Park, California, 1989, p xv.

9.33 **Jeffrey C. Berlant**. *Profession & Monopoly: a Study of Medicine in the United States and Great Britain,* University of California, Berkeley, 1975.

9.34 **Charlotte B. Hoelzel**, "Using Structural Power Sources to increase Infleunce", *J of A N*, Nov 1989, Vol 19, No 11, pp 10-15.

9.35 **Barbara Keddy**, *et al.* "The doctor-nurse relationship: an historical perspective", *J of A N*, Nov 1986, Vol 11, No 6, pp 758. This study shows that especially in relation to nursing administration, nurses prefer to work with people who get things done and can control uncertainty in the work environment by an intelligent use of resources.

9.36 **Emily Mumford**, *Medical Sociology: Patients, Providers and Policies,* Random House, New York, 1983, p 302.

9.37 **Vivian Griffin**. "Preferred Level and Award of Nurse Pre-Registration Program", October, 1989 p 14.

9.38 **Patricia Benner**, *From Novice to Expert: Excellence and Power in Clinical Nursing Practice,* Addison-Wesley, Menlo Park, 1984. (A minor point regarding terminology, Florence Nightingale would not have approved of the use of 'novice', with its obvious religious connotations, and 'expert' sounds a bit shady, as though it is necessary to state the obvious.)

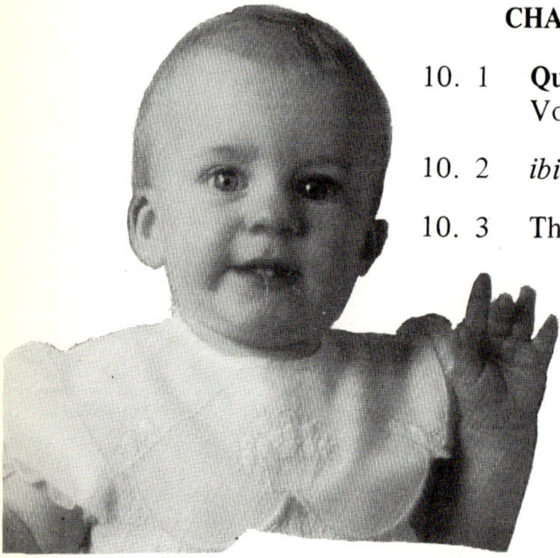

CHAPTER 10

10. 1 **Queensland Parliamentary Debates**, 1922, Vol. CXL, p 1858.

10. 2 *ibid,* p 1858.

10. 3 This oral evidence was collected throughout the State from interviewing 91 women who were mothers, midwives, child welfare nurses or doctors between 1910 and 1945. For more detail of this evidence, the methodology used in the collection and collation of the evidence and where the tapes will be stored see **W.A. Selby**, 'An Historical Study of the Impact on Women of the Queensland Labor Governments' Maternal and Infant Welfare Policies 1915-1957', Ph.D. Thesis, (Griffith University, Brisbane, forthcoming 1991). Fictitious names will be used in this paper.

10. 4 For example see **M.J. Thearle and H. Gregory**, 'Choices for Childbirth: Midwifery in Nineteenth and Early Twentieth Century Queensland', (Brisbane 1988), unpublished manuscript; **H.C. Murphy**, 'History of Maternal and Child Welfare Service, Queensland', *Queensland Health: Journal of the Department of Health and Home Affairs,* Vol. 1, No. 4, (June 1963); **R. Patrick,** *A History of Health and Medicine in Queensland 1824-1960,* (Brisbane 1987), p. 158-164, 374-380; **M.J. Thearle**, 'Dr Alfred Jefferis Turner 1861-1947: His Contribution to Medicine in Queensland', M.D. Thesis, unpublished, (Brisbane 1987, Chapter 7; **F.M.C. Forster,** *Progress in Obstetrics and Gynaecology in Australia*, (Sydney 1967).

10. 5 **Annual Reports of Infant Welfare 1926 to 1937**, *Queensland Parliamentary Papers,* 1927 to 1938. See in particular the 8th Annual Report of Infant Welfare 1933/34, *Queensland Parliamentary Papers,* Session of 1934, Vol. 1.

10. 6 **R. Ward,** *The Australian Legend*, (Oxford 1966).

10. 7 *Queensland Parliamentary Debates*, 1922, Vol. CXL, p 1854.

10. 8 Report from Director of Maternal and Infant Welfare Services to Senior Commonwealth Medical Officer, 8.7.1947, Queensland State Archives, Location No. A/31677.

10. 9 See 'A Bill to Provide for the Early Notification of Birth', Queensland State Archives, Location No. A-31673.

10.10 Memo from James Stopford to all Ministers 21.12.1925, Queensland State Archives, Location No. A-4730, (Hospitals, maternity 25:10587).

10.11 Correspondence re The Golden Casket 1923-30, Home Secretary's Office, Queensland State Archives, Location No. A-4678.

10.12 Maternal and Child Welfare: Staffing 1934-41, Correspondence with Home Office, Queensland State Archives, Location No. A-31679.

10.13 Copy of Statement made by William McCormack, Home Secretary, announcing the Maternity Act, 13.12.1922, Queensland State Archives, Location No. A-4730.

10.14 'Motherhood and Child Welfare Scheme', unsigned memo, 1926, Queensland State Archives, Location No. COL-236.

10.15 Annual Report of Maternal and Child Welfare Services 1939-40 in Annual Report of the Director-General of Health and Medical Services, *Queensland Parliamentary Papers,* Session of 1940.

10.16 Copy of opening speech for the Bundaberg and Gin Gin Maternity Hospitals made by Edward Hanlon, 1932, Queensland State Archives, Location No. COL-363.

10.17 *The Evening News*, Rockhampton, 29.10.1923.

10.18 Continual references are made to this slogan in all the archival documents. For example, see Queensland State Archives, Location No. COL-363.

10.19 **Oueensland Parliamentary Debates**, 1944-45, CLXXXIII, p 1547.

10.20 Interview Tape No. 90.

10.21 Register of Queensland Nursing Homes 1904-1926, Queensland State Archives, Location No. A-4722.

10.22 Letter from Secretary of Nurses Registration Board to Under Secretary, 6.5.1916, Queensland State Archives, Location No. A-5075 (Nurses 16:04306).

10.23 Interview Tape No. 19.

10.24 Interview Tape No. 87.

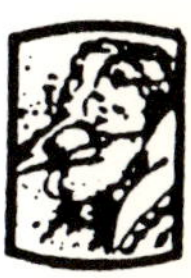

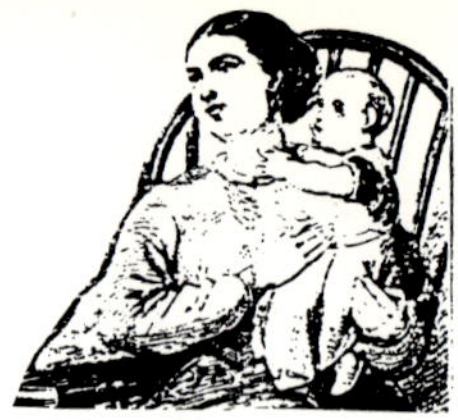

CHAPTER 10 (continued)

10.25 Interview Tape No. 9.

10.26 Home Office Memo, unsigned, Queensland State Archives, Location No. A-3568 (Hospitals, generally 30.9985).

10.27 **Report from Director of Maternal and Infant Welfare Services,** 8.7.1947, p. 3.

10.28 *Queensland Parliamentary Debates*, 1922, Vol. CXL, p. 1870.

10.29 Interview Tape No. 71.

10.30 Interview with Dr A.D.D. Pye, General Medical Superintendent for all Hospitals governed by the Brisbane and South Coast Hospitals Board 1933-67, 11.8.1989. Dr Pye trained at Sydney University 1920-25.

10.31 **E. Sydney Morris**, 'An Essay on the Causes and Prevention of Maternal Morbidity and Mortality', *The Medical Journal of Australia*, 12.9.1925, p. 307, my emphasis.

10.32 *ibid,* p. 308-9.

10.33 *ibid,* p. 321.

10.34 **R. Marshall Allan**, 'Report on Maternal Mortality and Morbidity in the State of Victoria', *Medical Journal of Australia,* 2.6.1928, p. 683.

10.35 Letter from R. Cilento to Minister of Health and Home Affairs, 4.10.1939, Queensland State Archives, Location No. A-31677.

10.36 Annual Report of Supervision of Private Hospitals, in Annual Report of Health and Medical Services in Queensland for 1937/38, *Queensland Parliamentary Papers*, Session of 1938, Vol. II.

10.37 Interview Tape No. 90.

10.38 **P. Cilento**, *Lady Cilento. My Life*, (Brisbane 1987), p. 101, **A. Jefferis Turner** , 'Experiences in Preventive Medicine', *Medical Journal of Australia*, 12.11.1938, p. 812.

10.39 See for example **J. Donzelot**, *The Policing of Families*, (New York 1979); **J.J. Matthews,** *Good and Mad Women: The Historical Construction of Femininity in Twentieth Century Australia,* (Sydney 1984), **K.M. Reiger**, *The Disenchantment of the Home: Modernising the Australian Family 1880-1940*, (Melbourne 1985).

CHAPTER 10 (continued)

10.40 **6th Annual Report on Infant Welfare 1931-32**, *Queensland Parliamentary Papers,* Session of 1932, Vol. 1, p. 1.

10.41 **9th Annual Report on Infant Welfare 1934-35**, *Queensland Parliamentary Papers,* Session of 1935, Vol. 1, p. 2.

10.42 **3rd Annual Report on Infant Welfare 1928-29**, *Queensland Parliamentary Papers,* Session of 1929, Vol. 1, p. 2.

10.43 **8th Annual Report on Infant Welfare 1933-34**, *Queensland Parliamentary Papers,* Session of 1934, Vol. 1, p. 2.

10.44 Interview Tape No. 71.

10.45 Interview Tape No. 90.

10.46 Interview Tape No. 29.

10.47 Interview Tape No. 42.

10.48 Interview with Dr F. Arden, Brisbane, 22.11.1989.

10.49 **D. Gordon,** *Health, Sickness, and Society. Theoretical Concepts in Social and Preventive Medicine,* (St Lucia 1976), p. 180-193.

CHAPTER 11

11. 1 **Elliott, Isabelle M.** Ashford History of Surgical Dressings. London, 1964.

11. 2 **Pearn J.** The Sylvia Stretcher. A perspective of Sister Elizabeth Kenny's contribution to the first-aid management of injured patients. *Med J Aust* 1988, 149. 636-638.

11. 3 A Coast Chronicle. Sydney. The Prince Henry Hospital.

11. 4 **Ryan JA.** History of Queensland Ambulance Service 1892-1950, and a History of the Rockhampton Ambulance Brigade 1901-1950. Rockhampton, Queensland Ambulance Transport Brigade (Rockhampton Centre), 1950.

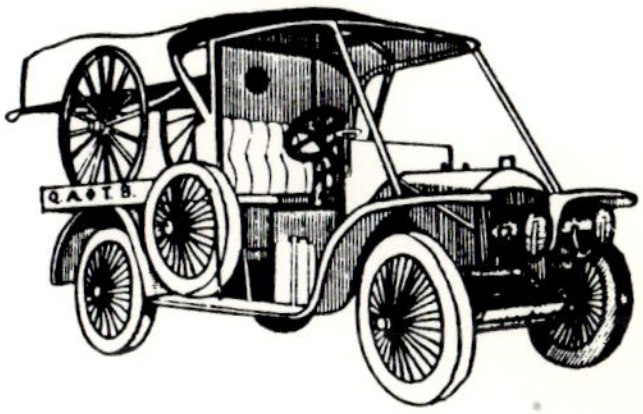

CHAPTER 12

12. 1 **Mulcahy, Monsignor Joseph.** Silver Jubilee of the Catholic Club, Mackay, 1915-1940, p. 17.

12. 2 **Kerr, J.** Pioneer Pageant, A History of Pioneer Shire Council, 1980, p 26.

12. 3 **Wright BD, Manning RJ, Hayes TP.** The First Fifty Years, History of St Patrick's Christian Brothers' College, Mackay, 1979, p. 5.

12. 4 **Kerr, J.** Pioneer Pageant, A History of Pioneer Shire Council, 1980, p 206.

12. 5 *Mackay Mercury,* 20th January 1879.

12. 6 **Wright BD.** Mater Hospital, Mackay, 1927-1987, p. 52.

12. 7 *Mackay Mercury*, 6th May 1885.

12. 8 *Mackay Mercury,* 6th May 1885.

12. 9 *Mackay Mercury*, 9th May 1885, 12th May 1885, 13th May1885.

12.10 *Mackay Mercury*, 12th September 1885.

12.11 **Table** (pp. 240-41) shows details of the deaths recorded at the Mackay Orphanage from the beginning of 1881 until closure at the end of 1885. Causes of death vary, but show a marked preponderance towards diseases of the heart. An obituary in the Sydney *Catholic Weekly* (undated) following Father Bucas' death in 1930 (aged 90 years), mentioned his association with the Orphanage, and its removal to Rockhampton because of disease, stating that the cause of the children's debility and death was now thought to be most likely due to hookworm infestation.

In an article, 'The Saga of the Australian Leech Worm', **Dr John Thearle** stated that 'the first recorded case of hookworm disease was described in Queensland in 1889 by Dr J.B. Hogg'. He cites the case of two sisters sent from Cairns to Brisbane three years later suffering from the disease. It is noteworthy that a number of the deceased from Mackay Orphanage had been placed therein from tropical areas further north – Townsville, Port Douglas, and notably, Cooktown.

Since Dr A.H. Cutfield retired from practice in Mackay in November 1889 to return to England (where he practised at Ross-on-Wye until 1925), it is probable that he had no knowledge of hookworm disease, though he was familiar (cf. letter 29.1.1885) with malarial cachexia, which he considered to be the main cause of ill health in the Orphanage children. When one considers the strange causes of death attributed to children in the Mackay district in the latter half of the nineteenth century – debility, miasmas, tabes mesenterica – one wonders just how prevalent hookworm infestation was during that era.

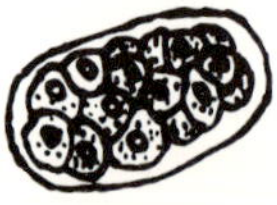

INDEX

A

A (contd)

B

B (contd)

C

C (contd)

D

D (contd)

E

F

I (contd)

J

K

L

L (contd)

M

M (contd)

N

N (contd)

O

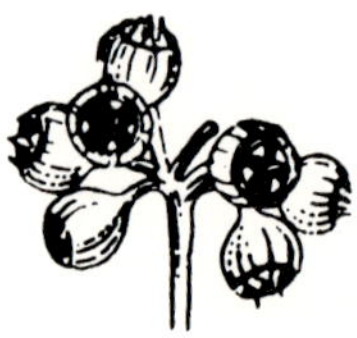

P

Q

R

S

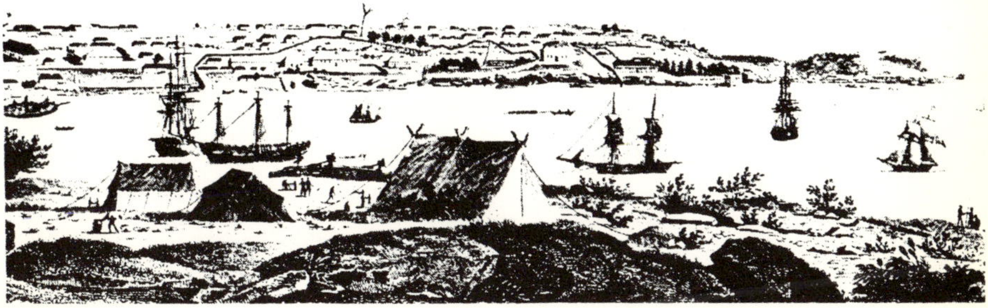

THE COVER

The cover *montage* captures some of the themes contained in this book. In it, the artists – Paul Ramsden and Bronwyn Searle – have highlighted some of the essential topics in the wider context of health care at frontiers in Australia. Such frontiers have been those of the land itself; of the identification of disease and its cure; of the rise of technology to help in the reduction of ill health; and of the attitudes of health professionals who strive to reduce the incidence and effects of disease.

The *montage* is composed of several disparate elements. The portrait (male) in the bottom right quadrant is of Dr Thomas Henry Huxley (1825-1895), and is adapted from a portrait by Alphonse Legros in The Royal Society, London. Huxley was a surgeon, explorer and biologist who spent a significant period of his early life in Australia. He explored and collected at Lord Howe Island, on the Darling Downs of Queensland and in Papua New Guinea. He went on to become President of The Royal Society in London.

The hand-carried wheeled stretcher ambulance portrays the way in which patients were transported to hospital prior to the introduction of motor ambulances in the first decade of the twentieth century. The artists have used as their models, two bearers from the Manly Ambulance Unit (of Sydney), shown wearing their 'lion tamer' uniforms of 1903.

The hookworm eggs are portrayed as seen under the microscope, and are adapted from an original hand-drawn sketch in a notebook kept by Dr Alfred Jefferis Turner of Brisbane, and entitled 'Ova as passed in stool, seen under a high power'. The hookworm eggs symbolize the preventive medicine campaigns which were a major feature of preventive medicine programmes in Northern Australia in the first decade of the twentieth century.

The group of tents is taken from a photograph entitled 'Innisfail – Government Hospital, 1885', and highlights the conditions of patient care, and the working conditions for nurses in former times at Australian frontiers. The temperature charts are the work of Dr Carl Reinhold Wunderlich (1815-1877) who published his work 'The Behaviour of Body Temperature in Disease' in Leipzig in 1868, and show the resolution of the fever of lobar pneumonia 'by crisis' (left hand chart),and that seen in bronchopneumonia 'by lysis' (right hand chart).

The woman examining the child's throat is modelled on an early photograph of Dr Eleanor Elizabeth Bourne, seen examining a child's throat at a School Medical Service examination at Charleville in 1912.

JHP